T0371606

Integrated Management of Complex Intracranial Lesions

Integrated Management of Complex Intracranial Lesions

Open, Endoscopic, and Keyhole Techniques

Edited by
Vijay Agarwal

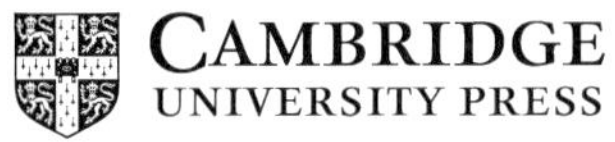
CAMBRIDGE
UNIVERSITY PRESS

CAMBRIDGE
UNIVERSITY PRESS

University Printing House, Cambridge CB2 8BS, United Kingdom

One Liberty Plaza, 20th Floor, New York, NY 10006, USA

477 Williamstown Road, Port Melbourne, VIC 3207, Australia

314–321, 3rd Floor, Plot 3, Splendor Forum, Jasola District Centre, New Delhi – 110025, India

103 Penang Road, #05–06/07, Visioncrest Commercial, Singapore 238467

Cambridge University Press is part of the University of Cambridge.

It furthers the University's mission by disseminating knowledge in the pursuit of education, learning, and research at the highest international levels of excellence.

www.cambridge.org
Information on this title: www.cambridge.org/9781108782838
DOI: 10.1017/9781108908610

© Cambridge University Press 2021

This publication is in copyright. Subject to statutory exception and to the provisions of relevant collective licensing agreements, no reproduction of any part may take place without the written permission of Cambridge University Press.

First published 2021

Printed in the United Kingdom by TJ Books Limited, Padstow Cornwall

A catalogue record for this publication is available from the British Library.

Library of Congress Cataloging-in-Publication Data
Names: Agarwal, Vijay, 1980– editor.
Title: Integrated management of complex intracranial lesions : open, endoscopic, and keyhole techniques / edited by Vijay Agarwal.
Other titles: Open, endoscopic, and keyhole techniques
Description: Cambridge, United Kingdom ; New York, NY : Cambridge University Press, 2021. | Includes bibliographical references and index.
Identifiers: LCCN 2021008906 (print) | LCCN 2021008907 (ebook) | ISBN 9781108830034 (hardback) | ISBN 9781108908610 (ebook)
Subjects: MESH: Brain Neoplasms – surgery | Craniotomy – methods | Neuroendoscopy – methods
Classification: LCC RD594 (print) | LCC RD594 (ebook) | NLM WL 358 | DDC 617.4/81–dc23
LC record available at https://lccn.loc.gov/2021008906
LC ebook record available at https://lccn.loc.gov/2021008907

ISBN 978-1-108-83003-4 Hardback
ISBN 978-1-108-90861-0 Cambridge Core
ISBN 978-1-108-78283-8 Mixed Media

Cambridge University Press has no responsibility for the persistence or accuracy of URLs for external or third-party internet websites referred to in this publication and does not guarantee that any content on such websites is, or will remain, accurate or appropriate.

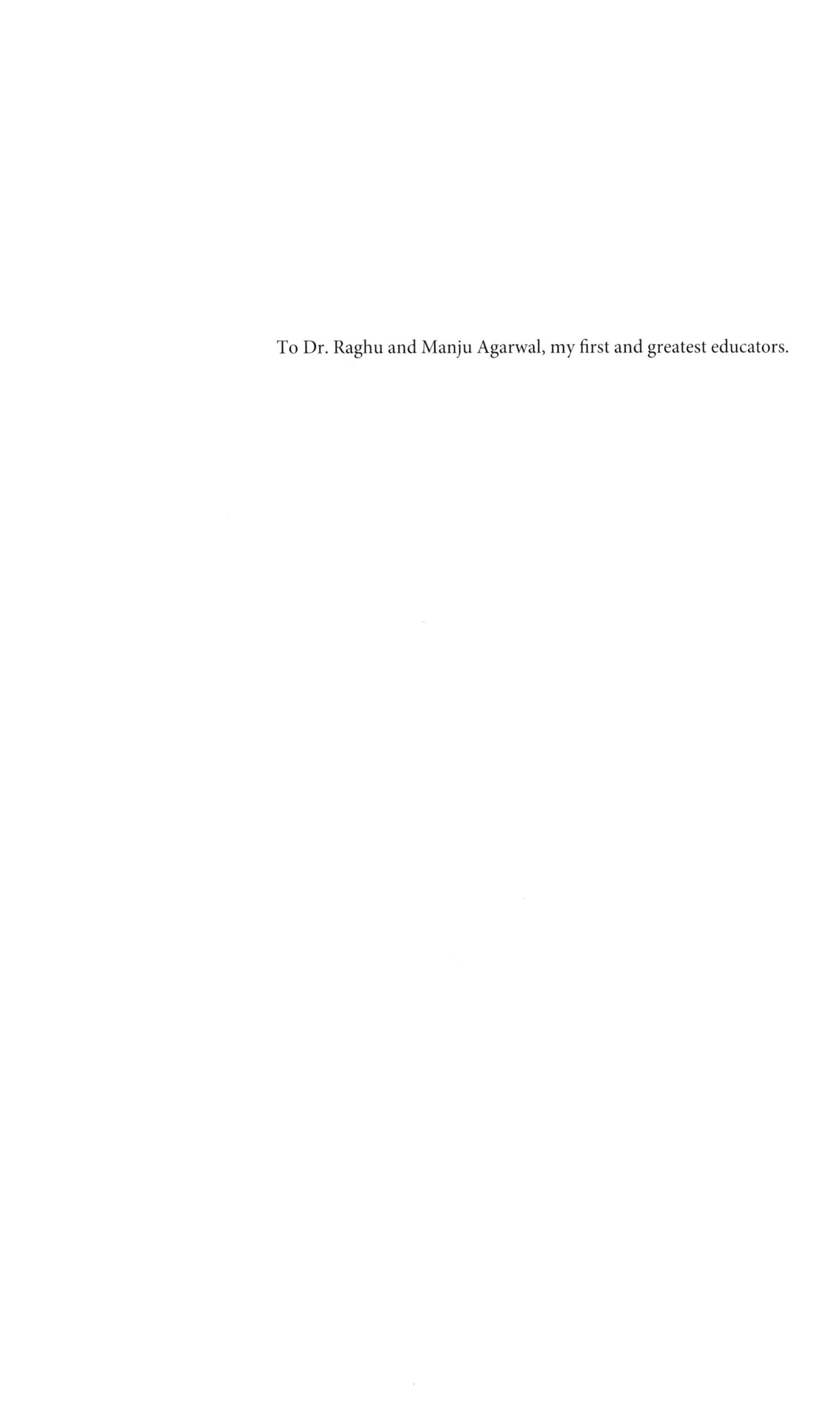

To Dr. Raghu and Manju Agarwal, my first and greatest educators.

Contents

This book provides access to an online version on Cambridge Core, which can be accessed via the code printed on the inside of the cover

Contributors

Vijay Agarwal
Chief, Division of Skull Base and Minimally Invasive Surgery; Associate Director, Residency Training Program; Assistant Professor, Department of Neurological Surgery; Montefiore Medical Center, The University Hospital for the Albert Einstein College of Medicine

Manish K. Aghi
Department of Neurological Surgery, University of California San Francisco

Zaid Aljuboori
Department of Neurological Surgery, University of Washington

Leopold Arko IV
Department of Neurological Surgery, Weill Cornell Medical Center

Daniel L. Barrow
Department of Neurosurgery, Emory University

Robert G. Briggs
Department of Neurosurgery, University of Southern California

Steven Carr
Department of Neurological Surgery, University of Missouri

C. Michael Cawley
Department of Neurosurgery, Department of Radiology and Imaging Sciences, Emory University

Ankush Chandra
Department of Neurological Surgery, University of California San Francisco

Andrew K. Conner
Department of Neurosurgery, University of Oklahoma

Dale Ding
Department of Neurosurgery, University of Louisville

Murray Echt
Department of Neurological Surgery, Montefiore Medical Center the University Hospital for the Albert Einstein College of Medicine

Ivan El-Sayed
Department of Otolaryngology – Head & Neck Surgery, University of California San Francisco

Griffin Ernst
Department of Neurosurgery, University of Oklahoma

Andrew M. Erwood
Department of Neurosurgery, Emory University

Allan Friedman
Department of Neurosurgery, Duke University

Takanori Fukushima
Department of Neurosurgery, Duke University

Abigail Funari
Department of Neurological Surgery, Montefiore Medical Center the University Hospital for the Albert Einstein College of Medicine

James A. Garrity
Department of Ophthalmology, Mayo Clinic

Chad A. Glenn
Department of Neurosurgery, University of Oklahoma

Lain Hermes González Quarante
Department of Neurosurgery, Clínica Universidad de Navarra

Amit Goyal
Department of Neurosurgery, University of Minnesota

Jonathan A. Grossberg
Department of Neurosurgery, Department of Radiology and Imaging Sciences, Emory University

Emily Guazzo
Department of Otolaryngology, University of Queensland and Griffith University

Brian M. Howard
Department of Neurosurgery, Department of Radiology and Imaging Sciences, Emory University

Adam J. Kimple
Department of Otolaryngology / Head & Neck Surgery, University of North Carolina

Kevin Li
Department of Otolaryngology, Montefiore Medical Center the University Hospital for the Albert Einstein College of Medicine

Michael J. Link
Department of Neurosurgery, Mayo Clinic

Darlene Lubbe
Department of Otolaryngology, University of Cape Town

James G. Malcolm
Department of Neurosurgery, Emory University

Viraj J. Mehta
Department of Ophthalmology, Mayo Clinic

Pradeep Mettu
Department of Ophthalmology, Mayo Clinic

Michael A. Mooney
Department of Neurosurgery, Harvard Medical School/Brigham and Women's Hospital

Eric Moore
Department of Otolaryngology/Head & Neck Surgery, Mayo Clinic

Peter Morgenstern
Department of Neurological Surgery, Mount Sinai

Howard Moskowitz
Department of Otolaryngology, Montefiore Medical Center the University Hospital for the Albert Einstein College of Medicine

Hamzah Mustak
Department of Ophthalmology, University of Cape Town

Mohammed Nuru
Department of Neurological Surgery, University of California San Francisco

Kyle P. O'Connor
Department of Neurosurgery, University of Texas Health Sciences Center at Houston

Ali H. Palejwala
Department of Neurosurgery, University of Oklahoma

Ben Panizza
Department of Otolaryngology, University of Queensland

Panayiotis Pelargos
Department of Neurosurgery, University of Oklahoma

Gustavo Pradilla
Department of Neurosurgery, Emory University

Daniel Price
Department of Otolaryngology, Mayo Clinic

Rima S. Rindler
Department of Neurosurgery, Emory University

Hayder R. Salih
Department of Neurosurgery, Neurosurgery Teaching Hospital, Baghdad, Iraq

Hikari Sato
Department of Neurosurgery, Duke University

David Schoppy
Department of Otolaryngology, Kaiser Permanente Moanalua Medical Center

Theodore H. Schwartz
Department of Neurological Surgery, Weill Cornell Medical Center

Arturo Solares
Department of Otolaryngology, Emory University

Robert F. Spetzler
Department of Neurosurgery, Barrow Neurological Institute

Madeleine Strohl
Department of Otolaryngology, University of California San Francisco

Michael E. Sughrue
Center for Minimally Invasive Neurosurgery, Sydney, AU

Charles Teo
Center for Minimally Invasive Neurosurgery, Sydney, AU

Philip V. Theodosopoulos
Department of Neurological Surgery, University of California San Francisco

Brian D. Thorp
Department of Otolaryngology / Head & Neck Surgery, University of North Carolina

Jamie Van Gompel
Department of Neurosurgery, Mayo Clinic

Kumar Vasudevan
Department of Neurosurgery, Emory University

Brian J. Williams
Department of Neurosurgery, University of Louisville

Adam M. Zanation
Department of Otolaryngology / Head & Neck Surgery, University of North Carolina

Foreword

"If you change the way you look at things, the things you look at change."
Wayne Walter Dyer, American philosopher

Stone tools were used by early hominids to perform one of the earliest surgical procedures of which we have evidence: perforating the skull to let out demons or to release insanities resulting from head injuries. The oldest trephinations, from 10,000 BCE, have been found in Northern Africa. There is no evidence these ancient humans performed surgery on the brain, and thus these instances cannot be regarded as the true beginning of the field of neurosurgery. Yet it took Homo sapiens 290,000 years of natural selection to be able to trephine the skulls of other Homo sapiens and only 11,000 to develop modern neurosurgery, replete with all the tools and knowledge we now have at our disposal.

American medicine has done a remarkable job of increasing the quantity of life. Now we are faced with the challenge of improving the quality of that prolonged life. We all hope to live long lives, but none of us want to live to be 100 years old if it means we cannot move, suffer from pain, are severely disabled, or have lost the memories we spent a lifetime creating. Indeed, we face many ongoing challenges in the neurosciences, and those challenges must be addressed by scientists and physician-scientists in all departments and centers. Among the many successes of modern neurosurgery is the development of surgical exposures of intracranial pathology that have reduced the need to manipulate and retract neural tissue.

All neurosurgical trainees benefit from microsurgical and skull base surgical training. The skills of spine, pediatric, tumor, peripheral nerve, functional, and trauma neurosurgeons are enhanced by exposure to microsurgical training and the anatomical basis of skull base exposures. The benefit of illumination and magnification provided by the operative microscope and the principle of removing extraneous, disposable tissue, such as bone from the base of the skull, to minimize or eliminate retraction and manipulation or the brain can be applied to all subspecialties of neurosurgery and is one of the many principles that separate neurosurgery from other surgical disciplines.

In this volume, Dr. Agarwal has assembled world experts from the disciplines of otolaryngology and neurosurgery to provide a comprehensive treatise on the current state of the art in the surgical exposure of pathology of the base of the human skull.

We must thank, most of all, our patients, who have put their faith and trust in not only our surgical but our decision-making skills.

Daniel L. Barrow, MD
Pamela R. Rollins Professor & Chairman
Director, Emory/MBNA Stroke Center
Department of Neurosurgery
Emory University School of Medicine
Atlanta, Georgia

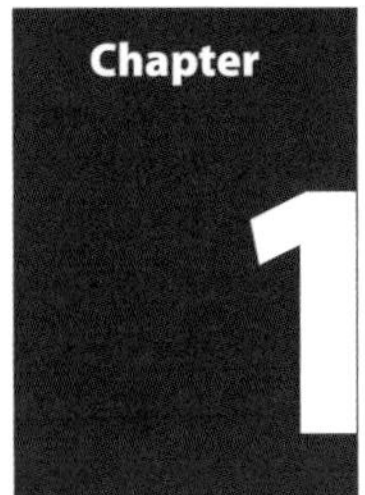

Combined Endonasal Transethmoidal, Transcribriform, and Endoscope-Assisted Supraorbital Craniotomy

Leopold Arko IV, Peter Morgenstern, and Theodore H. Schwartz

Introduction and Indications

Traditional transcranial approaches to the anterior skull base provide wide exposure but often require significant retraction of the brain and manipulation of neurovascular structures that lie between the surgeon and the pathology. The bifrontal, extended-subfrontal, or frontobasal approaches necessitate the sacrifice of the superior sagittal sinus, which can lead to brain edema or venous infarct. Minimally invasive routes have been developed to curtail the practice of brain retraction and provide a means of access to the pathology that, in well-selected cases, may reduce the need to cross the plane of cranial nerves or arteries.

The *extended endonasal approach* (*EEA*) is a global term used to describe a variety of approaches that utilize the nasal sinuses as corridors to reach a variety of locations along the midline and parasagittal skull base (1). When exposing the anterior skull base or frontal fossa, the ethmoid sinuses and the frontal sinus can be opened by removing the cribriform plate. This so-called transethmoidal, transcribriform approach allows for the resection of midline anterior skull base lesions without the need to sacrifice the superior sagittal sinus or retract the frontal lobe (2, 3). Other benefits of this approach include direct visualization and cauterization of the ethmoidal arteries for tumor devascularization, direct exposure of the cribriform plate (which is often invaded by tumors), and direct access and wide exposure to lesions that may have invaded the nasal sinuses. A vascularized nasal septal flap is easily obtained from this approach and helps decrease the rate of cerebral spinal fluid (CSF) leaks. However, given the breadth of the anterior skull base and the large size of the defect created, additional support may be needed to prevent CSF leaks in this area.

The transethmoidal, transcribriform approach is limited anteriorly by the frontal sinus, laterally by the lamina papyracea, and posteriorly by the planum sphenoidale (Table 1.1; Figure 1.1).

Table 1.1 Indications and limitations of the endonasal transethmoidal, transcribriform approach, supraorbital approach, and combined approach

Approach	Indication	Advantage	Disadvantage	Medial-to-lateral limitation	Anterior-posterior limitation
Endonasal transethmoidal, transcribriform	Medially centered anterior skull base lesions with nasal extension	Direct visualization of tumor, access to blood supply	CSF leak risk, patient loss of smell	Lateral to middle orbital line	Frontal sinus, posterior planum sphenoidale
Supraorbital	Anterior skull base tumors with lateral extension and without nasal extension	Direct visualization of tumor	Lack of access to vascularized flap, difficulty if pathology invades into the diploë of the skull base	Cribriform plate, crista galli, lateral and inferior sphenoid wing	Frontal sinus, invasion into frontal sinus, posterior to sphenoid wing
Combined	Extension beyond the lamina papyracea, extension into nasal sinus	Increased direct access to tumor, minimal brain retraction	Long operative time, patient loss of smell, CSF leak	Lateral and inferior sphenoid wing	frontal sinus, invasion into frontal sinus, posterior to sphenoid wing

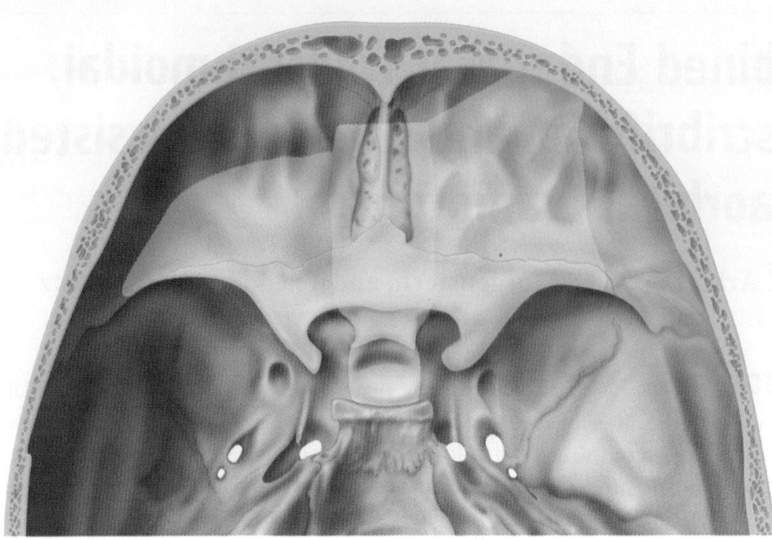

Figure 1.1 Axial overview of the cranial skull base outlining the area reached using the combined extended endonasal approach (EEA) and endoscopic-assisted supraorbital approach. The green shaded area represents the area exposed during an EEA, and the blue shaded area represents the area directly exposed during a supraorbital approach. The area with color overlap represents areas exposed equally well with either approach.

Complete removal of the lamina papyracea combined with a limited superomedial orbitectomy can provide further lateral extension, but the orbit itself cannot be mobilized beyond a few millimeters (4). Expansion of the approach through the sphenoid can aid in improving visualization of lesions that extend posteriorly. Removal of the tuberculum sellae provides further access to the medial optic nerve, chiasm, and lesions that expand into the third ventricle (5).

For pathology that does not lie completely within the confines of the area exposed by the transethmoidal, transcribriform approach, additional exposure can be provided by combining the EEA with a separate transcranial approach (6). In some cases, depending on the pathology and its location, only a supraorbital approach is required, which can be further expanded using endoscopic assistance. This approach provides direct access to the anterior cranial fossa floor and decreases the need for brain retraction. Using angled endoscopes, access to the anterior olfactory groove, intrasellar space, inferior optic nerve, interpeduncular space, medial middle fossa, and anterior third ventricle can be obtained through the supraorbital approach (7).

For some anterior cranial fossa lesions, the supraorbital approach is limited. Lesions extending far to the contralateral side can be difficult to resect, even with angled endoscopes. Laterally extending the frontal sinuses can limit the medial portion of the craniotomy. This can be overcome by cranializing the frontal sinus or packing the open portion of the sinus; however, the risk of pneumocephalus or CSF leak may not warrant this approach if sinus repair or packing is necessary. Lesions extending far anterior into the frontal sinus can also be difficult to reach, as are lesions that are either lateral or inferior to the sphenoid ridge. In addition, lesions that grow through the cribriform plate cannot be resected solely using the supraorbital approach, due to limitations on drilling the cribriform plate and crista galli (4).

Combining supraorbital endoscope-assisted craniotomy with the transethmoidal, transcribriform approach can help overcome some of the limitations of using a single approach. The EEA is the best approach for the removal of lesions that extend intranasally and are located along the cribriform plate, and for repairing the defect. The supraorbital approach can then be added to remove lesions extending anteriorly to the frontal sinus or extending laterally beyond 1 cm of the lamina papyracea (LP). Pathologies that most commonly fall into this category include olfactory groove meningiomas, esthesioneuroblastomas, and squamous cell carcinomas.

Other operative concerns to consider before choosing a combined approach include the extent of the lesion into the frontal sinus. Bilateral frontal sinus invasion still would be best removed with a bifrontal craniotomy. This would allow for a large pericranial flap harvest for skull base repair. Frontal sinuses are difficult to repair with a nasal flap.

Histology should also be considered during this process. For instance, en bloc resections, which may be necessary for some malignancies, cannot be obtained through this route. If the pathology is highly vascular, preoperative embolization should be considered. In addition, an EEA will likely eliminate olfaction and gustation, and patients should be counseled on this sensory loss.

Patient Positioning and Preparation

When conducting the combined approach, the surgeon can choose to perform the individual approaches sequentially or perform both approaches simultaneously. Typically, with either sequence, the patient will be placed in a rigid Mayfield head holder. The head can be fixed in a single position for both approaches with 15–30 degrees of extension, ipsilateral rotation, and abduction toward the contralateral shoulder (Figure 1.2A). The amount of rotation should be just enough to center the operative eyebrow at the highest point of the surgical field and permit comfortable endonasal access. The navigational system is then registered. The patient receives perioperative antibiotics with a broad enough spectrum to cover the nasal sinus flora. We generally use vancomycin and a second-generation cephalosporin. Perioperative antiepileptics and dexamethasone can also be administered. A lumbar drain may be placed, depending on the size of the expected defect, and intrathecal fluorescein (0.2 ml of 10% fluorescein with 10 ml of CSF or preservative-free saline) can help identify intraoperative CSF leaks (8, 9). If fluorescein is injected, the patient should be premedicated with 50 mg of intravenous diphenhydramine in addition to dexamethasone. Areas near the umbilicus and also near the lateral portion of the thigh are prepped for the harvesting of fat and fascia lata grafts, respectively.

Surgical Technique

Endonasal Transethmoidal, Transcribriform Approach

In preparation for the sinus procedure, the middle turbinates and the ethmoidal arteries are injected with 1% lidocaine with epinephrine (1:100,000 dilution). A large nasal septal flap should be harvested at the beginning of the dissection, as previously described (10). Bilateral, or "Janus," flaps may be helpful, depending on the expected size of the defect (11). There are five vertical structures in the nasal cavity that can be removed in a graded fashion, depending on the required size of the exposure. These include the septum in the midline, each of the middle turbinates, and each lamina papyracea. An uncinectomy is performed to reveal the maxillary sinus ostium using a sickle blade. This fully exposes the ethmoid bulla, allowing for dissection lateral to the lamina papyracea. If even further lateral resection is needed, the lamina papyracea can be resected if the periorbita is not violated. Once lateral dissection of the ethmoids to the lamina papyracea is completed

(a)

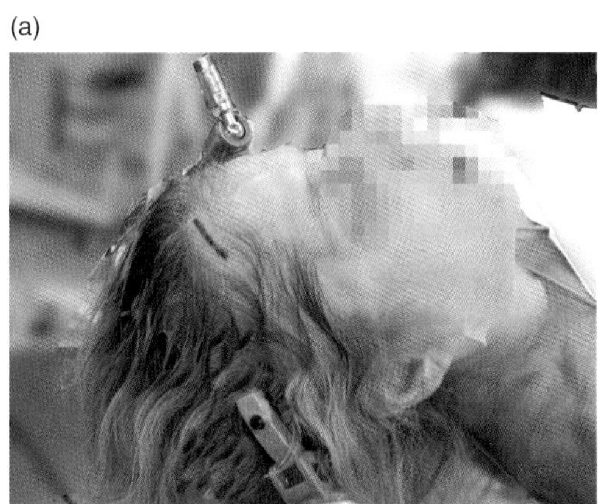

(b)

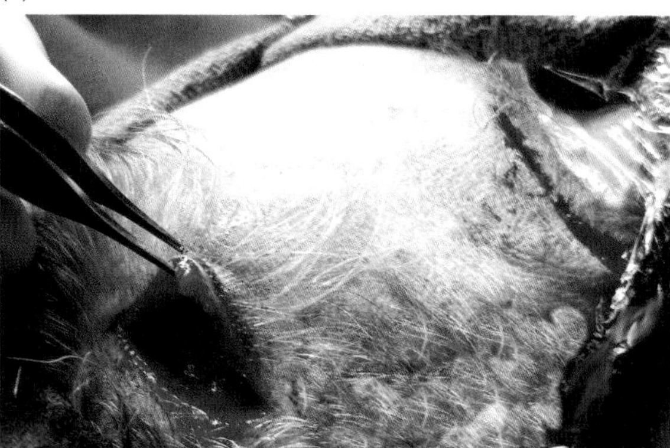

Figure 1.2 (A) Intraoperative photo showing the head position for combined supraorbital and EEA. Typical positioning requires 15–30 degrees of extension, ipsilateral rotation, and abduction toward the contralateral shoulder. (B) Visualization of a superior forehead incision for a pericranial graft along with a typical supraorbital incision.

bilaterally, submucosal dissection and resection of the upper third of the nasal septum are completed to form a large, single cavity. The anterior and posterior ethmoidal arteries are identified and coagulated. The olfactory epithelium and mucosa are removed following cauterization. High-speed drills are used to remove the fovea ethmoidalis, beginning anteriorly at the frontoethmoidal recess and progressing posteriorly to the sphenoid sinus. If the lesion overlies the planum sphenoidale or tuberculum sellae, the sphenoid sinus is then opened bilaterally. Laterally, the cribriform plate is drilled at the border with the lamina papyracea. The thick bone of the crista galli is drilled in the midline. The thin bone is then freed with curettes and removed with Kerrison and pituitary rongeurs. If the pathology is intradural, the dura can be opened once maximum exposure is obtained.

The lesion is then debulked internally, typically using bimanual suction. For firmer lesions, an ultrasonic aspirator (Cavitron, Valleylab, CO) or monopolar (Elliquence, Oceanside, NY) may be used. After adequate debulking, the capsule of the lesion is mobilized. Sharp dissection and cautery are used to free the capsule from vascular and neural structures such as the A2 branches.

Several options exist to close the defect. If bony margins are present, a "gasket-seal" closure can be performed (12, 13). An inlay of Duraform (Natus Neuro, Middleton, WI) can be used as a first layer. A fascia lata graft or Dura-Guard (Synovis Surgical, St. Paul, MN) piece is then cut so that it has a diameter about 1 cm larger than the skull defect. This graft is then laid over the opening. A piece of MEDPOR (Stryker, Kalamazoo, MI) is then cut to the size of the defect and countersunk into the defect just beyond the edge of the bone. The previously harvested nasoseptal flaps are laid so that they extend beyond the margin of the fascia lata or Dura-Guard (14). A sealant such as DuraSeal (Integra, Plainsboro, NJ) or Adherus (Stryker, Kalamazoo, MI) is then placed over the gasket seal. If the defect is large with no boney margins, an inlay-onlay of fascia lata can be performed and buttressed with a Foley balloon to provide extra support. The balloon stays in place for a few days and is then removed. The nasal cavity is then filled with Floseal (Baxter, Deerfield, IL), and NasoPore (Stryker, Kalamazoo, MI) is inserted into the nasal cavity.

Supraorbital Approach

The incision for the supraorbital approach is made from within the eyebrow, extending from the supraorbital notch to just past the insertion of the temporalis muscle, with care taken not to injure the supraorbital nerve. The exposure must be lateral to the frontal sinus and extend far enough to allow a burr hole to be made in the key hole of the pterion.

The side chosen depends on the location of the pathology. Approaching ipsilaterally to the greatest lateral extent of the pathology can be advantageous, particularly if the pathology extends laterally to the optic nerve. However, the medial optic canal can often be hidden given the low angle of approach. Therefore, if the pathology extends into the medial optic canal, a contralateral approach can often be advantageous (Figure 1.1) (15). An incision is made with a 15 blade in the middle of the eyebrow. Dissect sharply down through the frontalis and orbicularis oculi to the pericranium. The pericranium is incised in a U-shape fashion with the base of the "U" at the orbital ridge. Longer pericranial flaps can be harvested by dissecting the pericranium further posterior and making a second incision on the forehead (Figure 1.2B). This flap is useful when there is a large frontal sinus violation or inadequate closure from the EEA. The skin incision is then retracted with elastic stay retractors. The temporalis is dissected widely enough to reveal the key hole. A single burr hole is made in the key hole. A craniotome is then used to make as large a craniotomy as is allowed by the incision, which is typically 3 × 3 cm (Figure 1.3). The craniotome is stopped along the medial and lateral edges of the orbital bar. Thereafter, the orbital bar is removed with a chisel or an ultrasonic knife, while the periorbita is retracted and protected with a brain retractor. The bone flap is then removed. Some authors do not routinely remove the orbital rim, although this can increase the size of the opening, improve maneuverability, and increase upward exposure to reach the top of larger tumors.

The frontal lobe and dura are retracted and a microscope is used to view the orbital floor. A diamond drill is used to remove any prominent bone. The dura is then opened and flapped in a U-shape fashion with the base of the "U" at the orbit. CSF is evacuated to assist with brain relaxation. (One accessible area for CSF is the optico-carotid cistern.) Another option for brain

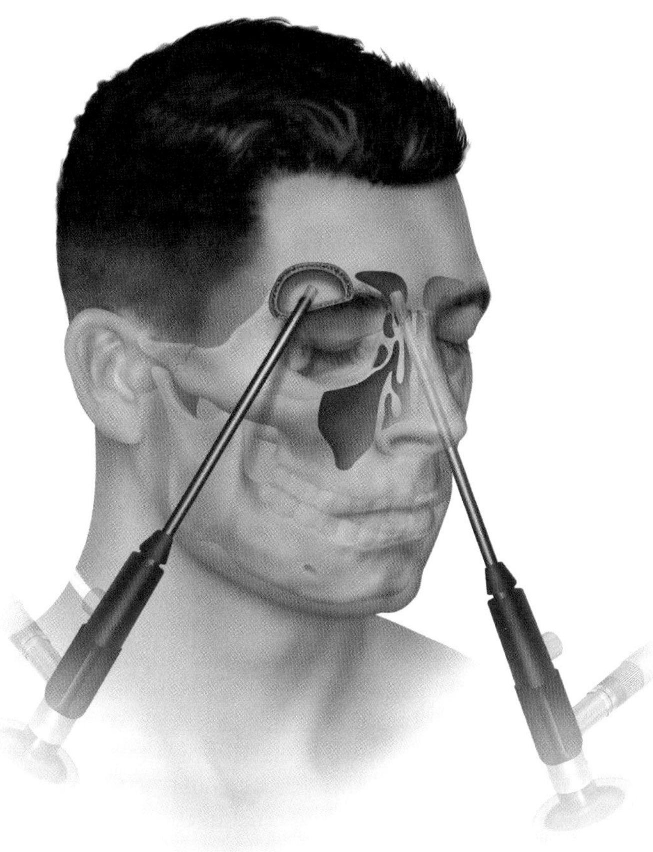

Figure 1.3 Schematic of size and location of supraorbital craniotomy along with the trajectory of the EEA

relaxation is to open the lumbar drain that was placed before the operation, although this is generally not necessary.

Depending on the surgeon's preference, initial dissection to the pathology can be performed with the aid of either a microscope or an endoscope. Endoscopic views, especially with a 45° scope, can provide a much wider view of the pathology. The scope can be held by a second surgeon or placed in a scope holder. At the very least, the endoscope can be used to inspect the surgical cavity for residual tumor if a microscopic resection is preferred. Once the lesion is resected, hemostasis is obtained in the cavity. The pericranial graft can be laid over any opening made in the frontal sinus.

The dura is closed and made watertight. If necessary, extra Duragen or Gelfoam can be placed over the dura to help with watertight closure. The bone flap is affixed with low-profile plates. The temporalis muscle is reapproximated by placing small tack-up holes along the superior temporal line. Bone cement can be used to cover any remaining gaps in the bone. The galea is closed with 3–0 vicryl sutures. The skin is closed with a 5–0 Prolene stitch in a subcuticular fashion without knots along the incision. The two ends of the Prolene stitch are knotted together over a Telfa dressing. The Prolene stitch is removed in 5–7 days.

Postoperative Care

Immediately post-surgery, the head of the patient's bed is elevated 30 degrees. Patients are given typical sinus precautions: no blowing of the nose, no use of straws, and a strict bowel regimen to prevent straining. Patient diets are advanced slowly to reduce the risk of vomiting. If a lumbar drain was placed, it is drained depending on the severity of intraoperative CSF leakage. For lesions extending into the sellar space, patients are placed on diabetes insipidus watch. In such cases, postoperative cortisol and pituitary function labs are also obtained. Patients without a CSF leak may get out of bed on the first day postoperation.

Case Presentation

A 53-year-old woman presented with nasal congestion. She was initially diagnosed with nasal polyp disease but began having tooth pain leading to a CAT scan of the head. This revealed a mass in the anterior skull base. A brain MRI further elucidated an enhancing mass of the anterior skull base on the right side (Figure 1.4). The mass extended intracranially from the back of the frontal sinus, anteriorly over the crista galli along the cribriform plate, and back to the anterior margin of the planum. The mass also extended down through the olfactory bulb and into the nasal cavity medial to the middle turbinate. Although esthesioneuroblastoma was considered in the differential diagnosis, the imaging was most consistent with olfactory groove meningioma.

A lumbar drain was placed before final positioning, and fluorescein (0.25 mL in all of 4% fluorescein diluted with 10 mL of CSF) was injected. The patient was placed supine with the head in a Mayfield head holder and registered with frameless stereotactic navigation. The planned approach was a right supraorbital craniotomy with orbital osteotomy performed simultaneously with an EEA and transethmoidal, transcribriform approach. The supraorbital approach allowed for a complete removal of the supratentorial intradural portion of the mass. This was accomplished by using both a microdissection technique as well as a 45-degree endoscope to see into the olfactory groove. A piece of autologous pericranium was used for a secondary repair of the dura. The previously harvested pericranium and frontalis muscle were used to cover the frontal sinus. The bone was replaced with low-profile plates and the skin was closed as previously described.

Next, the endoscopic approach commenced. A nasoseptal flap was developed on the left side and was tucked into the nasopharynx. The ethmoid was exposed so that the roof of the nasal cavity and the olfactory groove could be viewed bilaterally. Next, bilateral partial inferior turbinectomies and

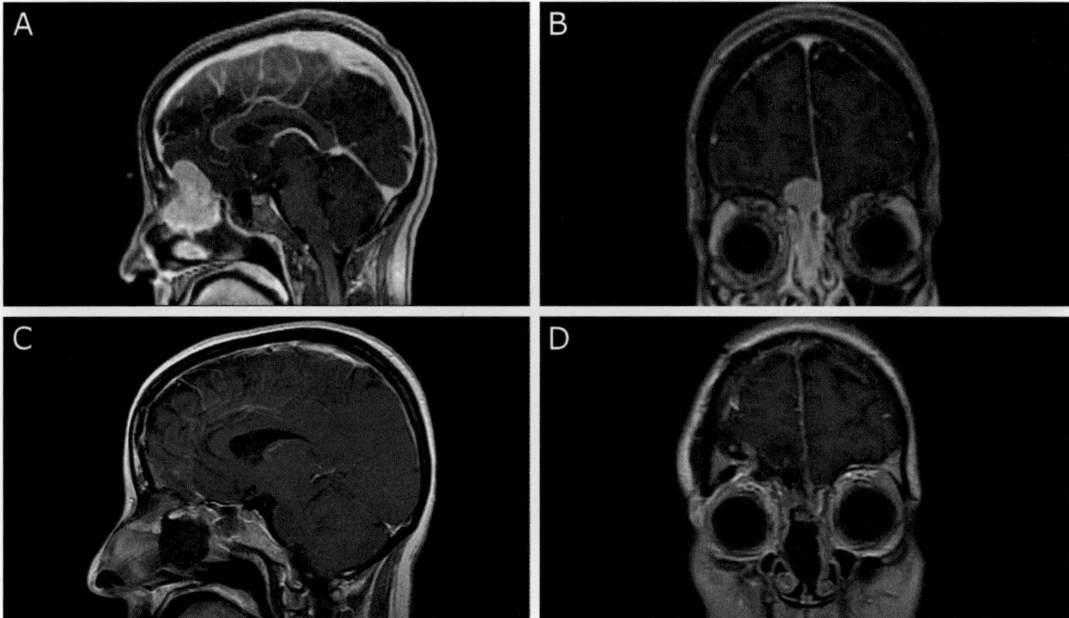

Figure 1.4 (A) Sagittal and (B) coronal view of a preoperative T1-weighted post-contrast image depicting a large enhancing mass compatible with an olfactory groove meningioma. The tumor extended far anterior against the frontal sinuses with extension into the nasal cavity. Patient underwent a combined approach. Postoperative post-contrast T1-weighted (C) sagittal and (D) coronal planes depict a complete resection.

bilateral uncinectomies were performed. A complete right-sided ethmoidectomy was then performed. The perpendicular plate of the ethmoid was removed under direct vision. The tumor was removed from the olfactory groove bilaterally. The dura was exposed all the way to the planum sphenoidale to ensure all the mass had been removed. A dural defect was noted. After removal of the perpendicular plate and the lateral lamella of the roof of the ethmoid sinus, the nasoseptal flap was rotated into the area of the defect. DuraSeal was sprayed into the area around the flap, followed by FloSeal. CSF/fluorescein leak was not observed after the repair. NasoPore splints were inserted into each nostril. Postoperative MRI films of the brain showed a gross tumor resection (Figure 1.4), and final pathology confirmed olfactory groove meningioma.

Conclusion

The combined endoscopic endonasal transethmoidal, transcribriform approach with endoscope-assisted supraorbital craniotomy is a minimally invasive approach that can be used as an alternative to the classic transcranial, transfacial, or combined craniofacial approaches to lesions of the anterior cranial fossa. This approach is best used for lesions that extend anteriorly to the frontal sinus, laterally beyond the lamina papyracea, and inferiorly into the ethmoid sinus. There are several methods for closing the skull base defect both from above and below with this approach, including pericranial graft, a vascular nasal septal flap, and a gasket seal with fascia lata.

Key Points

- The combined endoscopic endonasal transethmoidal, transcribriform approach with endoscope-assisted supraorbital craniotomy can be used for lesions that extend laterally beyond the lamina papyracea and inferiorly into the ethmoid sinus.
- This combined approach can be completed in one operative sitting or done sequentially, depending on the location of the lesion.
- The combined approach is limited anteriorly by the frontal sinus and posteriorly by the sphenoid wing.
- There are many different methods used to close the post-operative defect, including a pericranial flap, a vascular nasal flap, and a gasket seal closure.
- Patients must be counseled on the risk of CSF leak and the high likelihood of decreased olfaction following surgery.

References

1. Schwartz TH, Fraser JF, Brown S, Tabaee A, Kacker A, Anand VK. Endoscopic cranial base surgery: classification of operative approaches. *Neurosurgery*. 2008;**62**(5):991–1002.
2. Banu MA, Mehta A, Ottenhausen M, Fraser JF, Patel KS, Szentirmai O, et al. Endoscope-assisted endonasal versus supraorbital keyhole resection of olfactory groove meningiomas: comparison and combination of two minimally invasive approaches. *J Neurosurg*. 2016;**124**(3):605–20.
3. Jho HD, Ha HG. Endoscopic endonasal skull base surgery: Part 1 – The midline anterior fossa skull base. *Minim Invasive Neurosurg*. 2004;**47**(1):1–8.
4. Borghei-Razavi H, Truong HQ, Fernandes-Cabral DT, Celtikci E, Chabot JD, Stefko ST, et al. Minimally invasive approaches for anterior skull base meningiomas: supraorbital eyebrow, endoscopic endonasal, or a combination of both? anatomic study, limitations, and surgical application. *World Neurosurg*. 2018;**112**:e666–74.
5. Greenfield JP, Anand VK, Kacker A, Seibert MJ, Singh A, Brown SM, et al. Endoscopic endonasal transethmoidal transcribriform transfovea ethmoidalis approach to the anterior cranial fossa and skull base. *Neurosurgery*. 2010;**66**(5):883–92; discussion 92.
6. Knopman J, Sigounas D, Huang C, Kacker A, Schwartz TH, Boockvar JA. Combined supraciliary and endoscopic endonasal approach for resection of frontal sinus mucoceles: technical note. *Minim Invasive Neurosurg*. 2009;**52**(3):149–51.
7. Wilson DA, Duong H, Teo C, Kelly DF. The supraorbital endoscopic approach for tumors. *World Neurosurg*. 2014;**82**(1–2):e243–56.
8. Placantonakis DG, Tabaee A, Anand VK, Hiltzik D, Schwartz TH. Safety of low-dose intrathecal fluorescein in endoscopic cranial base surgery. *Neurosurgery*. 2007;**61**(3 Suppl):161–5; discussion 5–6.
9. Raza SM, Banu MA, Donaldson A, Patel KS, Anand VK, Schwartz TH. Sensitivity and specificity of intrathecal fluorescein and white light excitation for detecting intraoperative cerebrospinal fluid leak in endoscopic skull base surgery: a prospective study. *J Neurosurg*. 2016;**124**(3):621–6.
10. Hadad G, Bassagasteguy L, Carrau RL, Mataza JC, Kassam A, Snyderman CH, et al. A novel

reconstructive technique after endoscopic expanded endonasal approaches: vascular pedicle nasoseptal flap. *Laryngoscope*. 2006;**116**(10):1882–6.

11. Nyquist GG, Anand VK, Singh A, Schwartz TH. Janus flap: bilateral nasoseptal flaps for anterior skull base reconstruction. *Otolaryngol Head Neck Surg*. 2010;**142**(3):327–31.
12. Leng LZ, Brown S, Anand VK, Schwartz TH. "Gasket-seal" watertight closure in minimal-access endoscopic cranial base surgery. *Neurosurgery*. 2008;**62**(5 Suppl 2): ONSE342–3; discussion ONSE3.
13. Garcia-Navarro V, Anand VK, Schwartz TH. Gasket seal closure for extended endonasal endoscopic skull base surgery: efficacy in a large case series. *World Neurosurg*. 2013;**80**(5):563–8.
14. McCoul ED, Schwartz TH, Anand VK. Vascularized reconstruction of endoscopic skull base defects. *Oper Tech Otolaryngol Head Neck Surg*. 2011;**22**(3):232–6.
15. Singh H, Essayed WI, Jada A, Moussazadeh N, Dhandapani S, Rote S, et al. Contralateral supraorbital keyhole approach to medial optic nerve lesions: an anatomoclinical study. *J Neurosurg*. 2017;**126**(3):940–4.

Combined Endonasal and Transorbital Approach

Darlene Lubbe and Hamzah Mustak

Introduction

The concept of using endoscopy in the orbit was first proposed by Norris in 1983 (6). The inability to safely insufflate and create a working space, coupled with the available technology at the time, led to a loss of interest in this approach. Advances in imaging technology, illumination sources, and instrumentation have resulted in a renewed interest and the adoption of these technologies in orbital surgery.

Combining endoscopic transnasal and transorbital approaches allows for multiportal surgery, where instruments can reach difficult-to-access skull base areas with minimal collateral damage to normal tissues. Different surgical trajectories can be obtained and the use of standard zero-degree endoscopes and instruments allows for easier manipulation of the target lesion. Multistage surgery can often be avoided and lesions can often be removed en-bloc. Endoscopic transnasal approaches offer access to the central and medial areas of the skull base; however, the orbit limits access to the lateral skull base through this approach. Kris Moe popularized the concept of transorbital portals that overcome the obstacle of the orbital contents allowing for access to the superior and inferior lateral areas of the skull base (4,5). The transorbital approach takes advantage of the natural tissue planes and displacement of the globe and orbital soft tissues to create a portal for introduction of the endoscope and operating instruments. The drive for the development of minimally invasive surgery has seen a renewed interest in exploring the transorbital corridors, along with their advantages, limitations, and role in addressing intra-orbital pathology.

Endoscopic surgery involving the orbit can therefore be categorized according to whether the target lesion is within the orbit, adjacent to the orbit, and extradural or located intracranially requiring intradural dissection (Figure 2.1).

A combination of portals can often be used to approach a lesion and allows for the manipulation of the target from different directions and angles. (Figure 2.2).

Indications for Endoscopic Orbital and Multiportal Endonasal and Transorbital Approaches

Endoscopic Orbital Surgery: Intraconal and Extraconal Surgery

The endoscope is a useful tool for addressing lesions within the orbit and for managing disease affecting the bony walls of the orbit. The surgery is extradural and breaching the dura during these cases would be a complication of surgery, similar to breaching the dura during endoscopic sinus surgery. Endoscopic approaches for addressing orbital tumors are best suited for lesions that are extraconal and in the mid to posterior orbit. These lesions are approached in the subperiosteal plane and the periorbita is opened only once the tumor is identified tenting it. This approach limits orbital fat prolapse which would make surgical exposure more difficult. Transorbital surgery avoids the need for a craniotomy and removal of the roof of the orbit and reconstruction of the defect. The decision on which transorbital portal to use and whether to combine it with an endonasal approach depends on the location of the orbital lesion. If the lesion is located within the superior, lateral, or inferior orbit, a single portal transorbital approach is indicated. If the lesion is located within the medial orbit, a precaruncular or endonasal approach can be utilized, or a multiportal approach using both portals can be used to assist in lesion manipulation (Figure 2.3).

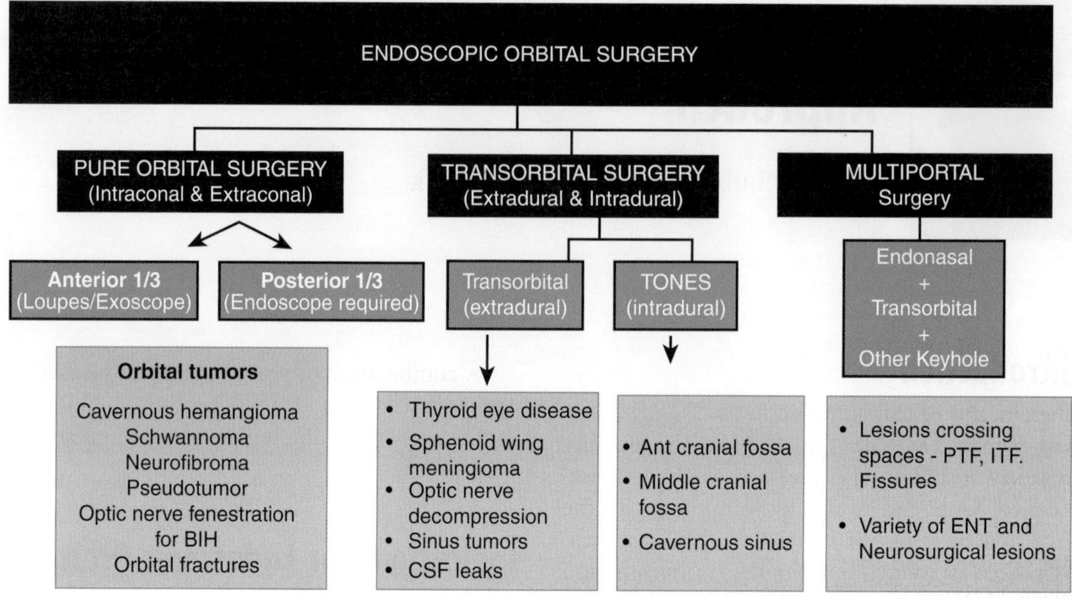

Figure 2.1 Algorithm showing endoscopic surgery involving the orbit categorized according to whether the target lesion is within the orbit, adjacent to the orbit, and extradural or located intracranially requiring intradural dissection

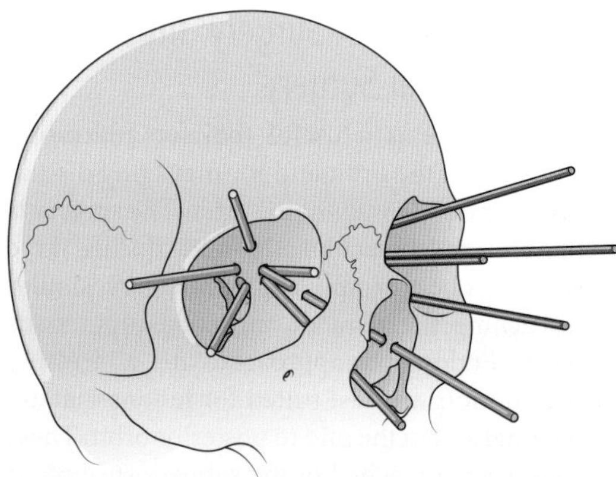

Figure 2.2 A combination of 10 portals can be used to approach a lesion and allows manipulation of the target from different directions and angle

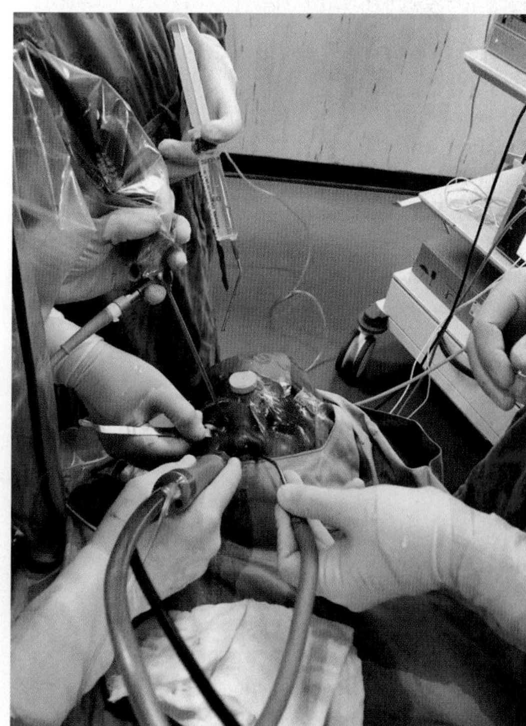

Figure 2.3 Multiportal approach using the precaruncular and binostril portals

Cavernous hemangiomas are one of the most common orbital tumors and often patients present with proptosis as the main complaint. The transorbital portal allows for a minimally invasive approach to these lesions, avoiding a craniotomy, an orbitotomy, or an extensive endonasal dissection, depending on the location of the lesion. Other advantages are that the patients can be discharged the same day, avoid the need for post-operative intensive care monitoring, and have no visible scar except for the temporary blepharoplasty incision, when used. These lesions can often be approached by at least two different transorbital portals and the approach selected depends on the relationship of the lesion to nearby structures. A decision needs to be made regarding the safest route of removal between the rectus muscles, and the relationship between the lesion and neurovascular structures must be understood and respected. Cavernous hemangiomas located in the medial orbit can be safely and quickly removed through a precaruncular transorbital approach (Figures 2.4 and 2.5).

Although the endonasal approach is seen as a minimally invasive approach, this approach requires extensive dissection of the sinuses, and often a septal window is required for instrument manipulation. This approach leaves the patient with potential nasal morbidity. The precaruncular approach avoids the need for reconstruction of the medial orbit since the lamina papyracea is left intact with no risk of secondary enophthalmos, and avoids nasal morbidity.

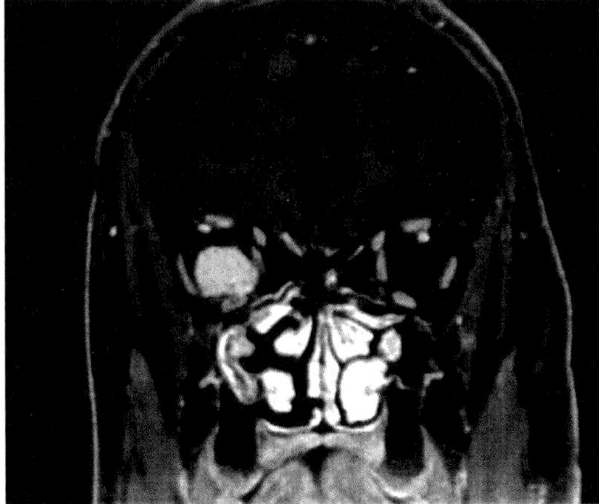

Figure 2.4 CT of a cavernous hemangioma located in the medial orbit

Endoscopic Transorbital Surgery (Extradural and Intradural)

Transorbital surgery by definition implies that the orbit is used as a portal to reach areas that abut the orbital contents. Often the eye is not pathologically involved and great care should be taken not to compromise a healthy eye. The surgical corridor created could remain extradural, or surgery can extend through the dura to address intracranial lesions. The eye is retracted either laterally, medially, superiorly, or inferiorly to help create the surgical pathway. It is usually not required to breach the periorbita unless the lesion involves the orbit itself and an extra- or intraconal dissection is required for complete surgical resection.

Transorbital (extradural) surgical portals create an access route to the paranasal sinuses adjacent to the bony orbit and areas of the skull base that are otherwise difficult to access. The inferior and superior orbital fissure, pterygopalatine fossa, and infratemporal and temporal fossa can all be accessed through transorbital portals.

The lateral frontal sinus and lateral sphenoid sinus can be difficult to access through transnasal routes in well-pneumatized sinuses. An endoscopic Lothrop operation will give good access to the frontal sinuses but if disease is located more lateral than the reach of available 70-degree instruments, another surgical route is required

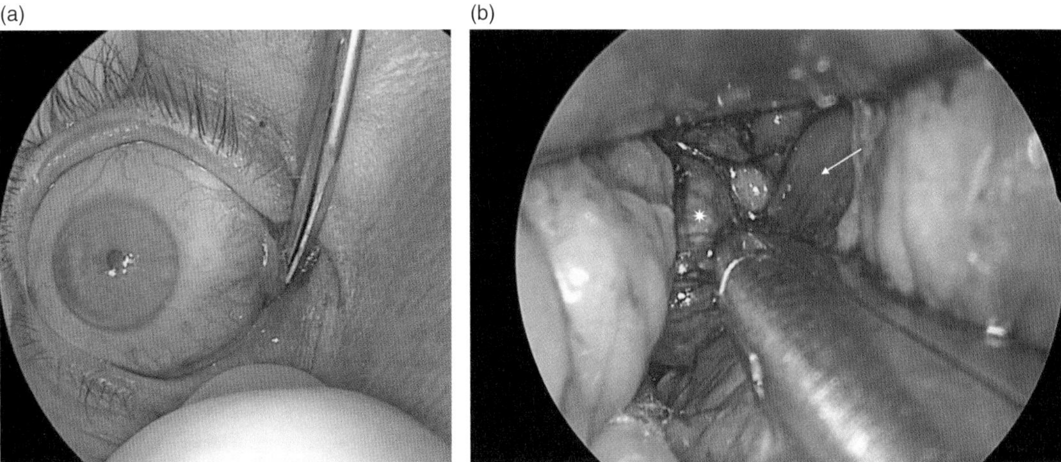

Figure 2.5 The lesion can be resected through a precaruncular transorbital approach.

to adequately address disease in this area, especially when dealing with malignant lesions. Frontal sinus pathology can therefore be addressed using a purely transorbital superior eyelid approach or can be combined with an endonasal approach to allow for multiportal surgery, whereby disease can be completely removed using minimally invasive techniques.

The lateral aspect of a well-pneumatized sphenoid sinus is traditionally accessed through an endonasal transpterygoid approach. This approach is often used to repair spontaneous cerebrospinal fluid (CSF) leaks secondary to lateral sphenoid sinus defects and to address encephaloceles in this area. Transorbital surgery offers an alternative pathway to access the lateral sphenoid sinus, often with a direct trajectory to the target lesion. Whereas the precaruncular transorbital approach offers a quick pathway to the sphenoid sinus and optic nerve, a contralateral precaruncular approach or an ipsilateral lateral transorbital approach gives access to the lateral aspect of a well-pneumatized sphenoid sinus. Examples of extradural lesions that can be accessed using a transorbital approach are listed in Table 2.1.

Transorbital neuro endoscopic surgery (TONES) implies the dura is purposely breached to reach lesions involving the anterior and middle cranial fossa. TONES cases should always be done in conjunction with a neurosurgeon to address the intracranial component of the tumor and for the repair of CSF leak. Surgery is performed through the corridor created, either by using an endoscope or a microscope, depending on the preference of the neurosurgeon. Indications and examples of cases that can be done using TONES are given in Table 2.2. The decision as to whether to use a TONES portal or multiple portals, combined with an endonasal approach, depends on the location of the pathology, the need for optic nerve decompression, and the composition of the surgical team.

Table 2.1 Examples of extradural lesions that can be addressed through transorbital portals

Superior approach
- Frontal sinus lesions – inverting papilloma, osteoma, mucocele, malignant lesions
- Superior orbital and orbital apex lesions
- Repair of CSF leaks involving the frontal sinus, orbital roof

Medial approach
- Ethmoidal vessels, optic nerve, lateral sphenoid sinus, cavernous sinus

Inferior approach
- Inferior orbital lesions / Inferior orbital fissure pathology
- Infraorbital nerve to foramen rotundum
- Orbital floor fractures / Blow-out fractures with entrapped muscle

Lateral approach
- Sphenoid wing meningioma – for removal hyperostotic bone, orbital tumor
- Superior orbital fissure or lateral aspect of optic nerve

Multiportal Surgery

Multiportal transorbital surgery offers access to the target lesion by combining any of the eight transorbital portals with the two nasal corridors. Other keyhole approaches that can be used in combination with the 10 previously described portals are a maxillary sinusotomy, frontal sinusotomy, and the supraorbital keyhole approach. Often, multiple approaches are possible, and the portal utilized depends on the location of the target lesion, the trajectory required, instrument availability, and surgeon experience. Figure 2.6 presents is a good candidate case for multiportal surgery. Possible approaches for complete resection include the following:

- Craniotomy / osteoplastic flap
- Transorbital approach
- Endoscopic Lothrop / Draf-3 operation
- Multiportal surgery combining a transorbital approach and an endoscopic Lothrop

Table 2.2 Indications for TONES

Superior approach
- Frontal meningiomas or other benign and malignant lesions of anterior cranial fossa
- Cerebrospinal fluid leak
- Optic nerve fenestration

Lateral approach
- Sphenoid wing meningiomas
- Lesions involving the middle or anterior cranial fossa
- Superior orbital fissure lesions
- Cavernous sinus laterally

Medial approach
- Anterior cranial fossa / cribriform plate
- Optic nerve
- Cavernous sinus

There is not necessarily one "correct" approach, but rather the approach should be tailored according to patient factors (e.g., age, comorbidities, aesthetic need), lesion factors (e.g., malignant or benign, access for instrumentation such as high-speed drills), and surgeon ability and comfortability. Multiportal surgery combinations are numerous and will continue to expand as new indications are found to address various skull base pathologies.

Both benign and malignant lesions involving the orbit and sinuses can be managed using this multiportal combination. It is important to remember that the same common principles apply during multiportal surgery – complete resection is required for malignant lesions and minimally invasive surgery is not indicated in cases where a tumor invades the skin or breaches the periorbita. External procedures with reconstruction and vascularized flaps may be indicated in these instances.

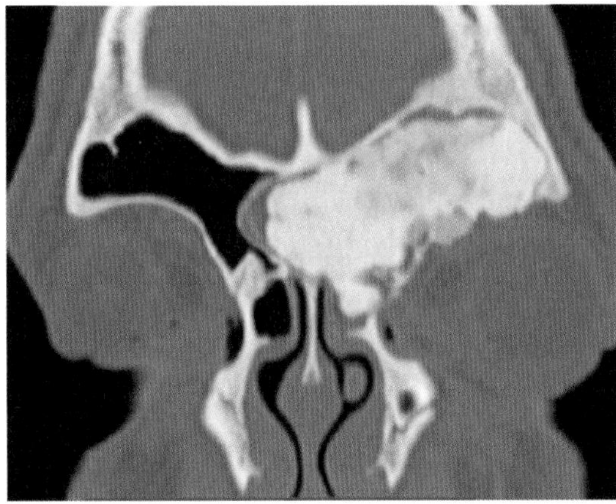

Figure 2.6 Giant osteoma of the left frontal sinus

Examples of multiportal combinations, common clinical scenarios, and the decision-making process behind the specific approaches are illustrated as follows.

Superior Eyelid +/- Endonasal Approach (One- or Two-Nostril Approach)

The superior eyelid approach alone provides sufficient access to the frontal sinus if there is no intranasal tumor component present (Figure 2.7). An endoscopic Lothrop (Draf-3) operation is useful when the frontal sinuses are completely accessible through an endonasal route. In this operation, the floor of both frontal sinuses is removed, and the frontal sinus inter-sinus septum is resected together with the superior nasal septum to create a wide communication between the frontal sinuses and the nasal cavity. The lateral aspect of a well-pneumatized frontal sinus can often be well visualized with a 70-degree endoscope, but it is not always possible to reach the lateral wall of the sinus with available instrumentation.

Multiportal surgery for frontal sinus lesions combines the superior eyelid approach with a unilateral endonasal approach for lesions not crossing the midline, or with a binostril approach for lesions crossing the midline. The binostril

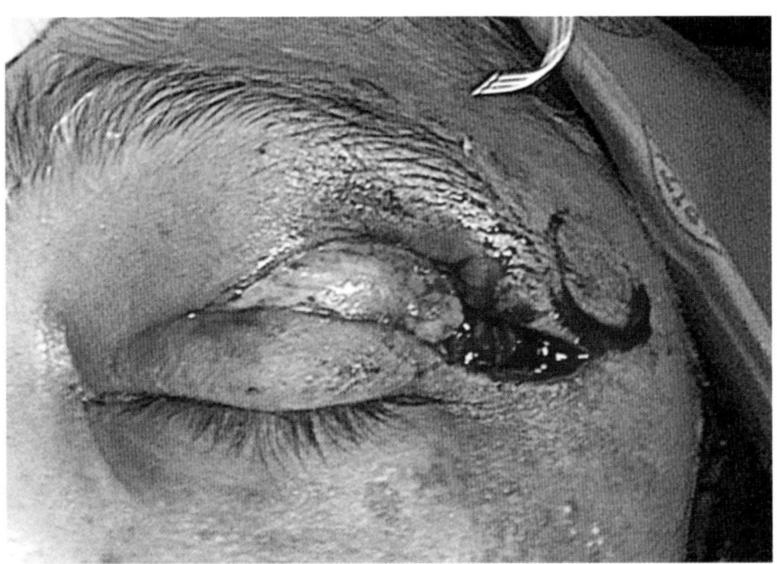

Figure 2.7 The superior eyelid approach alone provides sufficient access to the frontal sinus.

approach is used during a Lothrop operation, and the superior septectomy allows for multiple instruments to converge at the target lesion in the frontal sinus. Benign lesions such as osteomas, inverting papillomas, ossifying fibromas, as well as malignant tumors of the sinonasal cavity, can be addressed using these approaches. The combination of the transorbital and endonasal approaches avoids a craniotomy/osteoplastic flap operation and allows for normal function of the frontal sinuses post-operatively; it obviates the need for orbital reconstruction in most cases. The addition of the binostril approach allows for three surgical portals with a variety of multifunctional instruments being able to be manipulated through each port, thereby allowing multiple functions to be performed at the target area simultaneously (Figure 2.3).

Inferior Transorbital +/- Unilateral Endonasal Approach

The inferior subconjunctival approach can be used in isolation for lesions involving the inferior orbit; for access to the infraorbital nerve, inferior orbital fissure, or pterygopalatine fossa; or can be used combined with an ipsilateral endonasal approach for lesions involving the maxillary sinus or orbital floor. The multiportal approach allows for excellent access, visualization, and manipulation of lesions that cross surgical boundaries, such as an orbital lesion extending through the inferior orbital fissure into the pterygopalatine or infratemporal fossa (Figure 2.8). The infraorbital nerve can be followed back to the foramen rotundum, if required.

Medial Transorbital +/- Endonasal Approach (One or Two-Nostril Approach)

The medial (pre- or transcaruncular) approach can be used on its own (Figure 2.9) or can be combined with the endonasal approach (Figure 2.3) to address various lesions involving the orbit, anterior cranial fossa, cribriform plate, olfactory fossa, and ethmoid and sphenoid sinuses. This approach provides an excellent route to the optic nerve for medial optic nerve decompression. This procedure is often performed in conjunction with a superolateral approach for tumor resection, such as in the case of a sphenoid wing meningioma. The decision as to whether to use the precaruncular approach alone in optic nerve decompression, or a precaruncular combined with a unilateral or bilateral endonasal approach, depends on the associated orbital and sphenoid sinus

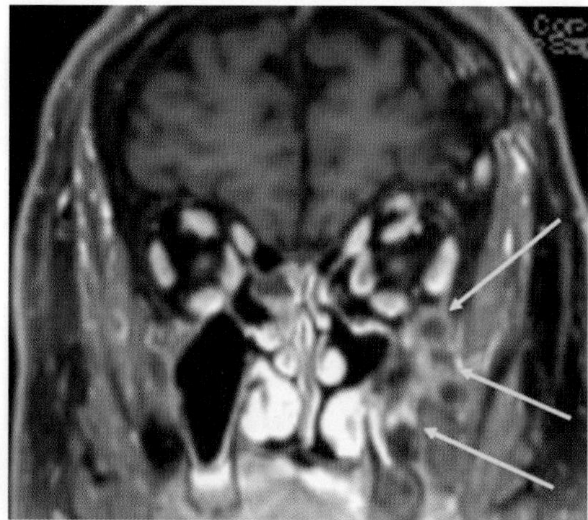

Figure 2.8 Plexiform neurofibroma crossing surgical boundaries; involving the orbit, inferior orbital fissure, pterygopalatine fossa

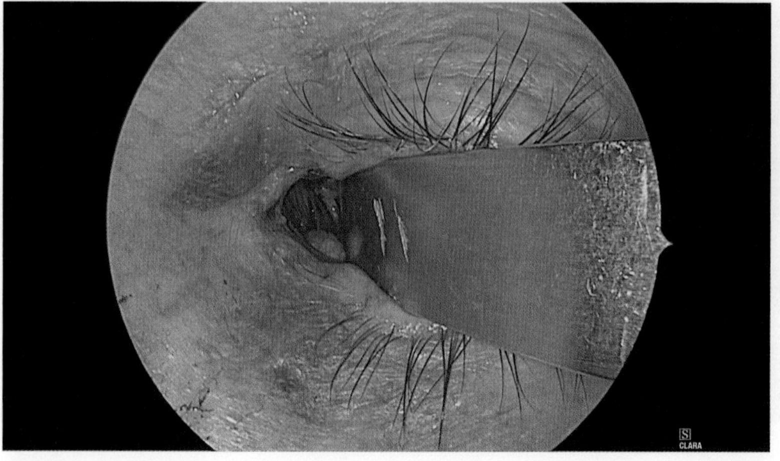

Figure 2.9 Precaruncular approach (left eye), with incision made between caruncle and medial canthus

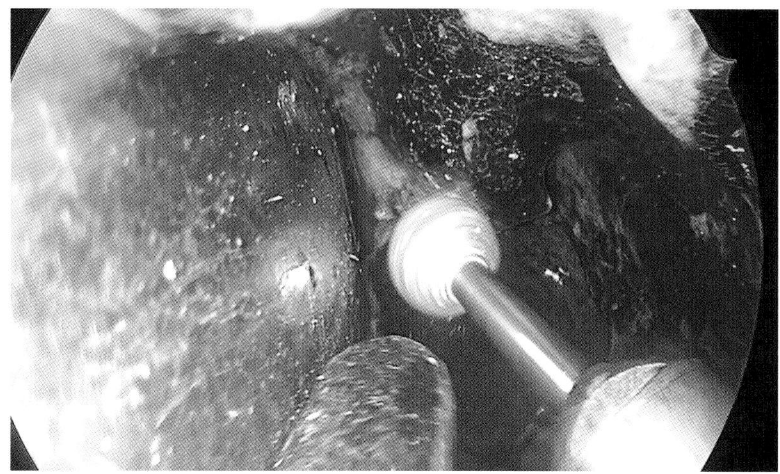

Figure 2.10 Using the precaruncular approach with a combined endonasal approach allows for retraction of the orbital contents (right eye) during medial optic canal decompression

pathology. In a proptotic eye, an endonasal approach to the optic nerve can often be difficult because of herniating periorbita anterior to the optic nerve. Using the precaruncular approach with a combined endonasal approach allows for retraction of the orbital contents, such as periorbital fat, thereby making the use of powered instrumentation in close proximity to the orbit safer (Figure 2.10). There are cases of tumors in the sphenoid sinus, such as is often seen in patients with sphenoid wing meningiomas, a multiportal approach to the optic nerve is necessitated to allow multiple instruments to converge on the target lesion. To provide both suction and irrigation whilst drilling the optic canal, two portals are often required to provide clear visualization of the optic nerve. Combining the precaruncular portal with an ipsilateral endonasal portal avoids the need to perform a posterior septectomy, as is required with a binostril approach during transsphenoidal surgery to the skull base for this indication.

The anterior and posterior ethmoidal arteries are easily and quickly ligated through a minimally invasive precaruncular approach (1). This is often required prior to tumor resection if the lesion is supplied by the ethmoidal vessels, which are branches of the ophthalmic artery. These vessels cannot be safely embolized during cerebral angiography, as is done with branches of the external carotid artery system. This approach is particularly useful in patients with severe epistaxis secondary to nasoethmoidal fractures and traumatic ethmoidal artery injury, where embolization of the ethmoidal arteries is not an option.

Cavernous hemangiomas located medially in the orbit are often approached using a binostril endonasal approach. However, this approach requires extensive sinus work, including a posterior septectomy/septal window, medial rectus muscle manipulation, and medial orbital wall reconstruction using a mucoperichondrial flap to prevent enophthalmos. If the lesion is too large to be resected through a precaruncular approach, an ipsilateral endonasal approach allows for manipulation of the lesion into the nasal cavity for easier removal.

The contralateral precaruncular approach can be combined with a 1 or 2 nostril approach for lesions involving the lateral aspect of the sphenoid sinus, such as Sternberg canal defects (3). Using a contralateral precaruncular approach allows for direct visualization of the skull base defect using a zero-degree endoscope and straight instrumentation, obviating the need for angled scopes and curved instruments as is used during the traditional transpterygoid approach.

Superolateral Transorbital + Endonasal Approach (One- or Two-Nostril Approach)

As discussed previously, endonasal or transorbital medial optic nerve decompression can be performed prior to resection of tumors involving the brain, orbit, or orbital walls. Decompressing the optic nerve is often required for lesions compressing the optic nerve at the level of the optic canal. Also, decompression of the nerve via an endonasal approach prior to tumor resection via a transorbital approach allows for increased space for the optic nerve in the sphenoid sinus, reducing the risk of iatrogenic optic nerve injury. Sphenoid wing meningiomas are a good example of a lesion that can be addressed using a multiportal approach, which includes an endonasal approach for medial optic nerve decompression, followed by a superolateral transorbital approach to resect the tumor and drill hyperostotic bone, which involves the superior and lateral orbital walls and the middle cranial fossa.

Overall, the decision as to whether a pure transnasal or transorbital or a combined multiportal approach should be used depends on the location of the target lesion, existing neurological deficits, functional status of the eye, experience of the surgeon, and availability of specialized instrumentation.

Patient Selection

Most benign lesions are well suited for the minimally invasive approach offered by an endoscopic transorbital surgery. The size of the lesion does not necessarily prohibit the use of this approach, since most benign lesions can be either decompressed (e.g., vascular malformations or dermoid cysts) or removed piecemeal through the minimal access corridor. Malignant lesions and benign pathologies that require complete excision, such as pleomorphic adenomas, are more restrictive in terms of suitability of the endoscopic approach, and in these cases, the risks and limitations of access need to be weighed against the risks and implications of an incomplete resection.

Several other factors relating to both the patient's anatomy as well as the pathology involved also need to be considered:

- Orbital configuration – Shallow orbits are less accommodating to applied pressure and therefore at higher risk of vascular and neurological injury as a result of the retraction required for the creation of a working corridor. Review of pre-operative imaging should include assessment of the orbital depth and volume.
- Location of the pathology – Lesions involving the anterior orbit are easily accessible through an open approach utilizing the same incisions. The endoscope loses its value for addressing lesions in this region.
- Extent of the lesion – Extensive lesions involving both the extradural and intradural compartments are better addressed with traditional wide access techniques such as a craniotomy. Using the TONES approaches to address extensive lesions involving these spaces would not justify the time and equipment resources required.

Decision-Making Algorithm

Sphenoid wing meningiomas provide a good illustrative example for the role of a combined endoscopic lateral orbit and transnasal approach (Figure 2.11) (2,4,5).

Morphologically, these tumors can be described as being en plaque or globoid. En plaque tumors exhibit a carpet-like growth pattern and can extend anteriorly to involve the orbit. Surgical resection is the treatment of choice; however, traditional approaches aimed at complete resection involve obtaining wide access through a craniotomy. Recent advances in multiportal endoscopic surgery, as well as radiotherapy treatment, have challenged this paradigm. The advantage of a minimally invasive surgery includes limiting the comorbidities associated with a craniotomy and the retraction of the intracranial contents.

While multiportal endoscopic surgery certainly has its advantages, it is not a universal surgical approach. The decision on which surgical approach to use is based on the degree of intracranial, orbital, and skull base involvement.

The superolateral transorbital approach provides wide surgical access without the need for a

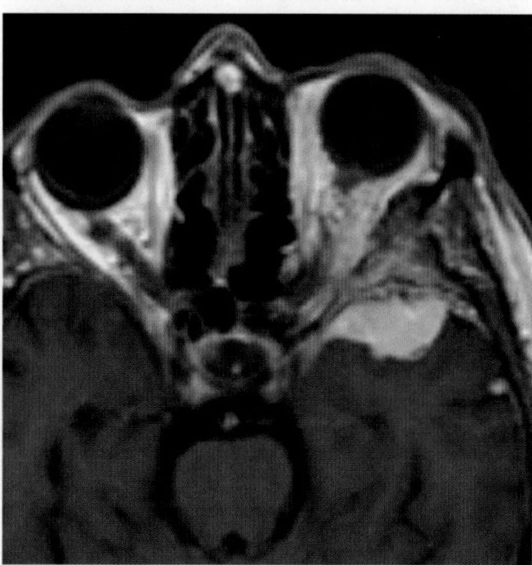

Figure 2.11 Sphenoid wing meningioma showing intracranial component, lateral hyperostotic bone, and orbital tumor component

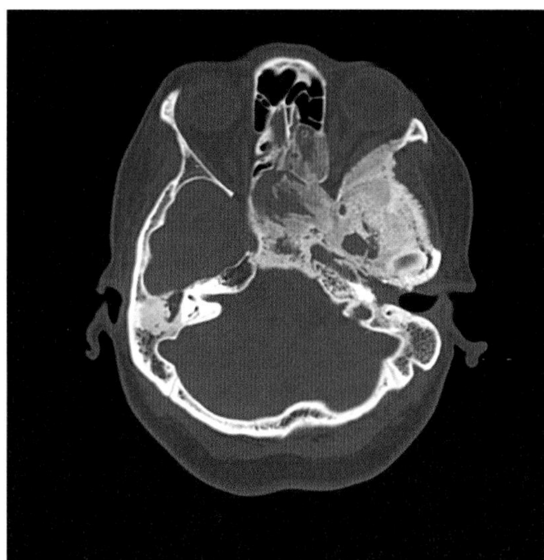

Figure 2.12 Large sphenoid wing meningioma requiring a craniotomy for more complete tumor resection

craniotomy. The bony orbital rim can either be removed or left intact depending on the space available for the introduction of the endoscope and instrumentation. The involved bone of the lateral orbital wall posterior to the rim is drilled away and creates a wide corridor for access to the lateral skull base and the middle cranial fossa. The approach, however, has limited medial access to the skull base. Combined multiportal surgery with transnasal access to the medial skull base may address this limitation, but where there is extensive involvement of the medial skull base, wider access through a craniotomy may be more appropriate (Figure 2.12).

Clinical Scenario

Patients with sphenoid wing meningioma often present with proptosis, visual loss, and/or eye pain. A craniotomy alone cannot always adequately address these symptoms, especially if the tumor involves the sphenoid sinus with medial involvement of the optic canal. Bony hyperostosis often involves the superior, lateral, and inferior orbital walls, and for adequate decompression, a multiportal approach to access these areas may be required (4). Combining a craniotomy with a transorbital and/or endonasal approach can help address proptosis and visual loss. Figure 2.12 demonstrates an advanced sphenoid wing meningioma with the involvement of the lateral and medial components of the sphenoid bone.

Contraindications to Doing Transorbital Surgery

Transorbital approaches take advantage of adnexal tissue planes to create a surgical corridor that allows for access to the skull base. Retraction required to create the corridors often exerts pressure on the globe. Specific contraindications thus are mostly related to conditions of the eye that may be affected. A history of intra-ocular surgery in the past 6 months is a relative contraindication due to the risk of wound rupture during retraction of the globe. Intra-ocular surgery in the last 6 weeks runs a high risk of wound dehiscence, and consultation with an ophthalmologist is important to decide on the optimal timing for subsequent transorbital surgery. Ocular conditions such as glaucoma (especially advanced glaucoma), corneal ectatic disease, scleritis, scleromalacia, high myopia, and retinal vascular disease are also considerations in deciding on whether to use the transorbital approach. The ocular disease severity needs to be weighed against the benefits of a transorbital approach. Adnexal and ocular surface infections such as conjunctivitis and dacryocystitis need to be ruled out or treated adequately prior to surgery.

Alternative Approaches

Lateral Orbitotomy

The lateral orbit is approached most commonly by an extended upper lid crease incision with dissection down to the bony orbital rim. If required, the bony rim can be drilled to provide wider exposure and access to the orbit. The rim is then reconstructed at the end of the procedure. Once the rim is removed, the trigone of the greater wing of the sphenoid can be removed either with a high-speed drill or rongeur. The endoscope or microscope can be used through the external corridor to address intracranial lesions. Once the bone is removed, the temporalis muscle and dura are exposed laterally. Good access is provided with this approach to deep orbital lesions. For intracranial lesions, the dura is opened and ultimately repaired at the end of the case using standard techniques. Fat and/or fascia lata grafts can be harvested from the abdomen and upper leg.

Craniotomy

Pterional Approach and Its Variations

The pterional approach is the gold standard approach to address sphenoid wing meningiomas or tumors involving the greater wing of the sphenoid. A description of the surgical technique is outside the scope of this chapter and will be discussed elsewhere. A disadvantage of this approach is the inability to reach a tumor located medially within the sphenoid sinus. Combining a pterional approach with an endonasal approach and medial optic nerve decompression addresses this limitation.

Unilateral Frontal Craniotomy and Bifrontal Craniotomy

For lesions involving the anterior cranial fossa, frontal sinuses, or superior orbit, a unilateral or bifrontal craniotomy is often used. The advantage of this approach is wide surgical exposure, especially if reconstruction is required. Major disadvantages of this approach include the brain retraction required, the risk to olfaction, and the risk of breach of the frontal sinuses.

Supraorbital Keyhole Approach

With this minimally invasive approach through the eyebrow or palpebral fissure, deep-seated lesions of the anterior skull base can be reached with minimal brain retraction. It is important to pay special attention to correct patient positioning and brain relaxation (e.g., cisternal decompression, lumbar drains, etc) to maximize corridors.

Endoscopic Endonasal Approaches

Endoscopic endonasal surgery provides good access to the nasal cavity, paranasal sinuses, medial orbit, and midline structures in the anterior skull base. For anterior skull base meningiomas, a major disadvantage of this approach is the high risk of cerebrospinal fluid leaks. The advent of the pedicled nasoseptal flap has reduced the risk of post-operative CSF leak, but transcranial approaches are often still favored above endonasal approaches, especially for the treatment of olfactory groove meningiomas. If the nasal septum is involved with tumor, a nasoseptal flap is not available for repair and an open approach with a pericranial flap may be favored to assist with the reconstruction of the large skull base defect.

Endoscopic Lothrop/Draf-3 Procedure

The lateral aspect of the frontal sinus cannot always be adequately reached, even with an endoscopic Lothrop operation. Although this area can be well visualized using a 70-degree endoscope, standard endoscopic sinus instruments often cannot reach the lateral wall of a well-pneumatized frontal sinus. It is therefore difficult to remove a tumor in this area using either curettes or powered instrumentation. Lesions that commonly involve this area include mucoceles, osteomas, inverting papilloma, squamous cell carcinomas, as well as other anterior cranial fossa lesions that invade the frontal sinus. Combining an endoscopic Lothrop operation with a superior eyelid approach provides good access to the lateral aspect of the frontal sinus with easy manipulation of lesions involving this area. It also allows for frontal sinus function to be preserved by allowing aeration and drainage of the sinus.

Endoscopic Transpterygoid Approach

The lateral aspect of a well-pneumatized sphenoid sinus can be approached using a transpterygoid approach. With this approach, it is useful but not essential to approach the sphenoid sinus from the contralateral nostril to get the correct trajectory to the skull base, usually for Sternberg canal defects or encephaloceles. The advantage of this approach is that it is minimally invasive compared to a standard craniotomy. The disadvantage is that there is often post-operative numbness of the palate secondary to extensive dissection of the pterygopalatine fossa, coupled with the fact that the sphenopalatine artery is often sacrificed on the ipsilateral side of the dissection, necessitating a contralateral mucoperichondrial flap to be used. The transorbital approach allows for an ipsilateral flap to be used.

Preoperative Planning

Suggested Pre-operative Imaging

Stereotactic navigation protocoled computed tomography (CT) of the orbits, skull base, and brain should be requested in all cases and assists with the assessment of the degree of bony infiltration by a tumor. Navigation-assisted surgery is especially helpful to maximize and confirm the degree of optic canal decompression and removal of hyperostotic bone in the sphenoid wing meningioma group of patients. Magnetic resonance imaging (MRI) with and without contrast assists with tumor delineation and is especially helpful for assessing the extent of intracranial and orbital tumor involvement. Navigation assists in planning the optimal surgical route and helps with real-time intraoperative guidance (Figure 2.13). Cerebral angiography and embolization should be performed in select cases to assist with the resection of vascular tumors.

Preoperative Patient Evaluation Checklist

- General assessment to determine fitness for general anesthesia
- Specific attention paid to the use of anticoagulant therapy
- Ophthalmic assessment – including history and timing of any previous ocular surgery, visual function assessment, and presence of established optic atrophy (which carries a guarded visual prognosis). Conditions that may be a contraindication to endoscopic orbital/transorbital surgery should be noted.

Surgical Technique

Pertinent Surface Anatomy in Transorbital Surgery

An understanding of the adnexal structures relevant to each of the four transorbital corridors is important to avoid disrupting the physiological dynamics necessary for the maintenance of the ocular surface. The *medial canthus* comprises the structures that form the medial border of the palpebral fissure. The *caruncle* is a triangular, pink, soft tissue structure that is found at the medial convergence of the upper and lower eyelids. Anterior to the caruncle and running within the medial most aspect of the upper and lower eyelids are the *lacrimal puncti* and their respective canaliculi. The canaliculi in turn drain into the *lacrimal sac*, which is bordered anteriorly by the anterior limb of the medial canthal tendon and posteriorly by the posterior limb, inserting onto

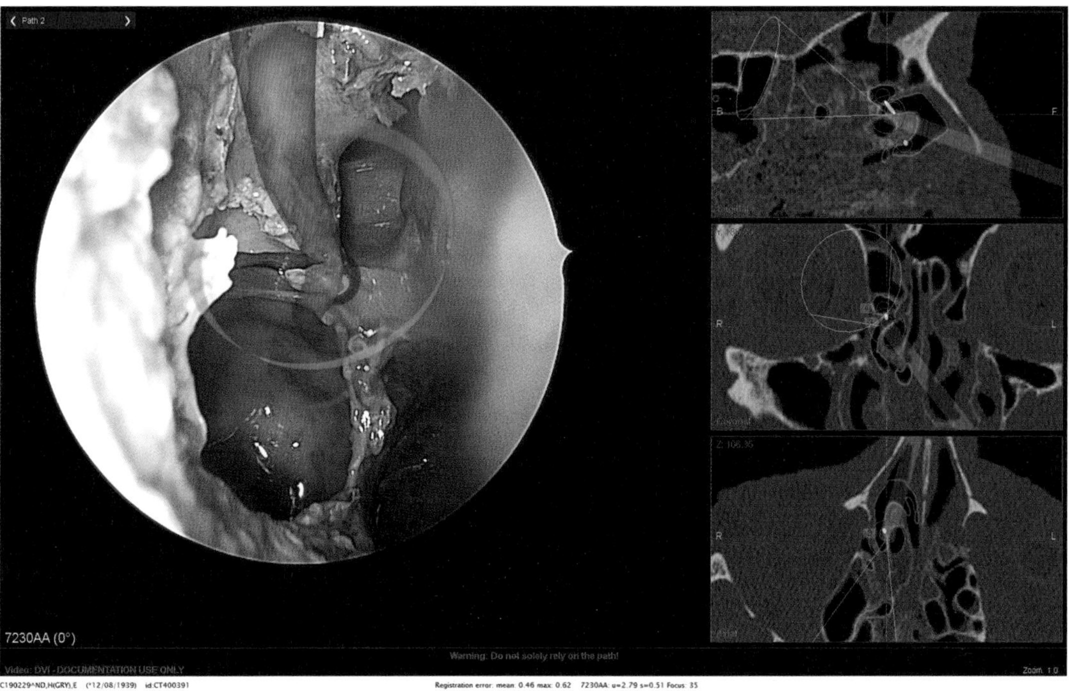

Figure 2.13 Navigation assists in planning the optimal surgical route and helps with real-time intraoperative guidance.

the posterior lacrimal crest. During incision of the caruncle in a medial approach, it is important to direct the dissection in a posterior-medial direction to avoid injury to the lacrimal sac and the posterior crest of the medial canthal tendon.

The *upper eyelid crease* is formed by the insertion of the *levator palpebrae muscle* onto the tarsal plate. The crease forms an ideal location for the placement of cosmetically hidden surgical incisions. An upper eyelid crease incision passes through the skin and orbicularis muscle before emerging on the convergence of the septum and *levator aponeurosis* as they insert onto the upper tarsal tissue. Dissection carried out in the sub-orbicularis plane superiorly emerges onto the periosteum of the orbital rim and the *arcus marginalis*. Excessive superior traction can stretch the levator aponeurosis resulting in aponeurotic ptosis.

Fibrous soft tissue connections extending from the upper and lower tarsus form the upper and lower crux of the *lateral canthal tendon*, respectively. These merge together to form a common tendon which then inserts onto a bony protuberance on the inner aspect of the lateral orbital rim known as *Whitnall's ligament*. The upper and lower lids meet to form the *lateral canthus*. The angle and height of the lateral canthus play an important role in maintaining the eyelid position and optimizing the directional flow of tears. Disruption of the lateral canthal anatomy can result in lateral ectropion, with symptomatic pooling of tears and epiphora.

The lower eyelid transconjunctival approach can be divided into pre-septal and post-septal. The tarsus of the lower eyelid is shorter than the tarsus of the upper eyelid by an average of 4 mm. Extensions from the inferior rectus muscle form the capsulopalpebral fascia, also known as the levator aponeurosis. The orbital septum merges with the capsulopalpebral fascia to insert onto the lower end of the tarsal plate. The pre-septal plane is favored in transorbital endoscopic approaches, as it avoids fat herniation, which makes access challenging.

Patient Positioning

The patient is placed in a supine position with the head slightly flexed as in standard FESS surgery. Total intravenous anesthesia is preferred in order to optimize the surgical field and endoscopic view. The nasal cavity is prepared using nasal packing or surgical patties soaked in a mixture consisting of 2 ml of adrenaline (1:1000) and oxymetazoline placed within the middle meatus.

Endoscopic Orbit Incisions

Pre- and Transcaruncular

Surgery is performed with the patient under either general or monitored anesthesia care. The medial orbit is infiltrated transconjunctivally with 1–2 ml of 2% lidocaine hydrochloride solution with adrenaline (1:100,000). The area is then prepared and draped in the usual sterile fashion. Stevens or sharp Iris scissors are used to create a vertical incision through the lateral fourth of the caruncle. The incision is carried for 8–10 mm both superiorly and inferiorly through the conjunctiva to create a wide window of exposure. The incision can be created medial to the caruncle (precaruncular), but an incision in the body of the caruncle heals well and provides a landmark to align the closure. The condensed fibrous layer just deep to the caruncle is incised in the direction of the posterior lacrimal crest using sharp dissection. Blunt dissection with closed scissor tips is used to palpate the posterior lacrimal crest and is then held firmly against the medial orbital wall 1–2 mm posterior to the posterior lacrimal crest. This establishes the plane for continued dissection to allow exposure of the periosteum immediately posterior to the posterior lacrimal crest. The plane of this dissection passes between the medial orbital septum and Horner's muscle. If the integrity of the septum is maintained, it can decrease the tendency for fat to spill into the surgical field. The periosteum along the posterior lacrimal crest is then widely incised with either needle cautery and/or a sharp periosteal elevator. A wide periosteal incision can allow the periosteum to act as a membrane to confine the orbital fat and improve exposure. Dissection should continue posteriorly in the subperiosteal plane. The periosteum is elevated superiorly and inferiorly to obtain a wide anterior aperture. The anterior and posterior ethmoidal arteries are identified and can either be spared or cauterized with bipolar cautery depending on the extent of dissection needed (Figure 2.14). The gentle stretching associated with medial orbital content retraction, as well as the superior and inferior subperiosteal dissection, allows for wide exposure of the medial wall extending to the orbital apex.

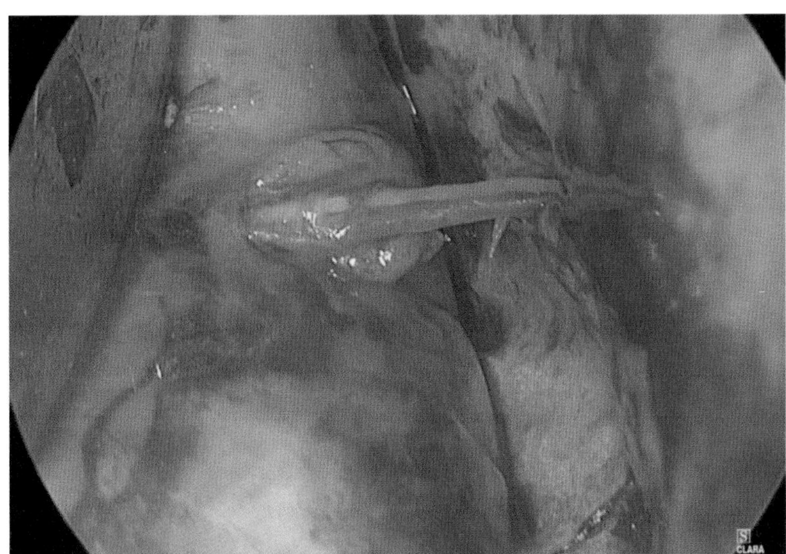

Figure 2.14 Anterior ethmoidal artery and nerve (right eye)

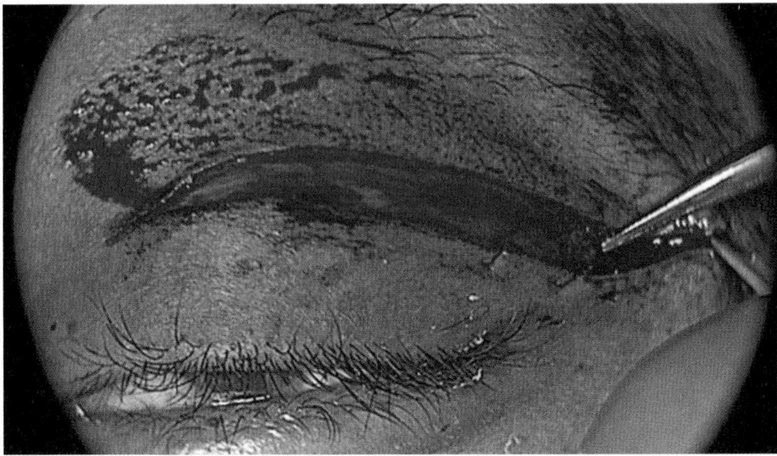

Figure 2.15 Superior eyelid incision made in natural crease line (as for blepharoplasty), sparing the lateral canthus of the eye

Superior Lid Crease with Lateral Extension

The skin incision in the upper lid is designed in a curvilinear fashion with the medial portion convex superiorly and the lateral portion in line with the lateral canthus. The incision is placed in a natural supra-tarsal skin crease. If a natural crease line is not seen the incision line is determined according to the measurements of the lower edge of a standard upper blepharoplasty: 10 mm above the lash line in the central part of the lid and 6–7 mm above the lateral canthus. The incision can be extended laterally onto the lateral orbital rim to improve the surgical access (Figure 2.15). The upper-eyelid incision is made using a No. 15 scalpel blade in a medial to lateral direction with gentle traction of the skin.

Dissection is carried through the skin and underlying orbicularis muscle into the sub-orbicularis space leaving the orbital septum intact. Dissection in this plane is directed superiorly and laterally to access the supra-periosteal plane over the superolateral bony rim. The periosteum is sharply split along the middle and approximately 1 cm above the edge of the orbital rim using a scalpel or needle cautery. A sharp periosteal elevator is then used to develop the sub-periosteal dissection plane (Figure 2.16a). A sub-periosteal dissection is directed back toward the orbital rim and then the tissue is reflected from the bony border with sweeping motions of the elevator. The periosteum is then dissected from the lateral and posterior surface of the superolateral rim. If the periosteum is disrupted, the

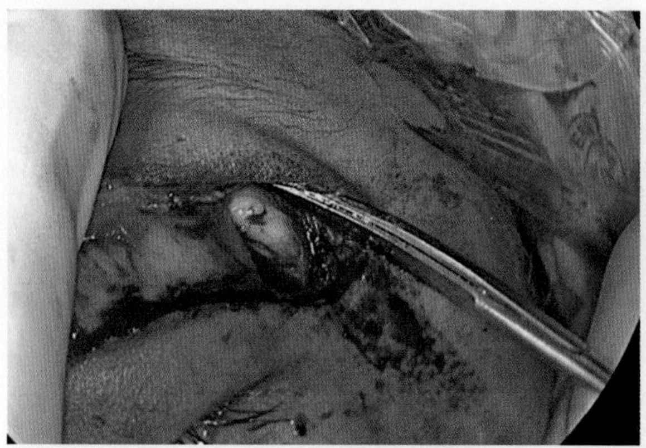

Figure 2.16a Tissue is cut above the orbital rim to avoid damaging the levator muscle

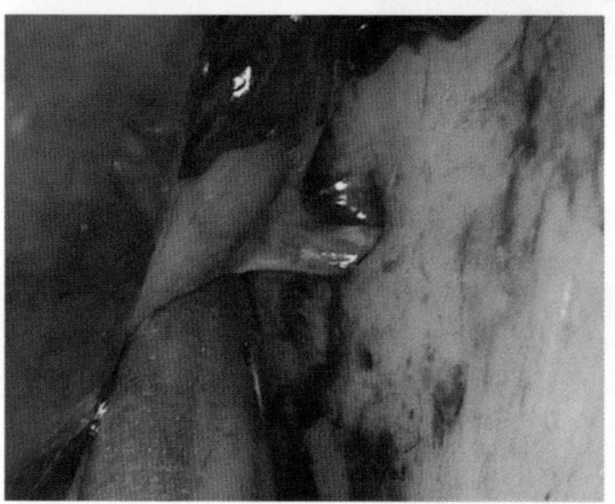

Figure 2.16b A neurovascular bundle in the lateral aspect of the left eye (recurrent branch of the middle meningeal artery), 1 cm anterior to the superior orbital fissure

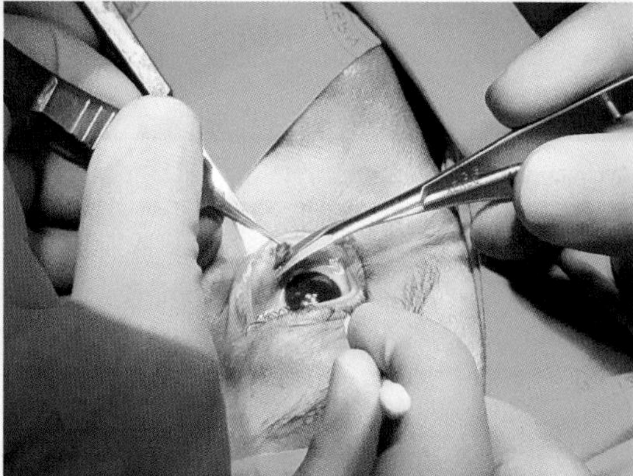

Figure 2.17 The lower eyelid is retracted anteriorly with a Desmarres lid retractor, and the transconjunctival incision is made using a Stevens scissor approximately 4 mm below the inferior border of the tarsus

lacrimal gland and orbital fat may prolapse into the surgical field. The sub-periosteal dissection can then be carried posteriorly to expose the reflection of the superior and inferior orbital fissure. Perforating neurovascular bundles can either be preserved or cauterized and dissected, depending on the pathology, target site, and exposure required (Figure 2.16b).

Inferior Transconjunctival

The lower eyelid is retracted anteriorly with a Desmarres lid retractor, and the transconjunctival incision is made using a Stevens' scissor approximately 4 mm below the inferior border of the tarsus (Figure 2.17). The incision is then extended across the horizontal length of the eyelid and can be extended through the caruncle if additional exposure is needed.

Blunt and sharp scissor dissection are performed until the inferior orbital rim is visualized. If desired, a 4-0 silk traction suture can be placed through the lower lid retractors to enhance exposure. The plane of dissection is within or just posterior to the plane of the orbital septum, which keeps the orbital fat posterior to the surgical field. The assistant should retract the anterior lamella away from the plane of dissection with the Desmarres retractor. The arcus marginalis at the inferior orbital rim should be identified. The periosteum is incised with a No. 15 Bard-Parker blade or the monopolar cautery along the inferior orbital rim. The subperiosteal dissection is initiated with the periosteal elevator. The thicker edge of the periosteum at the arcus marginalis can be grasped with forceps to aid in the dissection. A malleable retractor is inserted to gently retract the orbital contents superiorly once a subperiosteal pocket is formed. Keeping the periorbita intact during the dissection will facilitate maintaining wide exposure to the entire orbital floor (Figure 2.18). Closure of the periorbita is usually not required.

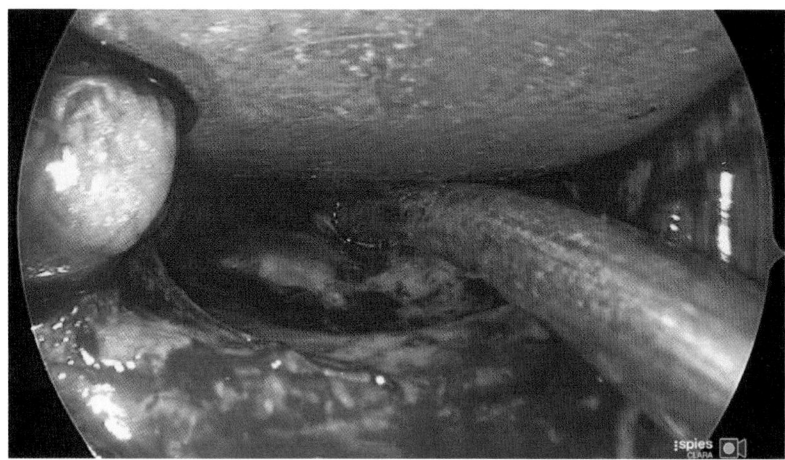

Figure 2.18 Inferior subconjunctival approach with access to inferior orbit and floor of orbit

Technical Nuances

Avoiding Complications and Converting to Open Surgery

A thorough pre-operative assessment and clear surgical plan are the first steps to minimizing intra-operative complications. The most common reason for abandoning a transorbital pathway is poor visualization within the dissection space due to herniation of orbital fat. Care must be taken to respect the anatomical planes and preserve the integrity of the periorbita. Uncontrolled bleeding in the operative field can also obscure the operative field. In the lateral orbital wall, failure to address perforating vessels prior to transecting them can make hemostasis challenging as the vessels tend to retract into the bone. Appropriate hemostatic aids such as bone wax and Floseal should be readily available in the operating room.

The decision to convert to open surgery is dependent on the surgical experience of the team, as well as the nature of the pathology and the ability to address it adequately using these minimally invasive approaches. A multidisciplinary team is useful during these surgeries and in pre-operative planning. While attractive, minimally invasive approaches have their limitations and knowledge of the limitations in relation to the pathology, available team members and surgical experience are integral to avoiding operative complications.

Post-operative Care

- Intra-operative antibiotic prophylaxis should be administered in all patients. A dose of systemic corticosteroids such as dexamethasone (8 mg) is also administered, which helps reduce post-operative inflammation.
- Precautions are taken to prevent post-operative nasal bleeding, such as the use of intra-operative hemostatic compounds and placement of a nasal balloon, if required.
- The precaruncular and inferior conjunctival wounds do not require suturing. The patient is given a regimen of steroid-antibiotic combination ophthalmic ointment or drops administered every 6 hours for the first 2 weeks. The superolateral eyelid incision is closed in a standard layered fashion, and a corrugated drain is placed for the first 24 hours to prevent hematoma formation.
- Patients who have had intradural surgery should be admitted to a high acuity care floor or ICU depending on the degree of resection, patient stability, and risk of complications.
- Patients who have had extradural surgery can be nursed in the general hospital ward.
- The patient should keep the head elevated for the first week post-operatively. Observations for the first 24–48 hours include:
  - Neurological observations at least every 4 hours for transorbital intradural cases
  - Ophthalmic assessment at least every 4 hours, including pupil assessment, gross visual assessment, and motility

Follow-up

- Initial follow-up should be around 7–10 days post-operatively. The purpose of the visit is to exclude wound sepsis and sutures, if present, can be removed.

- Six-week follow-up allows for the first comparisons to pre-operative measurements to be made, such as:
  - Visual function
  - Exophthalmometry measurements
  - Ocular motility
  - Assessment of upper eyelid function and position
- Repeat imaging can be performed at 3–6 months to assess for any residual disease.
- Cases should be managed by a multidisciplinary team including an oncologist, where appropriate. Patients may require adjunctive therapy and the optimal timing for this needs to be discussed.

Clinical Pearls

- It is important to maintain the subperiosteal dissection for transorbital approaches. Breaching the periorbita early will result in prolapse of orbital fat into the working corridor compromising visualization.
- The surgical team must be cognizant of the amount of force used in retraction. Prolonged forceful retraction on the eye can result in retinal vascular occlusions and traumatic optic neuropathy. It is useful to monitor the pupil for dilatation as well as a change in the pupil shape. Should this occur, then retraction should be stopped and instruments removed immediately until the pupil shape returns to normal.
- In the lateral approach, the thick area of the bony rim that accommodates the lacrimal gland can be drilled away to create space for the working corridor.

Key Points

- Endoscopic orbital and transorbital approaches have evolved to allow improved multiportal access to the skull base and anterior and middle cranial fossa.
- Development of a multidisciplinary team is useful in terms of establishing the skills required to address the range of pathologies that involve overlapping anatomical areas.
- Multiportal minimally invasive surgery improves on the morbidity associated with wider open approaches; however, these approaches may be restrictive in terms of adequate access. This depends on the pathology requiring treatment. It is important that the risks and benefits of the various approaches be considered in order to optimize clinical and radiographic outcomes.

References

1. Cornelis MMK, Lubbe DE. 2016. Pre-caruncular approach to the medial orbit and landmarks for anterior ethmoidal artery ligation: a cadaveric study. *Clinical Otolaryngology*. **41**(6):777–81.
2. Lubbe Darlene E, Moe Kris S. 2019. 16 transorbital approaches to the sinuses, skull base and intracranial space. In *Endoscopic Surgery of the Orbit Anatomy Pathology and Management*. BS Bleier, SK Freitag, R Sacks, eds. 1st ed. New York; Stuttgart; Delhi; Rio de Janeiro: Thieme.
3. Lubbe DE, Douglas-Jones P, Wasl H, Mustak H, Semple PL. 2020. Contralateral precaruncular approach to the lateral sphenoid sinus: a case report detailing a new, multiportal approach to lesions, and defects in the lateral aspect of well-pneumatized sphenoid sinuses. *Ear, Nose, & Throat Journal*. **99**(1):62–7.
4. Lubbe D, Mustak H, Taylor A, Fagan J. 2017. Minimally invasive endo-orbital approach to sphenoid wing meningiomas improves visual outcomes: our experience with the first seven cases. *Clinical Otolaryngology*. **42**(4):876–80.
5. Moe KS, Lubbe DE. 2019. 20 transorbital neuroendoscopic surgery of the skull base and brain. In *Transnasal Endoscopic Skull Base and Brain Surgery*. AC Stamm, J Mangussi-Gomes, eds. Stuttgart: Georg Thieme Verlag.
6. Norris JL, Cleasby GW. 1981. Endoscopic orbital surgery. *American Journal of Ophthalmology*. **91** (2):249–52.

Chapter 3

Combined Endonasal and Transoral Endoscopic Approach to the Craniovertebral Junction

Adam J. Kimple, Brian D. Thorp, and Adam M. Zanation

Introduction and Indications

Accessing the craniovertebral junction is a challenge. It is located deep within the head and neck, and is surrounded by vital structures. Additionally, injuring non-vital structures such as the palate can have devastating consequences on speech and swallowing. Surgical access to this region is needed for both intradural and extradural lesions, including chordomas (1,2), meningiomas (3,4), osteoradionecrosis (4,5), basilar aneurysms (6), and other degenerative diseases (7-9). Traditionally, access has been obtained by utilizing transoral approaches; however, as technology and advances in transnasal endoscopic surgery have developed, the transnasal approach has increased in popularity. Currently, surgical teams frequently use transnasal endoscopy to access the entire ventral skull base, the upper cervical vertebrae, and even the middle cranial fossa and jugular foramen (7,10). Transnasal routes allow direct access to the craniovertebral junction and less morbidity to the tongue, temporomandibular joint, and palate (11). Despite the advances in this technique due to improved knowledge and equipment, the patient's anatomy ultimately defines and limits the extent of these procedures (12). The inferior reach of the transnasal approach is limited by the hard palate, nasal bones, and overlying nasal soft tissue (Figure 3.1). Once this limit is reached, additional inferior access can be gained in a stepwise manner, with ultimate exposure obtained using a combined endonasal-transoral approach.

Caudal exposure to the craniovertebral junction is limited by the nasal bone and overlying soft tissue and the hard palate (Figure 3.1). The nasopalatine line (NPL) helps estimate the extent of caudal exposure to the craniovertebral junction and is drawn from the inferior edge of the nasal bones to the posterior border of the palatine bone. The NPL intersects the plane of the hard palate to form the nasopalatine angle (NPA) (12). The NPL and NPA allow an estimate of the caudal access afforded using straight endoscopes and instruments; however, this has been noted to overestimate the degree of caudal access (12). As discussed previously, additional caudal exposure may be obtained by extending the head (12), although the surgeon must consider the pathology and stability of the cervical spine before considering this action, as head extension in patients with a destabilized spine can result in catastrophic consequences. Using a transnasal approach with straight instruments, we are typically able to access the entire clivus and superior aspect of the first cervical vertebrae (C1). When additional caudal access is required, our next step is to retract the palate using a Penrose drain that is passed through the mouth and pulled up through the nose (13). The additional caudal access gained from this maneuver is minimal, due to the fact that the osseous boundaries of the nasal bone and the hard palate are not changed; however, we nevertheless feel this technique helps to protect the mucosal surfaces of the soft palate from iatrogenic, intraoperative injury.

For pathology involving C1 or the second cervical vertebrae (C2), additional caudal extension is required. In these situations, we will frequently drill through the posterior aspect of the hard palate while leaving the periosteum and mucosa of the oral surface of the hard palate intact. In our experience, this maneuver has minimal morbidity compared to splitting the palate, and it can considerably improve exposure to C1 or C2, as manipulation of the posterior edge of the hard palate increases the NPA (Figure 3.1; green dashed line). By keeping the entire soft palate and the periosteum of the oral surface of the hard palate intact, we reduce the risk

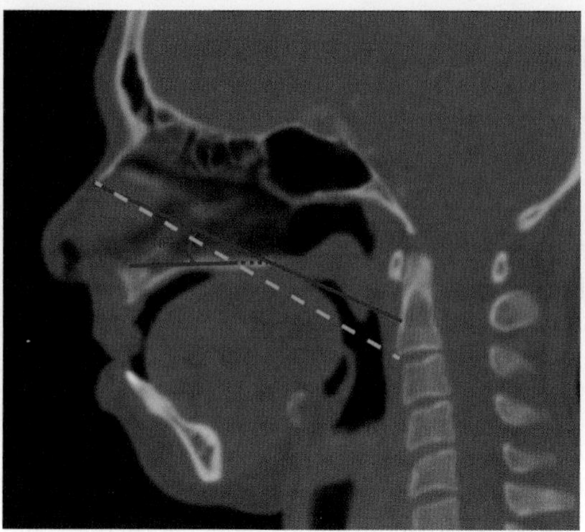

Figure 3.1 Depiction of the nasopalatine angle and the extent of caudal exposure. The inferior extent of an endonasal approach to the spine can be estimated by the use of the nasopalatine angle. A line is connected along the superior surface of the maxillary and palatine bone in the midsagittal plane (long red line). This is intersected by a line that extends from the caudal aspect of the nasal bone to the posterior edge of the palatine bone (short red line). The extension of this line estimates the inferior extent of dissection with zero-degree instruments and telescopes. The posterior edge of the palate can be removed while maintaining the oral mucosa to allow further caudal exposure (green dashed line).

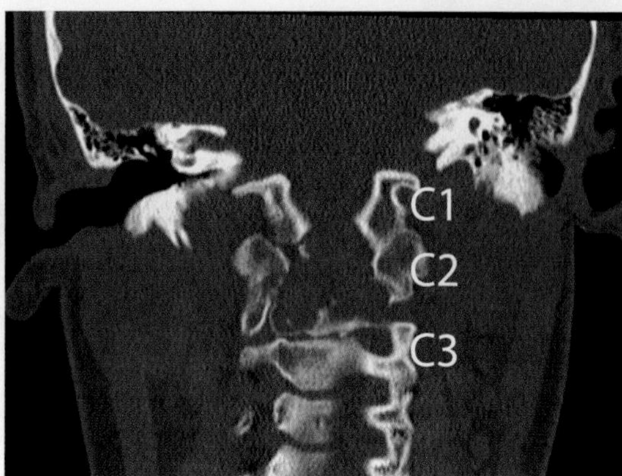

Figure 3.2 Computed tomography of the coronal plane of the cervical spine in a 15-year-old with a giant-cell tumor with extensive erosion of C1 and C2. The inferior extent of the tumor precluded a transnasal approach; however, a combined endonasal-transoral approach provided excellent visualization and working room for surgical removal of the tumor.

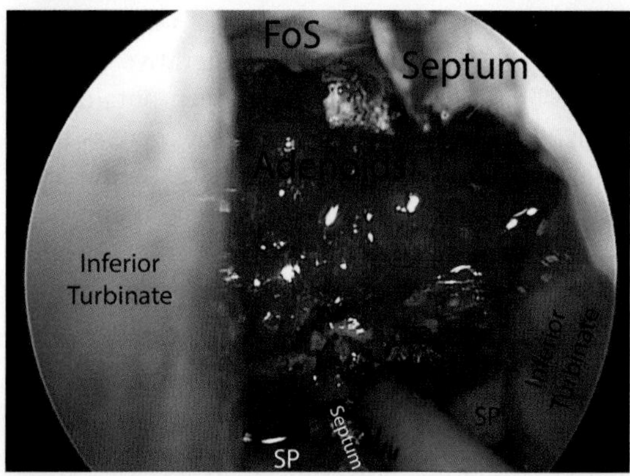

Figure 3.3 Transnasal visualization of the posterior nasopharynx. The posterior nasopharynx is bound laterally by the inferior turbinates, inferiorly by the soft palate (SP), and superiorly by the floor of sphenoid (FoS). A posterior septectomy was performed to allow for bilateral access.

of velopharyngeal insufficiency and have not noted any swallowing difficulties, nasal regurgitation, or changes in speech upon post-operative evaluation.

Surgical Technique

At our institution, we initially approach tumors of the craniovertebral junction using a transnasal approach. To gain additional caudal exposure, we extend this approach by removing the posterior component of the hard palate. If our caudal limit is reached, we utilize angled telescopes (45 degrees) to further increase caudal visualization. Detailed technical work is difficult when using the angled scope, particularly when utilizing a two-surgeon, four-hand approach, although this approach may be reasonable when limited caudal extension is needed. However, if significantly more caudal exposure is needed, a combined endonasal-transoral approach can considerably improve exposure.

For a combined endonasal-transoral approach, we typically orally intubate the patient and use a tonsil gag. This provides tongue retraction while keeping the endotracheal tube secure and out of the way. For prolonged cases, the tongue gag should be intermittently relaxed to allow perfusion of the tongue, typically every 20 minutes. A tracheostomy can be performed, although we do not routinely advocate for tracheostomies for the sole purpose of increasing caudal exposure.

To illustrate our approach, we present a case involving a 15-year-old female with a giant-cell tumor centered around C1 and C2 (Figure 3.2). The patient previously had a posterior stabilization. We proceeded with a transnasal approach and performed a posterior septectomy (Figure 3.3). The adenoid pad was then split using the suction bovie and pushed laterally to expose the

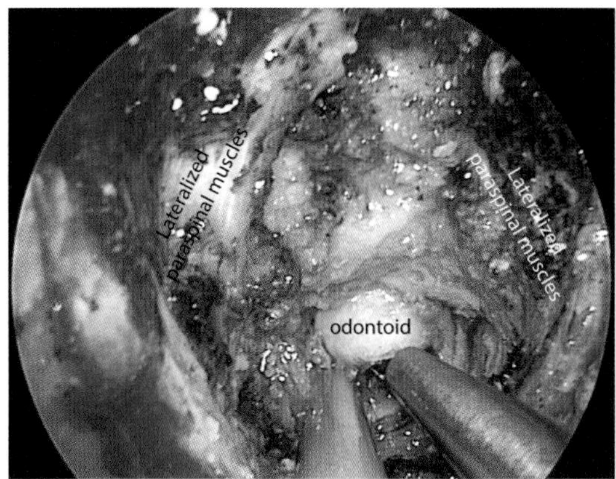

Figure 3.4 Visualization of the cervical vertebrae. The cervical vertebrae were visualized following dissection of the adenoids and paraspinal muscles. The odontoid process of C2 is prominently pictured.

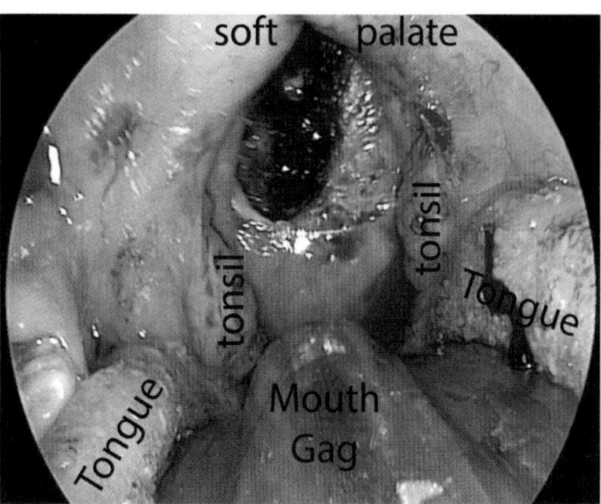

Figure 3.5 The transoral approach increases caudal exposure. Significant caudal exposure is gained from the transoral approach. A mouth gag is placed to retract the tongue. Using the transnasal approach, the inferior edge of the defect is visualized and can be extended by at least 1 cm.

fascia overlying the paraspinal muscles. The suction bovie was then used to split the paraspinal muscles, which were pushed laterally to expose the periosteum overlying the cervical vertebrae. We were then able to palpate the vertebrae, and the overlying fascia and periosteum were split to identify C1 and C2 (Figure 3.4). Because we did not have adequate caudal extension even with the palate retracted, we also used the oral corridor in a combined endonasal-transoral approach to increase caudal exposure.

A mouth gag was inserted to retract the tongue, enhancing exposure to C1 and C2 (Figure 3.5). We then continued the defect in the posterior nasopharynx inferiorly to the inferior border of C2. This exposure allowed us to remove the tumor using a combination of drills and cold instrumentation. Additionally, one of the advantages of the combined endonasal-transoral approach is that it enables us to close the wound by primary intention. We closed the oropharyngeal mucosa with interrupted 3-0 Vicryl sutures (Figure 3.6). We allowed the lateralized adenoid/nasopharyngeal mucosa to return to its native position medially and healed the defect by secondary intention. At a one-year follow-up exam, the patient was doing well, with no evidence of tumor recurrence.

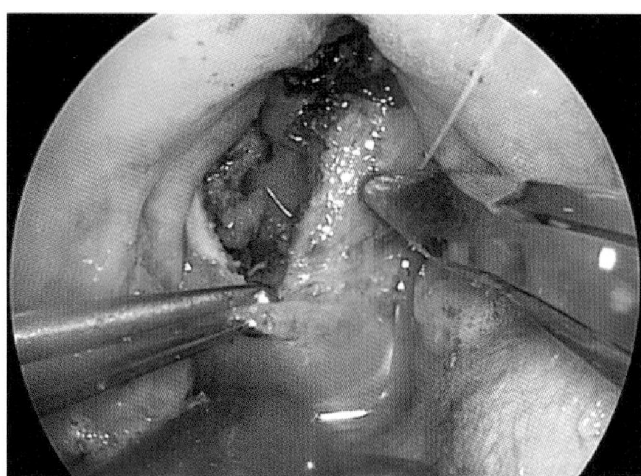

Figure 3.6 Wound closure following endoscopy using the combined endonasal-transoral approach. In addition to improved caudal exposure, the combined endonasal-transoral approach allows the surgeon to perform a primary closure, complete advanced tissue re-arrangement, and even potentially achieve a vascularized tissue inset.

Conclusion

The combined endonasal-transoral approach offers considerable access to the clivus up to C3 and allows for primary closure of the oropharyngeal defect (Figure 3.6). Additionally, access via the transoral corridor allows for advanced tissue rearrangement and allows for a microvascular anastomosis and vascularized flap inset if warranted. In general, we feel that a palatal split does not significantly improve access compared to the endoscopic combined endonasal-transoral approach described here. The palatal split adds a considerable amount of recovery time and has the potential to permanently damage swallowing function. We typically advocate for a palatal split for patients who require a maxillary swing to access the lateral extension of disease or for the superior exposure and instrument mobility that may be required for a cerebrospinal fluid (CSF) leak or other complex intradural pathology.

Overall, the combined endonasal-transoral approach should be a component of the armamentarium of skull base surgeons. It allows excellent visualization and surgical access to a variety of lesions from the clivus to C3.

Key Points

- When feasible, an endonasal approach to the craniovertebral junction decreases postoperative swallowing difficulties.
- The caudal extent of an endonasal approach can be enhanced with a transoral approach.
- The transoral corridor allows for advanced tissue rearrangement and allows for a microvascular anastomosis and vascularized flap inset, if warranted.

References

1. Rahme RJ, Arnaout OM, Sanusi OR, Kesavabhotla K, Chandler JP. Endoscopic approach to clival chordomas: the northwestern experience. *World Neurosurg.* 2018;**110**:e231–e8.
2. Labidi M, Watanabe K, Bouazza S, Bresson D, Bernat AL, George B, et al. Clivus chordomas: a systematic review and meta-analysis of contemporary surgical management. *J Neurosurg Sci.* 2016;**60**(4):476–84.
3. Shah RN, Surowitz JB, Patel MR, Huang BY, Snyderman CH, Carrau RL, et al. Endoscopic pedicled nasoseptal flap reconstruction for pediatric skull base defects. *Laryngoscope.* 2009;**119**(6):1067–75.
4. Graffeo CS, Dietrich AR, Grobelny B, Zhang M, Goldberg JD, Golfinos JG, et al. A panoramic view of the skull base: systematic review of open and endoscopic endonasal approaches to four tumors. *Pituitary.* 2014;**17**(4):349–56.
5. Tan SH, Ganesan D, Rusydi WZ, Chandran H, Prepageran N, Waran V. Combined endoscopic transnasal and transoral approach for extensive upper cervical osteoradionecrosis. *Eur Spine J.* 2015;**24**(12):2776–80.
6. Drazin D, Zhuang L, Schievink WI, Mamelak AN. Expanded endonasal approach for the clipping of a ruptured basilar aneurysm and feeding artery to a cerebellar arteriovenous malformation. *J Clin Neurosci.* 2012;**19**(1):144–8.
7. Gempt J, Lehmberg J, Grams AE, Berends L, Meyer B, Stoffel M. Endoscopic transnasal resection of the odontoid: case series and clinical course. *Eur Spine J.* 2011;**20**(4):661–6.
8. Goldschlager T, Hartl R, Greenfield JP, Anand VK, Schwartz TH. The endoscopic endonasal approach to the odontoid and its impact on early extubation and feeding. *J Neurosurg.* 2015;**122**(3):511–18.
9. Lemos-Rodriguez AM, Sreenath S, Unnithan A, Doan V, Recinos PF, Zanation A, et al. A new window for the treatment of posterior cerebral artery, superior cerebellar artery, and basilar apex aneurysm: the expanded endoscopic endonasal approach. *J Neurol Surg B Skull Base.* 2016;77(4):308–13.
10. Kassam A, Snyderman CH, Mintz A, Gardner P, Carrau RL. Expanded endonasal approach: the rostrocaudal axis. Part II. Posterior clinoids to the foramen magnum. *Neurosurg Focus.* 2005;**19**(1):E4.
11. Seker A, Inoue K, Osawa S, Akakin A, Kilic T, Rhoton AL Jr. Comparison of endoscopic transnasal and transoral approaches to the craniovertebral junction. *World Neurosurg.* 2010;**74**(6):583–602.
12. de Almeida JR, Zanation AM, Snyderman CH, Carrau RL, Prevedello DM, Gardner PA, et al. Defining the nasopalatine line: the limit for endonasal surgery of the spine. *Laryngoscope.* 2009;**119**(2):239–44.
13. Mummaneni PV, Haid RW. Transoral odontoidectomy. *Neurosurgery.* 2005;**56**(5):1045–50.

Combined Endoscopic Endonasal and Transcervical Approach

Ivan El-Sayed, David Schoppy, and Madeleine Strohl

Introduction

The parapharyngeal space (PPS) and infratemporal fossa (ITF) are distinct locations in the head and neck that have been historically difficult to access with surgery. With the development of improved endoscopic tools and the refinement of surgical techniques, these regions have become increasingly more accessible. This chapter presents a review of the pertinent anatomy of the PPS and ITF, a brief differential of lesions known to present in these locations, and a discussion of several different surgical approaches to access the region. Endoscopic endonasal, transoral, and transcervical approaches are detailed, along with a review of general indications, utility, and microsurgical anatomy.

The PPS and ITF are intimately related, with the ITF situated just lateral and superior to the more medial PPS. The PPS extends from the skull base superiorly to the hyoid bone inferiorly. The posterior fascia of the carotid sheath or prevertebral space forms the posterior boundary of the PPS, and this space extends anteriorly to the pterygomandibular raphe (1,2). The medial border of the PPS is the buccopharyngeal fascia and superior constrictor, while the PPS extends laterally to the inner fascia of the masticator space and deep lobe of the parotid gland. This space is classically divided into pre- and post-styloid compartments. The prestyloid compartment contains the deep lobe of the parotid gland, parapharyngeal fat, a portion of the mandibular division of the trigeminal nerve (V3), and the internal maxillary and ascending pharyngeal arteries (1). The poststyloid compartment contains the carotid artery, jugular vein, cranial nerves IX–XII, the sympathetic chain, and lymphatic tissue. These anatomic relationships are generally useful in narrowing the differential for lesions involving the PPS. Pleomorphic adenomas, other deep lobe parotid/salivary tumors, lymphomas, and lipomas can be found in the prestyloid compartment, while neurogenic tumors (such as paragangliomas and schwannomas) are some of the most common masses found in the poststyloid compartment. However, there are a wide variety of lesions, including various vascular tumors, vascular malformations, other neurogenic tumors, and inflammatory lesions that can present in the PPS (3,4).

The ITF is situated lateral and superior to the PPS and is bounded by the lateral pterygoid plate, posterior wall of the maxillary sinus, the ramus of the mandible and the temporalis muscle, the styloid process, and the tympanic portion of the temporal bone (5,6). Contents of the ITF include the maxillary artery, a portion of the mandibular branch of the trigeminal nerve (V3), the pterygoid musculature, and the pterygoid venous plexus (5). The most common lesions found in the infratemporal fossa include juvenile nasopharyngeal angiofibromas, adenoid cystic carcinomas, inverted papillomas, and schwannomas, though a range of masses can involve the infratemporal fossa, most commonly by extension from adjacent spaces (7–9).

One useful classification system for lesions of the infratemporal fossa integrates the location of the lesion, the potential approaches to the lesion, and the potential morbidity associated with a lesion in that anatomic space and necessary dissection for resection. The El-Sayed classification scheme for infratemporal fossa lesions is divided into A, B, C, and D categories. A "Type A" lesion is a limited lesion in the anterior infratemporal fossa/pterygoid fossa, medial to the lateral pterygoid plate and anterior to the eustachian tube. This can be usually resected with one approach, typically through a transnasal corridor including a maxillary antrostomy or post-lacrimal medial maxillectomy. A "Type B" lesion of the infratemporal fossa extends behind the posterior edge of the pterygoid plates and pterygoid musculature and necessitates a pre-lacrimal medial maxillectomy, Caldwell-Luc approach, or Endoscopic Denker's, possibly including a transseptal binaural approach for optimal exposure. A "Type C" lesion extends even more posteriorly into the posterior parapharyngeal space and/or the carotid space. Resection of a Type C lesion necessitates an endonasal approach used for a Type B lesion along with a transcervical approach to expose and have access to the carotid artery and jugular vein. A "Type D" lesion extends both posteriorly and inferiorly, below the level of the palatal line, and necessitates an endonasal approach used to resect a Type B lesion along with a transcervical approach to not only expose and be able to control the great vessels but additionally to free and resect the inferior extent of the tumor from adjacent structures.

Management of PPS and ITF Lesions

Initial Evaluation

Historically, a neck mass, pain, and/or dysphagia were the most common symptoms associated with lesions of the PPS (10). Lesions in the ITF can present in a variety of ways given the heterogeneous etiology and secondary involvement of the ITF by lesions extending from adjacent compartments. Unilateral nasal obstruction or facial swelling and pain are some of the more common symptoms that can eventually lead to an evaluation for an infratemporal or skull base mass (7,9).

Imaging

A CT with IV contrast has historically been used as an initial imaging study in the evaluation of parapharyngeal space lesions and can help delineate the principal anatomic compartment of the lesion and provide some information with regard to vascularity and bone involvement (10). MRI is commonly recommended in the evaluation of PPS and ITF masses, as it can provide soft tissue detail that may aid narrowing the differential and defining the scope of the lesion (11,12).

Biopsy

Seeking a tissue diagnosis through a fine needle aspirate (FNA) has been advocated as an important step in preoperative planning (13). While the non-diagnostic rate of FNA for parapharyngeal space lesions has been reported around 30–40%, the diagnostic accuracy of an FNA when compared with surgical pathology has been reported to range from 73% to 92% (14,15). Image guidance, specifically CT-guided FNA biopsy, has been reported to provide a non-diagnostic rate of 21% with a positive predictive value (PPV) for identifying benign lesions of 90% and a PPV for malignant lesions of 75% (16).

Combined Endoscopic Endonasal-Transcervical Approach

Patient Selection

Patient selection is dependent on the tumor pathology, location, and degree of invasion. Good candidates for this approach include 1) tumors situated in the infratemporal fossa above the floor of the maxillary sinus, with extension into the parapharyngeal space or approximating the great vessels, or 2) tumors that extend below the plane of the maxillary sinus. Benign tumors that can be shelled out or taken with close margins are ideal candidates for this approach. Tumors that invade the great vessels or with significant cranial nerve (i.e., cranial nerves 10 and 12) or mandibular involvement are not good candidates for this approach. Tumors that invade the inferior parapharyngeal space extending far below the maxillary floor should be considered for a transoral approach instead.

Pre-operative Planning

The patient should undergo imaging with magnetic resonance imaging to assess soft tissue and possible perineural extension, and computed tomography to evaluate bone. Vascular involvement should be carefully evaluated, as well as contralateral and intracranial extension. Biopsy or fine-needle aspiration of the mass will aid in planning and counseling. The airway should be assessed to determine if there will be difficulty with intubation, trismus, or post-operative edema. In general, there is minimal edema of the airway after a combined endoscopic transcervical approach, and a tracheotomy is typically not necessary.

Surgical Technique

The patient is brought to the operating room, and an oral intubation is performed. A shoulder roll is placed to expose the neck, and the head is placed on a gel headrest for stability. The image guidance system is fixed to the head so that it will move with the head when it is rotated, improving accuracy. The patient is prepped and draped with the nares, ipsilateral cheek, and neck exposed. The skin is marked with a modified Blair incision in the preauricular crease and along a skin crease to the tip of the ipsilateral hyoid bone 2 finger breadths below the mandible (Figure 4.1). The skin is injected with 1% lidocaine and 1:100,000 epinephrine. The nasal cavity is prepped with 4% cocaine pledgets, and a greater palatine block is performed bilaterally. A skin incision on the ipsilateral side of the tumor is made along the neck portion in a marked skin crease with a 15 blade. The incision is extended through the platysma and subplatysmal flaps are elevated to the mandible. If more exposure is needed, the preauricular incision can be completed to allow the parotid to be freed for exposure of the posterior mandible. An inferior flap is elevated about 1 cm for closure. The greater auricular nerve is preserved, and the anterior border of the sternocleidomastoid muscle dissected from the mandible down to the mid-point. The submandibular gland is elevated along its inferior border toward the mandible and the posterior belly of the digastric muscle is identified. Figure 4.2 shows a view of the transcervical anatomy. The muscle is dissected free from the hyoid to the skull base, and the parotid gland is elevated superiorly along its inferior surface. Next, the carotid artery and cranial nerves 11 and 12 are identified and preserved. The stylomandibluar ligament is then palpated and lysed to free the mandible and allow for further retraction. The great vessels and nerves are then dissected up to the skull base bone, which can be confirmed by palpation and image guidance. The styloid process may need to be freed and resected to allow for

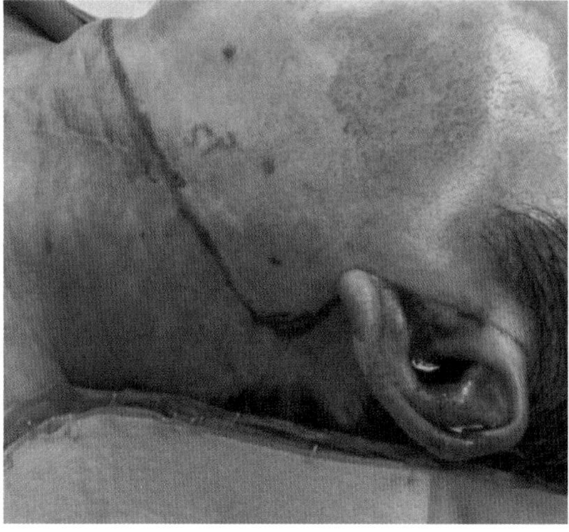

Figure 4.1 The skin is marked with a modified Blair incision in the preauricular crease and along a skin crease to the tip of the ipsilateral hyoid bone two fingerbreadths below the mandible

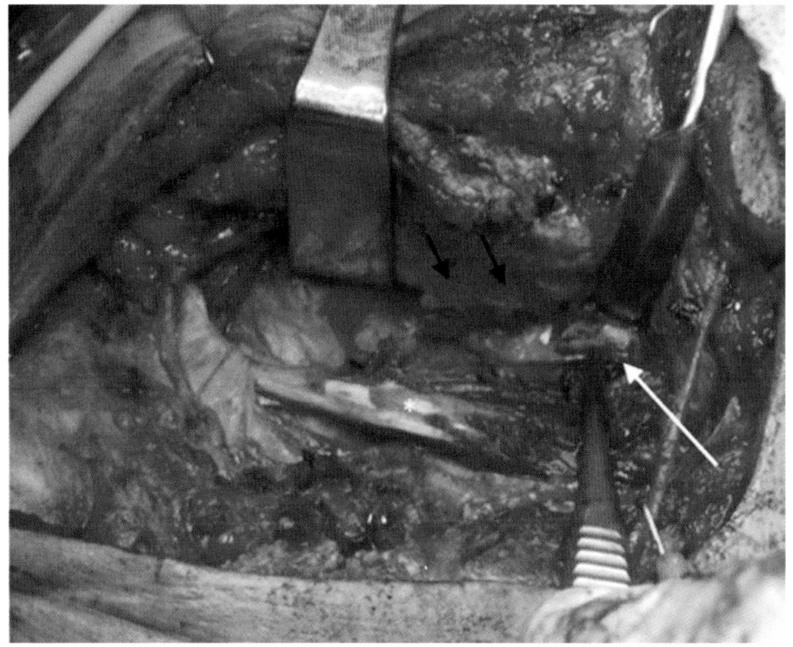

Figure 4.2 Transcervical view of anatomy. White arrow indicates the styloid process. Double black arrows indicate the back edge of the mandible.

exposure. Half-inch by 3-inch pledgets are lined along the carotid and nerves at the skull base, to protect them during endonasal dissection. If the tumor is identified at this point, its inferior surface and posterior borders can be dissected free. Anteriorly within the ITF, the medial pterygoid muscle can be identified as it attaches to the mandible and is followed superiorly, and then is dissected free at the anterior border. The pterygoid plates can be palpated as a landmark.

Next, the transnasal approach is undertaken. A zero-degree endoscope is inserted into the nasal cavity. The inferior turbinate on the ipsilateral side is resected. The uncinate and ethmoid bulla are identified after medialization of the middle turbinate. A backbiting forcep is used to open the uncinate along its inferior border, and the uncinate is then removed. The maxillary antrum ostium is widened. The ethmoid bulla can be removed to define the medial wall of the orbit. The posterior maxillary antrum wall is followed back to identify the sphenopalatine artery posterior to the ethmoid crystallis.

Next, the medial maxillary wall is removed. Using monopolar cautery, an incision is made along the piriform aperture at the nasal vestibule and then from the maxillary antrum to the piriform aperture. Another mucosal incision is made along the floor of the nasal cavity across the entire length of the maxillary sinus on the medial maxillary wall. The anterior wall of the maxilla is exposed with a freer. Using a high-speed drill with a coarse diamond burr, the anterior maxillary wall is entered and the maxillary sinus is exposed. The medial wall is drilled along the superior edge of the inferior turbinate to expose the nasal lacrimal duct, and this is sharply transected. Next, the drill is used along the inferior aspect of the medial wall to the greater palatine artery, which is identified and controlled. The medial wall of the maxilla is removed. The sphenopalatine artery is then followed into the pterygoid fossa, and the posterior maxillary wall is removed with the drill and Kerrison rongeurs. The periosteum of the pterygoid and infratemporal fossa is incised and the buccal fat pad is identified.

At this stage, the pterygoid plates are identified. These plates may be fused together or have tissue between them. Endoscopic views are shown in Figures 4.3 and 4.4. The internal maxillary artery is identified laterally and ligated with endoscopic clips. The trans-pterygoid approach is

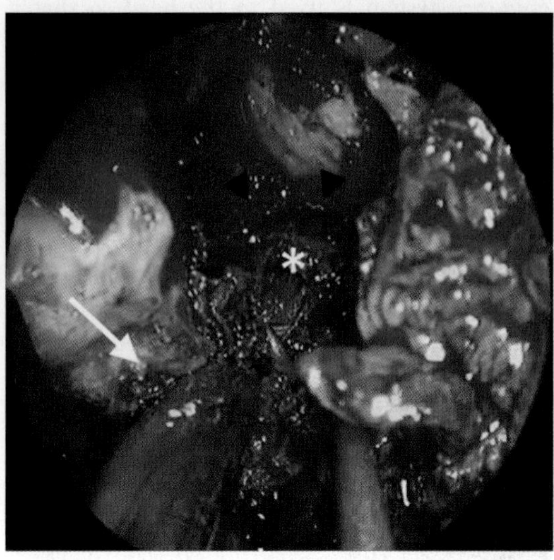

Figure 4.3 Endoscopic view. Asterisk is on a tumor at the foramen ovale. The white arrow is on the edge of the lateral pterygoid plate. Black arrowheads are along the expanded rim of the foramen ovale.

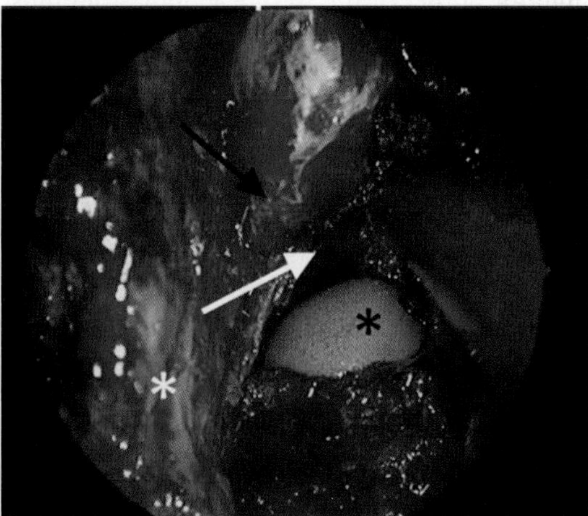

Figure 4.4 Endoscopic view. Black asterisk indicates the surgeon's finger from the transcervical exposure. White arrow indicates foramen ovale. Black arrow indicates the lateral pterygoid plate. White asterisk indicates the medial pterygoid plate.

performed in order to dissect the tumor from the eustachian tube. Removal of the lateral pterygoid plate exposes the V3 nerve exiting from the foramen ovale. The parapharyngeal space is located posterior to the masticator space, and removal of the lateral pterygoid plate positions the surgeon in the PPS. The eustachian tube is located medially just posterior to the pterygoid plates. The medial and lateral pterygoid muscles and buccal fat can be

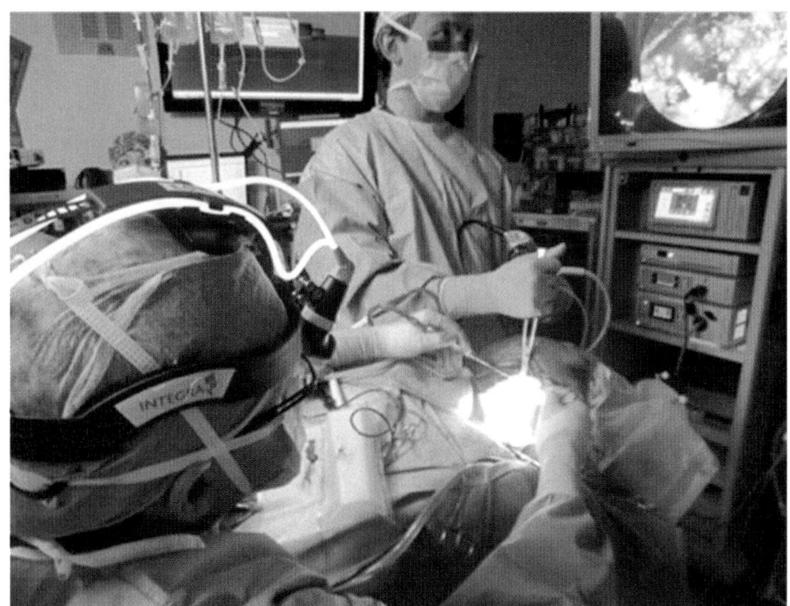

Figure 4.5 Intra-operative setup for a two-surgeon approach, with one surgeon working transcervically while the other works endonasally. Two screens allow both surgeons to operate independently and ergonomically.

dissected free and lateralized, if needed, to expose the PPS.

At this point, dissection can be continued through the neck as well, working to free the tumor posteriorly. Transnasally, the tumor's superior extent can be defined and freed, and the lateral and medial extent defined. The tumor can be dissected inferiorly into the neck and removed through this path, or removed piecemeal through the nose, depending on the pathology. Figure 4.5 shows the intra-operative setup for a two-surgeon approach, with one surgeon working transcervically while the other works endonasally. Two screens allow both surgeons to operate independently and ergonomically.

Discussion

A simultaneous, combined trans-nasal, trans-masticator, trans-pterygoid endoscopic approach, and transcervical approach can provide access to the PPS. This maneuver can avoid the need for more extensive procedures such as a mandibulotomy or trans-parotid approach with facial nerve dissection. Risks of the mandibulotomy approach include temporal mandibular joint pain and dysfunction, nonunion of the mandible, and the potential removal of a tooth. The trans-parotid approach can result in facial nerve stretch or injury. Utilizing endoscopic technology allows the combination of two corridors to be able to safely dissect the tumor. The transcervical approach allows for early identification of the carotid artery and important nerves. The transcervical approach adds approximately 30 minutes of surgical time and requires a second set of instruments, but may save time overall by allowing quicker trans-nasal work.

The trans-nasal approach is excellent for identifying and resecting lesions along the skull base up to the carotid canal. Anterior to the V3 nerve is predominantly the contents of the masticator space, and this area can be dissected relatively safely in an experienced surgeon's hands. Medial to the PPS are the constrictor muscles and pharynx, along with the tensor veli palatini muscle, which opens the eustachian tube. Surgery in this location could lead to eustachian tube dysfunction. Laterally, the space connects to the parotid gland and mandible ramus. Posteriorly, where the great vessels and cranial nerves 9, 10, 11, and 12 are located, is the most dangerous space, and the transcervical approach allows this area to be safely identified prior to starting the endonasal work.

Conclusion

The combined transcervical-transnasal approach provides access to the PPS at the skull base. The use of the two corridors is complementary and allows for full 360-degree access. This combined approach is useful for tumors extending high in the skull base and lying close and anterior to the great vessels, and for tumors that have inferior extension beyond that reachable through the nose alone.

Key Points

- The transcervical approach is a safe approach for identifying and protecting the carotid artery and cranial nerves prior to dissecting the tumor through a transnasal approach.
- The endoscopic endonasal approach provides important access to the superior aspect of the tumor.
- The inferior extension of the tumor can be dissected through the transcervical approach.
- The tumor can be removed through the neck or piecemeal through the nose.

References

1. Benet A, Plata Bello J, El-Sayed I. Combined endonasal-transcervical approach to a metastatic parapharyngeal space papillary thyroid carcinoma. *Cureus*. 2015;**7**:e285.
2. Lemos-Rodriguez AM, Sreenath SB, Rawal RB, Overton LJ, Farzal Z, Zanation AM. Carotid artery and lower cranial nerve exposure with increasing surgical complexity to the parapharyngeal space. *The Laryngoscope*. 2017;**127**:585–91.
3. Locketz GD, Horowitz G, Abu-Ghanem S, et al. Histopathologic classification of parapharyngeal space tumors: a case series and review of the literature. *European Archives of Oto-Rhino-Laryngology*. 2016;**273**:727–34.
4. Riffat F, Dwivedi RC, Palme C, Fish B, Jani P. A systematic review of 1143 parapharyngeal space tumors reported over 20 years. *Oral Oncology*. 2014;**50**:421–30.
5. Joo W, Funaki T, Yoshioka F, Rhoton AL Jr. Microsurgical anatomy of the infratemporal fossa. *Clinical Anatomy*. 2013;**26**:455–69.
6. Falcon RT, Rivera-Serrano CM, Miranda JF, et al. Endoscopic endonasal dissection of the infratemporal fossa: anatomic relationships and importance of eustachian tube in the endoscopic skull base surgery. *The Laryngoscope*. 2011;**121**:31–41.
7. Lisan Q, Leclerc N, Kania R, Guichard JP, Herman P, Verillaud B. Infratemporal fossa tumors: When to suspect a malignant tumor? A retrospective cohort study of 62 cases. *European Annals of Otorhinolaryngology, Head and Neck Diseases*. 2018;**135**:311–14.
8. Taylor RJ, Patel MR, Wheless SA, et al. Endoscopic endonasal approaches to infratemporal fossa tumors: a classification system and case series. *The Laryngoscope*. 2014;**124**:2443–50.
9. Tiwari R, Quak J, Egeler S, et al. Tumors of the infratemporal fossa. *Skull Base Surgery*. 2000;**10**:1–9.
10. Carrau RL, Johnson JT, Myers EN. Management of tumors of the parapharyngeal space. *Oncology*. 1997;**11**:633–40; discussion 40, 42.
11. Oakley GM, Harvey RJ. Endoscopic resection of pterygopalatine fossa and infratemporal fossa malignancies. *Otolaryngologic Clinics of North America*. 2017;**50**:301–13.
12. Eisele DW, Richmon JD. Contemporary evaluation and management of parapharyngeal space neoplasms. *Journal of Laryngology and Otology*. 2013;**127**:550–5.
13. Ohmann EL, Branstetter BFt, Johnson JT. The utility of fine needle aspiration to identify unusual pathology in a parapharyngeal mass. *American Journal of Otolaryngology*. 2011;**32**:82–4.
14. van Hees T, van Weert S, Witte B, Rene Leemans C. Tumors of the parapharyngeal space: the VU University Medical Center experience over a 20-year period. *European Archives of Oto-Rhino-Laryngology*. 2018;**275**:967–72.
15. Arnason T, Hart RD, Taylor SM, Trites JR, Nasser JG, Bullock MJ. Diagnostic accuracy and safety of fine-needle aspiration biopsy of the parapharyngeal space. *Diagnostic Cytopathology*. 2012;**40**:118–23.
16. Farrag TY, Lin FR, Koch WM, et al. The role of pre-operative CT-guided FNAB for parapharyngeal space tumors. *Otolaryngology*. 2007;**136**:411–14.

Combined Endoscopic Endonasal and Transcranial Approach to Complex Intracranial Lesions

Mohammed Nuru, Ankush Chandra, and Manish K. Aghi

Introduction

Transcranial approaches (TCA) and endoscopic endonasal approaches (EEA) to the anterior and central skull base are two common operative procedures employed in the modern treatment of skull base lesions. Independently, these techniques have been favored over other historical approaches such as craniofacial, transfacial, and midface degloving due to their inherent value in more cosmetically pleasing results, minimal invasiveness, shorter patient recovery times (1,2). Combined, these approaches add a new treatment solution to the neurosurgeon's armamentarium. They provide a relatively minimally invasive approach with maximal resection in indicated complex lesions – most commonly, large skull base tumors with possible vascular involvement rooted in the paranasal sinus region and extending far into the parenchyma of the brain. In this chapter, we will summarize the scope of each of these approaches to anterior and central skull base tumors and the limitations that the combined approach resolves.

Transcranial Approach to the Anterior and Central Skull Base

Transcranial approaches to the anterior and central skull base can be categorized and understood in several ways, such as relationship to the skull base (suprabasal, transbasal, subbasal), approach to the skull (anterior, anterolateral, lateral, posterior), and the bones traversed by the approach (pterional, orbitozygomatic). For the purposes of this chapter, we categorize the most commonly applied transcranial approaches according to the cranial fossae to which they provide the broadest access. We focus, in particular, on the anterior and middle fossae, for which transcranial approaches can be supplemented by the EEA (Figure 5.1).

Anterior Cranial Fossa

Transbasal (Subfrontal) Approach

The transbasal approach involves a bicoronal incision, anterior scalp reflection, anterior craniotomy, and frontal lobe retraction. This anterior approach is indicated for the exposure and resection of midline lesions of the anterior skull base with lateral extensions with or without vascular or nerve involvement, such as large fibrous pituitary adenomas (with minimal sphenoid sinus involvement), suprasellar tumors such as craniopharyngiomas (3), and anterior skull base meningiomas. For this approach, either a unilateral or bilateral craniotomy is used depending on the size and lateral extension of the lesion.

The standard transbasal approach is a time-tested procedure in the treatment of some midline tumors; however, it provides limited access to the paranasal sinuses, cribriform plate, and clivus. This is due to the overhang of the supraorbital notch, which necessitates a significantly greater frontal lobe retraction. Osteotomy extensions of the traditional approach reduce the level of retraction needed while increasing visibility to more posterior compartments (4,5). The anatomical positioning of the optic chiasm and size of the tuberculum sellae influence the decision-making process for this approach. To avoid visual complications, this approach should be avoided in the treatment of tumors in patients with a prefixed optic chiasm (Figure 5.2). The location of the optic chiasm in these patients shadows access to the sella turcica region. A large tuberculum sellae can also obstruct or reduce access to the sella turcica.

Interhemispheric Approach

The interhemispheric approach is indicated in the treatment of intracranially extending sellar tumors

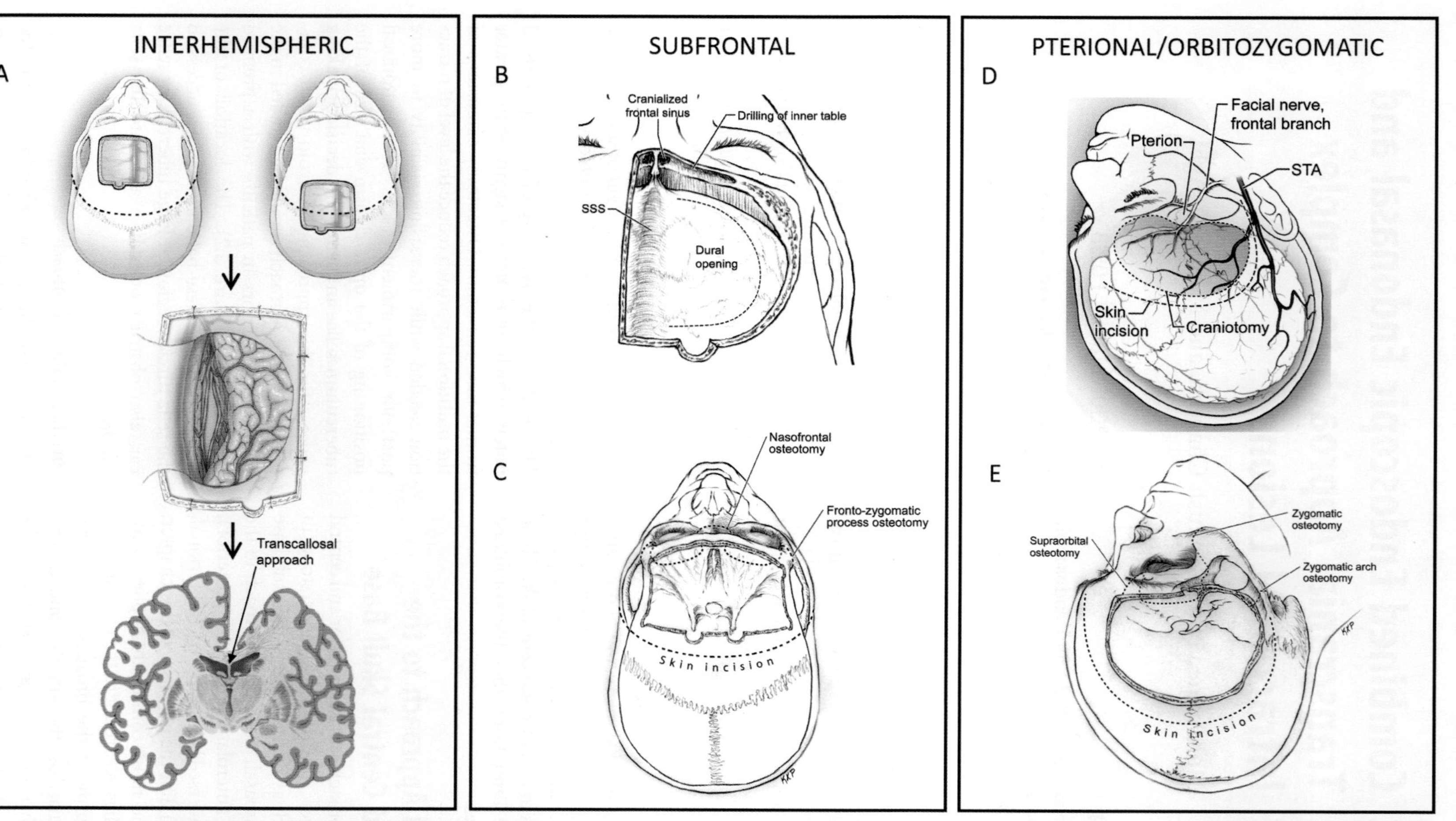

Figure 5.1 Transcranial approaches to the anterior or middle cranial fossa. Shown are diagrams depicting three common approaches to the anterior or middle cranial fossa with their associated skin incisions (shown with dashed lines), craniotomies, and parenchymal trajectories. **(A)** Interhemispheric approach to access tumors in the middle cranial fossa from above. Shown are steps including skin incision and bone flap (top row), which can be positioned in front of the coronal suture or centered around the coronal suture, depending on whether access is needed to the anterior or central portions of the third ventricle, brain retraction off the falx with exposure of anterior cerebral arteries that are also retracted (middle row), and a coronal view illustrating the callosotomy that is made to gain access to the lateral ventricle. **(B-C)** Shown are the skin incisions and craniotomy for the subfrontal approach for accessing the anterior cranial fossa through a (B) unilateral (top row) or (C) bilateral (lower row) approach. **(D-E)** Shown are the (D) pterional and its modification, the (E) orbitozygomatic craniotomy for accessing the middle cranial fossa from the side.

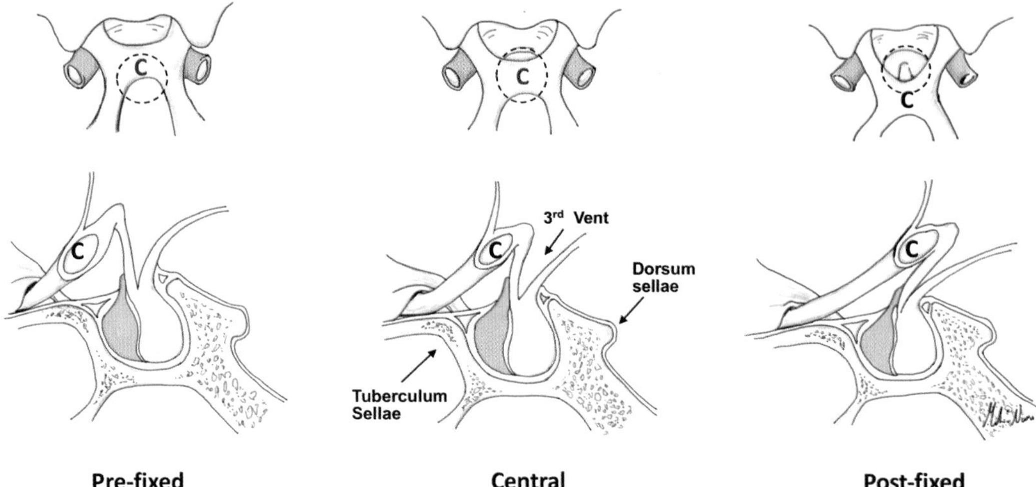

Figure 5.2 Locations of the optic chiasm and how they influence the choice of surgical approach. Shown are diagrams of axial and sagittal perspectives of the three variations in optic chiasm anatomy relative to the sella turcica region. From left to right are depictions of the pre-fixed, central, and post-fixed variants, respectively. In the pre-fixed variant, 10% of the optic chiasm is suspended over the tuberculum sellae. In this scenario, the optic nerve is shorter and the chiasm obstructs a subfrontal approach to pituitary adenomas; a subfrontal approach should be avoided in these patients. The next pair of images show a central orientation of the optic chiasm. Here, 80% of the chiasm is over the dorsum sellae. The last pair of images, to the right, displays the post-fixed variant. Here, the optic chiasm projects backward, and 10% of it hovers over the dorsum sellae. A longer optic nerve is observed in these patients. *C* = Optic chiasm. Depicted by the shaded area in yellow is the location of the underlying the diaphragma sellae.

and tumors originating in the third ventricle, such as craniopharyngiomas, colloid cysts, meningiomas, and hypothalamic gliomas (6,7). This approach is appealing because it avoids an excessive corticectomy and protects the white matter tracts.

The skin incision and craniotomy are made in reference to the coronal and sagittal sutures, depending on the approach (anterior, middle, or posterior transcallosal approach). Generally, the craniotomy is 6 × 4 cm, two-thirds anterior to the coronal suture, preferably over the non-dominant hemisphere, and with a medial limit of 1 cm over the sagittal suture. During the dural incision, great care should be taken to avoid damage to the superior sagittal sinus and large parasagittal veins. Damage can result in venous infarction of brain tissue and hemiparesis. The trajectory involves transcallosal incision and, in the case of laterally-extending lesions, may involve incision of the falx cerebri. The advantages of this approach include minimal corticectomy and minimal risks to the optic apparatus, hypothalamus, and carotid arteries. A contralateral approach to the affected cerebral hemisphere further minimizes retraction, especially for lesions that extend laterally. Furthermore, this is the only approach that provides bilateral exposure of the foramen of Monro and roof of the third ventricle (7). Complications of this approach include neuropsychological deficits associated with disruption of the corpus callosum, including memory, attentive, and motor-coordination deficits.

Middle Cranial Fossa

Pterional/Orbitozygomatic Approach

The orbitozygomatic approach is a modification of the pterional approach, incorporating osteotomies of the superior and lateral orbital ridges in one or more bone flaps. It is an anterolateral approach involving a standard pterional incision, anterior reflection of the scalp, lateral reflection of temporalis muscle, and craniotomy. The approach facilitates access to lesions of the anterior and middle cranial fossa, orbital apex, cavernous sinus, paraclinoid and parasellar regions, and basilar apex with minimal brain retraction (8). This approach is useful for tuberculum sellae and petrous apex meningiomas, clival lesions, lesions involving the lateral wall of the orbit, and lateral lesions in the middle cranial fossa (particularly those with vascular encasement or involvement) (9). After the craniotomy, the tumor is exposed via a transsylvian approach (Figure 5.3).

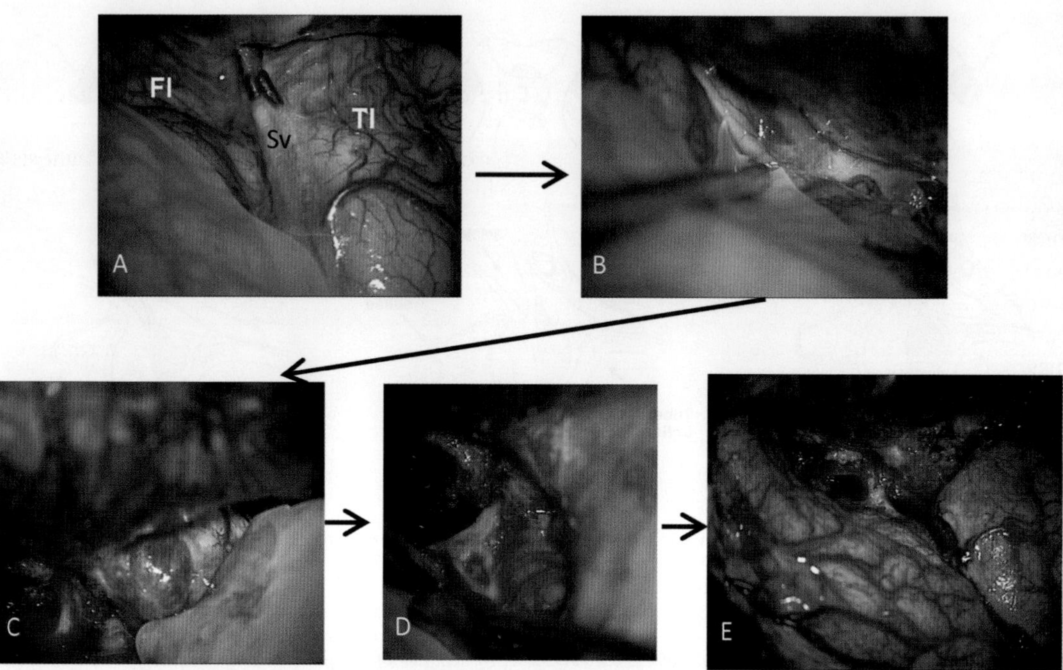

Figure 5.3 Giant pituitary adenoma seen through a right orbitozygomatic craniotomy and transsylvian exposure. Shown are images from a transsylvian exposure of a giant pituitary adenoma seen through an operative microscope. **(A)** Sylvian fissure prior to opening. **(B)** Opened sylvian cistern with carotid cistern in sight. **(C)** Tumor visualized from its right lateral surface between the frontal and temporal lobes with optic nerve draped over right lateral tumor surface. **(D)** View after initial tumor debulking. **(E)** View after additional tumor debulking. *FL* = Frontal lobe, *TL* = Temporal lobe, Sv= Sylvian vein.

One major advantage of the orbitozygomatic approach is that it often reveals normal anatomical structures, like the carotid bifurcation into anterior and middle cerebral arteries and the optic apparatus, before tumor debulking, which improves the safety of the approach. The orbitozygomatic approach also offers access to the third ventricle through the lamina terminalis, as well as the ability to fenestrate the lamina for CSF flow for further brain relaxation. Limitations of the orbitozygomatic approach include a lack of visualization of the ipsilateral wall of the third ventricle and hypothalamus during resection of tumors involving the third ventricle, such as craniopharyngiomas.

Subtemporal/Anterior Petrosal Approach

The subtemporal approach provides exposure from the anterior limits of the middle cranial fossa to the anterior portion of the petrous edge. It is a lateral approach involving a horseshoe incision beginning 1 cm anterior to the tragus, inferior reflection of the temporalis muscle, temporal bone craniotomy, and temporal lobe retraction. It provides optimal access to lesions associated with Meckel's cave, the tentorium, the incisura space, and the upper third of the clival region, as well as a lateral approach to the sella turcica region. Examples of resectable lesions accessible via this approach include petrous apex cholesteatomas, cholesterol granulomas, trigeminal nerve schwannomas, pituitary adenomas, and basilar apex aneurysms (10). An anterior petrosectomy is a modification that grants further posterior and medial access. Ultimately, it provides exposure to lesions of the petroclival region and ventral and ventrolateral aspects of the upper third of the brainstem. Indications for the subtemporal/anterior petrosal approach include posterior circulation aneurysms, midbrain and pontine intra-axial lesions, and intrapetrous lesions. Contraindications of this approach include purely clival tumors, tumors extending into cranial nerve foramina, lesions posterior to the internal auditory canal, and purely lower pontine and medullary lesions (11,12).

Endoscopic Endonasal Approaches to the Anterior and Central Skull Base

Endoscopic endonasal approaches to skull base pathology are primarily employed to gain subbasal access to lesions proximal to the midline of the skull base. Indicated pathologies include midline-localized lesions with minimal vascularization. Stemming from the traditional endoscopic transsphenoidal approach to sellar lesions (to gain access to pituitary adenomas, Rathke's cleft cysts, and craniopharyngiomas, for instance), expansion of the endoscopic endonasal approach has granted skull base surgeons additional access to anterior midline lesions (such as olfactory groove meningiomas, paranasal sinus cancers, and olfactory neuroblastomas) and posterior midline lesions (such as chordomas, tuberculum sellae meningiomas, and some petroclival meningiomas and juvenile nasopharyngeal angiofibromas) (13,14,15,16). Endoscopic endonasal surgeries are classified by their approaches relative to the sagittal (Figure 5.4) or coronal planes of the skull (17). Briefly, sagittal approaches are classified as transfrontal, transcribriform, and transplanar/transtubercular (anterior skull base approaches); transsphenoidal (central skull base approach); and transclival and transodontoid approaches (posterior skull base approaches).

The coronal classification of EEA expansions highlights the lateral extent of this approach. They provide greater resection potential for lesions that are more laterally located relative to the skull base midline. Lateral expansions of the anterior skull base fossa consist of the supraorbital and transorbital approaches, central fossa expansions consist of five transpterygoid approaches, and posterior fossa expansions consist of transcondylar and parapharyngeal approaches.

Surgical Considerations

It is critical that the surgical approach chosen best matches the goals of intervention discussed with the patient (tumor debulking/decompression, partial or complete resection, or tissue diagnosis). The decision-making process should also account for associated patient comorbidities and premorbid status, assessed by extensive neurological physical examination and imaging, and the role they may play in potential complications associated with a chosen approach. It should account for the surgical team's level of comfort with a given approach, which will influence the final patient outcome. Finally, the selection of surgical approach must be informed by the presentation of the lesion.

TCA and EEA possess unique strengths and limitations based on the location of the lesion relative to the skull base, the characteristics of the lesion (size, texture, firmness, and vascularity), the amount of sagittal and coronal extension, and the distribution between the intracranial and sinonasal compartments. The patient's anatomical variations (biological) or anatomical landmark alterations (from previous surgeries) should also be accounted for in the planning process – especially for the EEA. Anatomical variations include

- variations in the optic chiasm, including prefixed, central, or postfixed locations relative to the diaphragma sellae (Figure 5.2) (This affects the visual field defect seen in patients with pituitary adenomas [contralateral hemianopsia,

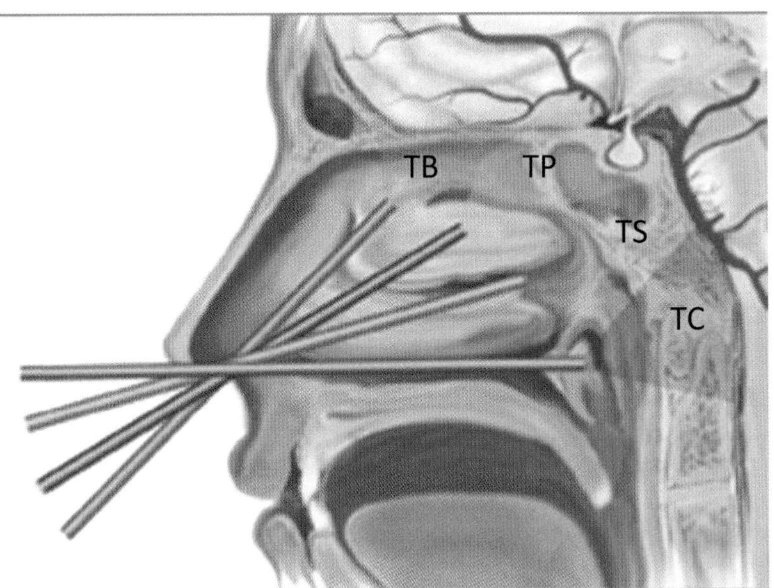

Figure 5.4 Approaches allowed through the endonasal corridor as seen in the sagittal plane. Shown are four surgical approaches to the anterior and middle cranial fossae enabled by the endonasal corridor. Namely, the transcribiform (TB), transplanum/transtuberculum (TP), transsphenoidal (TS), and transclival (TC) endoscopic approaches.

bitemporal hemianopsia, and monocular deficit, respectively] and influences the choice of craniotomy. Specifically, a subfrontal approach should be avoided in patients with a prefixed optic chiasm.);
- variation in sphenoid sinus shape (sellar, presellar, or conchal shape);
- presence of septal deviations; and
- configuration of the intercavernous sinus and distance between carotid arteries at the level of the sella.

These variations can be identified with preoperative CT or MRI. Patients with sellar or parasellar lesions should also undergo formal endocrinological evaluation and complete visual assessment prior to surgery (2).

Preoperative Considerations

In both approaches, MRI imaging should be used to assess the location of the lesion and the level of intracranial spread. Imaging studies should be performed in time to allow for the use of the images in intraoperative neuronavigation. CT imaging can also be employed to evaluate the air sinuses, the presence and extent of sinonasal and parasinus invasion, and the presence of CSF leaks. In the event of vascular involvement, CTA is preferred to MRA in visualizing the lesion's relationship to vascular structures of the brain, particularly to the carotid artery and venous outflow. In cases of significant vascular encasement, digital subtraction angiography (DSA) is preferred (5). The level of brain relaxation as well as intracranial pressure should be accounted for. A brain-relaxation strategy or protocol should be in place to reduce excessive retraction and its associated complications (see the section "Outcomes and Complications" later in this chapter). Li et al. (2016) outline common CSF diversion strategies and considerations that can ensure sufficient brain relaxation (18). Note that lumbar drains, if indicated, pose an increased risk of brain herniation, meningitis, and hydrocephalus.

Advantages and Limitations of EEA and TCA

EEAs are more technically complex, requiring proficiency in angled endoscope technique (if viewing structures around corners) and bimanual manipulation of surgical instrumentation (including straight and angled endoscopes, most commonly of 0 degrees and 45 degrees, respectively) with microsurgical technique. The endoscope provides the benefit of binocular, wide-angled visualization of the surgical site with undistorted depth perception. This is not the case in TCAs employing a microscope, as the microscope has a tendency to distort depth perception. EEAs are also relatively minimally invasive. They eliminate facial scarring, enable significantly shorter patient recovery times, impart less nasal trauma, and minimize neurovascular manipulation in indicated lesions. With regard to lesion resection, a piecemeal technique, as opposed to en bloc resection, is more common with EEAs. The characteristically narrower surgical corridors of this approach are more in line with piecemeal resection, a technique that may make it easier to obtain negative margins in anatomically challenging areas of the skull base.

Contraindications for this approach are large, laterally localized (or laterally-extending) lesions that are highly vascularized or receiving blood supply from major cerebral arteries (such as the anterior cerebral artery). Laterally located skull base tumors present a challenge due to anatomical and vascular boundaries (e.g., the medial orbital wall of the anterior skull base) and are a contraindication for a purely endonasal approach. Tumor encasement of the carotid artery, anterior cerebral artery, optic nerve, or chiasm are also contraindicated, mostly because of limited control in the event of injury to these vascular structures; in these cases, a suprabasal approach provides better control in resection.

Theoretically, TCAs allow access to lesions spanning the entire skull base, limited posteriorly by the clivus and foramen magnum. This approach lends itself best to broad, laterally extending lesions. Subbasal approaches like EEAs are limited laterally by the optic nerve, medial orbital walls, and internal carotid arteries, while TCAs are not limited by these structures. Subbasal approaches are better suited for the treatment of lesions with vascular involvement, as they provide excellent visualization and control of neurovasculature (particularly with an anterolateral approach, such as the orbitozygomatic approach). Reaching the retrosellar and clival areas extradurally can be challenging when using purely TCA. An extended EEA is better indicated for these lesions. Furthermore, the craniotomy approach and brain retraction result in increased patient recovery times. Intracranially spreading lesions can also result in the need for increased cortical retraction.

Outcomes and Complications (EEA versus TCA)

In indicated lesions, EEAs are favored over TCAs due to minimal neurovascular manipulation and the absence of brain retraction. A systematic review of literature comparing TCA and EEA outcomes for tuberculum sellae, olfactory groove, and planum sphenoidale meningiomas shows that TCAs are associated with increased rates of postoperative seizures (associated with retraction), hydrocephalus, and poorer visual outcomes compared with EEAs (19). However, EEAs are reported to have a higher incidence of postoperative CSF leakage (20). Patients are also at increased risk of meningitis from potential exposure to the aerodigestive tract. In our meta-analysis of pooled EEAs (49 patients) and TCAs (111 patients) for resection of tuberculum sellae meningioma, we reached a similar conclusion: EEA surgeries are associated with increased incidence of postoperative CSF leaks and improved visual outcomes (21). It should be mentioned that novel flap-repair techniques are being developed to decrease the incidence of postoperative CSF leakage (22,23). Vascularized nasoseptal flaps are the current gold standard in reconstruction, lowering the incidence of CSF leakage to 5% from 14.5% in some reports (24).

Possible complications of the extended TCAs include epiphora, damage to the lacrimal sac during osteotomy, and valvular collapse or saddle-nose deformity when the nasal bone is incorporated into the orbital bar. There is also an increased risk of exophthalmos when removal of the lateral orbital wall is necessary.

Combined Transcranial and Endoscopic Endonasal Approach

Brief History

Decades of advancements in endoscopic technology – such as the improvement of lenses, fiber optic illumination, videoscopes, techniques such as bimanual instrumentation, and bayoneted instruments – have enabled significant advances in combined transcranial-endoscopic endonasal approaches to intracranial lesions. Yuen et al. (1996) are credited as early pioneers of the combined transcranial-endoscopic endonasal approach, used in place of the transcranial-transfacial approach, for the treatment of olfactory neuroblastoma (25). In the last decade, more recent technological advancements such as neuronavigation, microvascular Doppler ultrasonography, ultrasonic aspirators customized for the endonasal approach, and vascularized flaps for reconstruction have set the stage for more extensive implementation of combined approaches to complex brain lesions.

Rationale and Advantages over Individual Approaches

Advantages of the combined transcranial and endoscopic endonasal approach compared to the TCA and EEA individually are:

- superior visualization (above and below) and neurovascular control for certain tumors in the event of neurovascular encasement;
- resection of far-extending intracranial tumors without limiting access to tumor infiltration of structures about the skull base;
- more accurate control of resection margins;
- less cortical retraction compared to a purely TCA, reducing the risk of postoperative seizures and postoperative cerebral edema;
- transcranial access to vascularized nasoseptal and turbinate flaps, which can be harvested endonasally and used to supplement pericranial flaps for a very thorough skull base reconstruction (26);
- eliminated need for invasive, extended TCAs to large, extending lesions, allowing for relatively shorter patient recovery times;
- improved tumor access in patients with a prefixed chiasm and sellar tumors with significant suprasellar extension compared to the TCA, which may present difficulty in visualization and separation of the tumor from tuberculum sellae (27);
- the combined strength of the lateral reach of the TCA with the visibility and minimally invasive nature of the EEA for central portions of the tumor; and
- that the combined approach is less surgically aggressive than either approach alone, reducing the risk of complications.

Patient Selection for Combined TCA and EEA

Table 5.1 lists examples of lesions described in the literature for which a combined approach was used. Preoperative considerations in patient selection are described here.

- Exclusive use of EEA is contraindicated in patients with a tumor involving the anterior wall of the frontal sinus, extensive dural involvement, carotid artery encasement, or extensive invasion of brain parenchyma (28,29). In such cases, the addition of a transcranial approach is necessary for optimum visualization and extraction of the tumor/lesion, as well as for control of heavily involved vasculature.
- The patient's surgical history can influence the risk of complications. A combined approach can reduce complications in patients with a history of fibrosis, edema, or surgery involving pedicled flaps, or who have lost important anatomical landmarks.
- Selecting which TCA to employ in tandem with which EEA relies heavily on the location of the lesion in the skull base (as detailed in the sections of this chapter describing the EEA and TCA). Furthermore, one must consider the level of neurovascular involvement. Generally, the preferred approach trajectory avoids major vascular manipulation or provides the best control for removal of lesions proximal to or surrounding neurovascular structures. Commonly applied combined approaches include the following:

• Transbasal + endoscopic endonasal approach
• Frontotemporal + endoscopic endonasal approach
• Pterional + endoscopic endonasal approach

Table 5.1 Summary of published examples of the use of combined transcranial-endoscopic endonasal approaches

	Lesions	Potential approach	Extent of removal	Description
1	Invasive olfactory neuroblastoma	Transbasal + transcribriform endoscopic endonasal approach (29)	GTR	Indicated for olfactory neuroblastomas with a broad lateral cranial base and sinonasal invasion
2	Retrochiasmatic craniopharyngioma	Staged orbitozygomatic + endoscopic endonasal approach (31)	GTR	Indicated for large tumors encasing the optic pathway, the supraclinoid carotid arteries, or the anterior/middle cerebral arteries at their origins
3	Giant pituitary adenoma	Transbasal + transsphenoidal endoscopic endonasal approach (32)	GTR	Indicated for giant pituitary adenomas with significant supra/parasellar extensions in the sagittal or coronal plane (33) or with a "dumbbell" or "hourglass" configuration
4	Giant clival chordoma	Retrosigmoidal + transclival endoscopic endonasal approach* (34)	NTR	Indicated for large clival chordomas and central skull base lesions extending into the posterior cranial fossa
5	Ethmoidal squamous cell carcinoma	Staged transbasal + transcribriform endoscopic endonasal approach (35)	GTR	Indicated for well-vascularized lesions with ethmoidal, sinonasal, and cribriform plate involvement with intracranial extension
6	Giant pituitary adenoma	Interhemispheric + transsphenoidal endoscopic endonasal approach (36)	GTR, STR	Indicated for large pituitary adenomas with superior extension into the lateral ventricle

The published examples fall between the years 2002 and 2014. Reported postoperative MRI scans (>9 months and <64 months) in all patients showed no evidence of tumor recurrence and confirmed gross total resection, with the exception of one patient in case series #6 with a subtotal resection that was reported to have a stable tumor residual at 63 months postoperation (both patients in this report refused radiotherapy treatment). Gross total resection (~100% removal); Near-total resection (>90% removal); Subtotal resection (50–90% removal).

*This is a combined posterior cranial fossa approach employed in the treatment of qualified lesions that border the distal central skull base (middle cranial fossa) and proximal posterior cranial fossa.

Operative Setup for Combined TCA and EEA

This approach requires two surgical teams and two operative fields (Figure 5.5) under the same round of general anesthesia. If staged approaches are employed for a pituitary adenoma, the patient must be observed closely in the time between the two surgical phases to ensure that residual tumor does not infarct and cause apoplexy.

The procedure can be staged to minimize approach-related morbidity (30) and surgeon fatigue. The transcranial surgeon and the operative microscope are positioned at the head of the patient, with the transsphenoidal surgeon standing to the right of the patient. A sterile drape can be placed to prevent cross-contamination of operative fields.

The patient is placed under general anesthesia with endotracheal intubation. Intravenous lines and arterial lines are established, the patient's eyes are protected with antibiotic ointment, and a Foley catheter is placed. A stereotactic neuronavigation system can be configured with preoperative MRI or CT scans (and merged scans for better bone and soft tissue delineation, if desired), and a lumbar drain can be placed to facilitate brain relaxation and postoperative CSF diversion. Fluorescein can also be administered through the lumbar drain for better visualization of the CSF defect during reconstruction (0.1 ml in 10 cc of CSF; preservative-free saline can also be injected over at least 10 minutes to minimize seizure risk).

The patient is positioned supine on the operating table with the head held in three-point fixation (e.g., using a Mayfield three-point head holder). The operating table should be flexed between 10 and 15 degrees to facilitate venous drainage. The patient's neck should be slightly extended to assist in frontal lobe relaxation from the base of the skull (29). If taking a frontotemporal or pterional transcranial approach, the head can be tilted contralaterally for ease of craniotomy and better visualization of the lesion. The scalp, mouth, and nose should be prepped with Povidone-iodine solution and draped. The lower abdomen should be prepped and harvested of fat for the reconstruction of the skull base following transsphenoidal treatment. Fascia lata from the thigh can also be harvested for transcranial reconstruction.

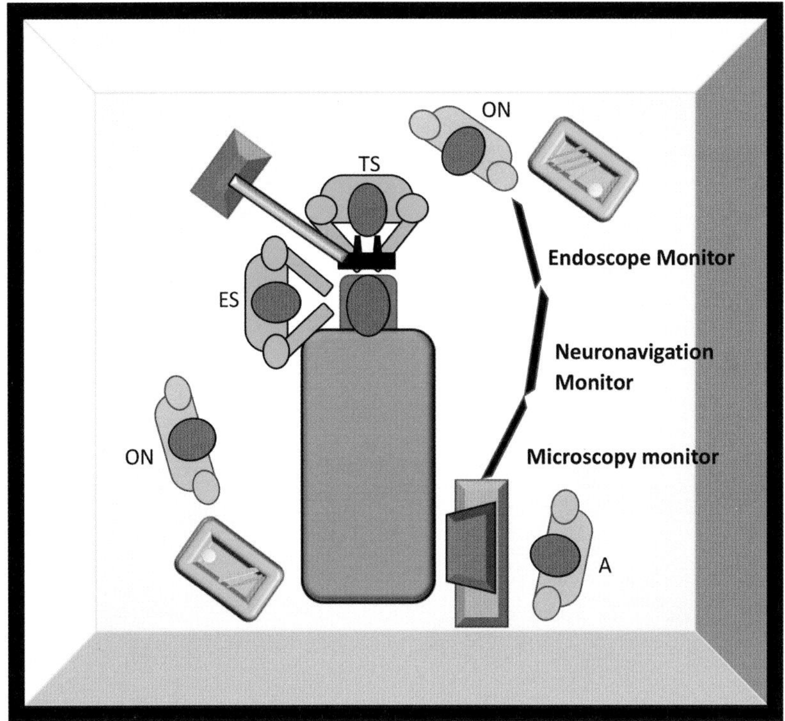

Figure 5.5 Schematic of operating room setup for simultaneous combined endonasal and transcranial approaches. Shown is an aerial perspective of the OR setup for a simultaneous combined approach. Monitor placement optimizes the endonasal surgeon's viewing angle of the microscope video feed in addition to the endoscope camera feed. The surgeons work with separate OR nurses and surgical utensils to minimize cross-contamination with the aero-respiratory tract from the endoscopic phase. In addition, a drape between the surgeons may be added to meet this end. TS = Transcranial surgeon, ES = Endonasal surgeon, ON = Operating room nurse, A = Anesthesiologist.

Decadron, antiepileptics, mannitol, and antibiotics should be administered prior to the first skin incision. To avoid epidural bleeding upon approach, mannitol can also be administered in a delayed fashion until after the craniotomy is complete and "tack-up" sutures have been placed.

Surgical Technique

Transbasal + Endoscopic Endonasal Approach Technique (Figure 5.6)

Transcranial Phase

- A bicoronal incision is made 1 cm anterior to the tragus on either side, and the scalp is reflected in a two-layer fashion. First, the galea is elevated, leaving the pericranium adhered to the skull. The pericranium is then elevated and reflected, with care taken not to disrupt the supraorbital neurovascular bundle and frontalis branch of the facial nerve lying in the superficial temporal fat pad.
- Frontal craniotomy is performed, employing an osteotome horizontally to disarticulate skull flap.
- The frontal sinus mucosa is cranialized; then the dura is opened and packed with Gelfoam soaked in antibiotics.
- The dural sac is opened by cutting into either side of the superior sagittal sinus, moving medially, with care taken to avoid bridging veins.
- The skull base deformity is sealed using the vascularized pericranial flap.

Endoscopic Phase

Prep

- A wet pad is placed in the patient's throat to prevent fluid drainage into the airway by way of the oropharynx.
- The nasal passage is prepped with pledgets soaked in 50% povidone-iodine solution, with care taken not to injure the nasal mucosa.

Nasal Step

- A rigid 0° endoscope is placed into the right nostril, parallel to the nasal floor, until the endoscope reaches the tail of the inferior turbinate.
- Cotton pledgets soaked in adrenaline are slid between the middle turbinate and the nasal

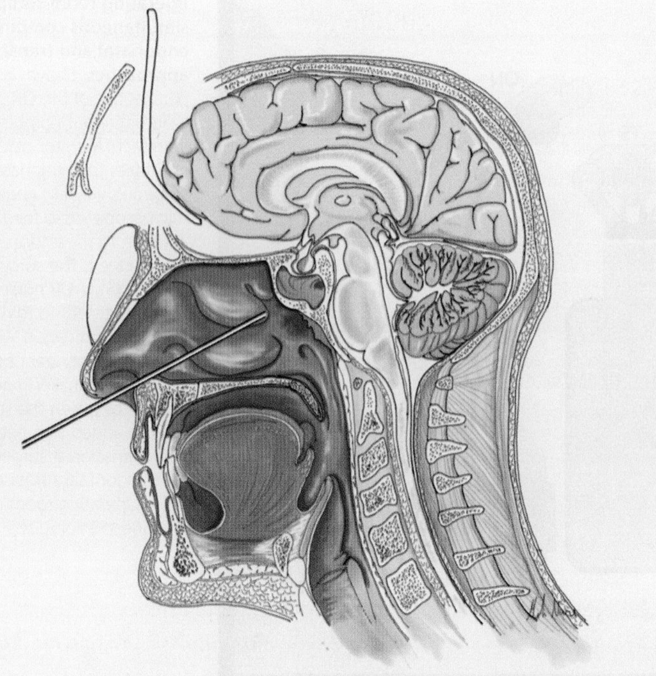

Figure 5.6 Illustration of exposure achieved with simultaneous combined endonasal and transcranial (subfrontal) approaches. Shown is an illustration of the exposure achieved from a frontal craniotomy, with frontal lobe retraction, and a transsphenoidal trajectory through the endonasal corridor.

septum. The middle turbinate is sharply luxated laterally to widen the surgical corridor.

Harvesting of Nasoseptal Flap

- The posterior incisions are made with care taken not to damage the septal cartilage.
- A unipolar electrocautery is used to make two horizontal incisions. The superior incision should start 1–2 cm below the superior aspect of the septum at the lateral side of the inferior portion of the sphenoid ostium. Take care to avoid the olfactory epithelium. The incision should extend medially to cross the rostrum of the sphenoid and then anteriorly to the nasal septum, ending directly across from the anterior edge of the inferior turbinate. The inferior incision should be made laterally beginning at the level of the posterior choana, extending medially following the free edge of the posterior nasal septum, continuing anteriorly along the maxillary crest, and ending parallel to the endpoint of the superior incision. The two incisions can then be connected by a vertical incision.
- A Cottle elevator is used to elevate the septal flap in an anterior-to-posterior fashion. A suction freer can then be used to elevate the nasal flap.
- The flap is then carefully tucked into the oropharynx until the reconstructive phase of the procedure, with care taken to avoid strangulation of blood supply to the flap (e.g., the posterior septal artery).

Sphenoidal Step

- An anterior sphenoidotomy is performed. First, the mucosa of the sphenoethmoidal recess is coagulated bilaterally. About 1 cm of the posterior part of the nasal septum is detached from the anterior wall of the sphenoid sinus and removed, facilitating binostril access.
- The sphenoid ostium is enlarged with a microdrill or bone punches.
- The sphenoid septum is then carefully removed with care taken to avoid damage to the mucosa, if tumor infiltration has not occurred.
- Anatomical landmarks are confirmed. An ultrasound Doppler probe can be used to confirm intercavernous and cavernous sinus locations. Boney landmarks include the carotid sinus and optical nerve bony prominences laterally, the tuberculum indentation anteriorly, and clival indentation posteriorly.

Sellar Step

- The second surgeon takes over control of the endoscope, freeing the first surgeon to proceed with the procedure bimanually, with one instrument placed in each nostril.
- The sella floor is opened and can be expanded laterally up to the carotid prominences, anteriorly up to the tuberculum, and posteriorly up to the clival indentations.
- Using a micro-Doppler, the location of the superior intercavernous sinus and carotid arteries are confirmed and avoided while performing the rest of the procedure.
- Both sellar dural layers are opened in a lateral-to -medial and superior-to-inferior fashion using a telescopic blade, with care taken to avoid the superior intercavernous sinus and carotid arteries.
- Proceed with lesion management using microneurosurgical techniques.

Orbitozygomatic + Endoscopic Endonasal Approach (Figure 5.7)

Transcranial Phase

- A curvilinear incision is made behind the hairline from the zygomatic arch (1 cm anterior to the tragus) to the mid-pupillary line. The scalp is reflected anteroinferiorly from the temporalis muscle and skull. Care is taken not to damage the nerve to the frontalis muscle and the supraorbital nerve coming out of the supraorbital foramen. A galeal-pericranial flap can be harvested for use during the reconstructive portion of the endoscopic phase.
- The temporalis fascia is cut through the superficial and deep layers and reflected anteriorly with the skin flap.
- Subperiosteal dissection is continued along the frontozygomatic process to expose the entire zygomatic process.
- A wedge of bone is dissected around the supraorbital nerve in the orbital rim and reflected with the periorbita and skin.

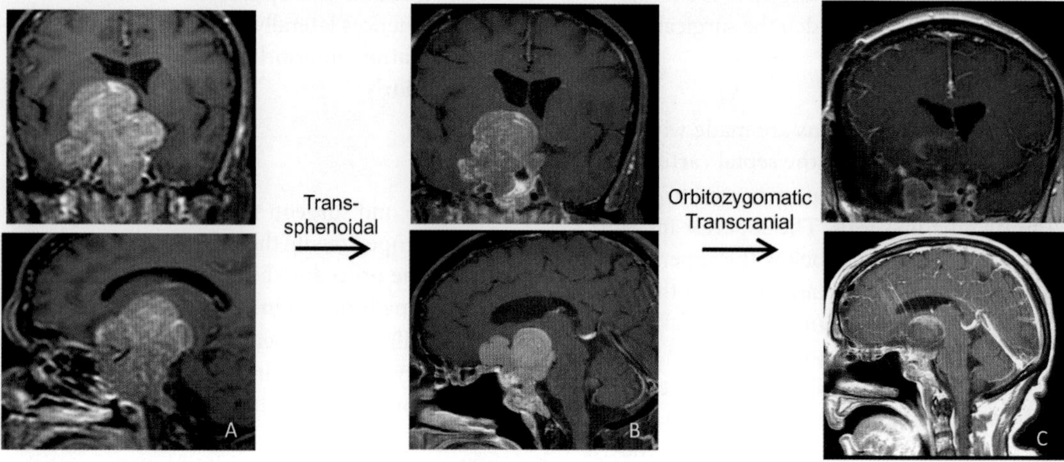

Figure 5.7 Example of a giant pituitary adenoma treated through staged endonasal and orbitozygomatic approaches. Shown are T1-weighted MRI scans (coronal and sagittal planes) from a staged transsphenoidal-transcranial removal of a large pituitary adenoma. Case was a 62-year-old female with more than 15 years of right-eye blindness and temporal field cuts in the left eye, presenting with headache. Labs revealed hypopituitarism. Preoperative scans (A) show a large right-sided dominant tumor compressing surrounding parenchyma and lateral ventricles above and invading Sinonasal space below. (B) Scan shows MRI after debulking and resection of tumor from Sinonasal cavity via endoscopic transsphenoidal approach. (C) Post-operative scan after transcranial resection via orbitozygomatic approach.

- The zygomatic arch is cut at the root of the zygoma and at the malar eminence and reflected inferiorly.
- The temporalis muscle is dissected from the skull in a superior-inferior fashion, preserving the deep temporalis fascia, and reflected inferiorly.
- The orbitozygomatic craniotomy is performed. The first burr hole is placed in the frontal bone behind the frontozygomatic suture. The second burr hole is placed behind the sphenosquamosal suture, 2 cm anterior to the posterior root of the zygomatic arch in the squamous temporal bone. The third burr hole is placed anterior to the temporal line at the level of the temporoparietal suture.
- The underlying dura is separated from the bone flap using a subperiosteal elevator.
- The burr holes are connected using a craniotome, and the bone flap is disarticulated using an osteotome, with care taken not to damage the periorbita or displace periorbital fat.
- The dura is dissected in a C-shaped fashion and reflected along the sphenoid wing.
- Based on the location of the lesion and access needs, proceed using either a transsylvian approach or a subcortical approach.

Endoscopic Phase

- Proceed using the steps described in the “Endoscopic Phase” of the section on the “Transbasal + Endoscopic Endonasal Approach Technique.”

Interhemispheric + Endoscopic Endonasal Approach (Figure 5.8)

Transcranial Phase

The incision and craniotomy are dependent on the chosen approach: anterior, middle, or posterior transcallosal. Prior to operation, consider any pathological modifications of the corpus callosum, septum pellucidum, or fornices complex, and perform a venous MR angiography to determine a position for the dural opening that best avoids bridging veins.

The surgery should be performed over the non-dominant hemisphere, if possible.

- For the anterior and middle approaches, a linear bicoronal incision is made just anterior to the coronal suture with care taken not to damage the temporalis muscle. For a posterior approach, position the patient in a prone position and perform the craniotomy

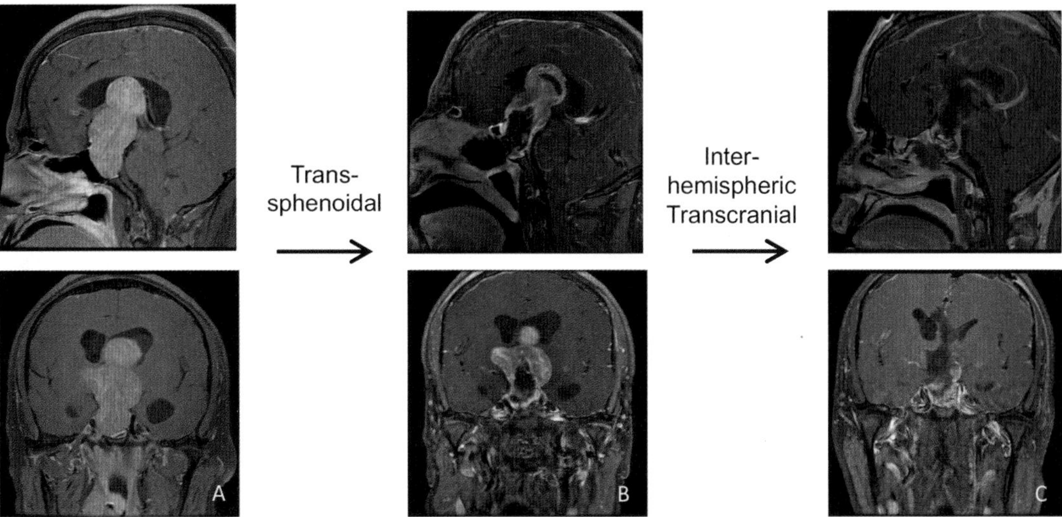

Figure 5.8 Example of a giant pituitary adenoma treated through staged endonasal and interhemispheric approaches. Shown are coronal and sagittal plane T1-weighted MRI scans from a staged transsphenoidal-interhemispheric resection of a large dumbbell-shaped tumor (A). Case was a 33-year-old male with a 3-year history of right-eye blindness and headache. (B) Scans after debulking and partial resection via a transsphenoidal approach from below. (C) Post-operative scan after transcranial resection of the intracranially extending portion of the tumor via an interhemispheric approach.

4–5 cm anterior to the confluence of sinuses (torcular herophili).

- For all approaches, create a 6 × 4 cm craniotomy by making two 1-cm burr holes over the sagittal sinus. In the anterior approach, the first burr hole is made 4 cm anterior to the coronal suture, while the second is positioned 2 cm posterior to the coronal suture. For the middle approach, the incision and craniotomy are positioned more posteriorly – the first burr hole at 2 cm anterior to the coronal suture and the second at 4 cm posterior to the coronal suture.
- A pedicled dural incision is created in a curvilinear fashion, and the dura is reflected, with care taken not to damage the superior sagittal sinus and bridging veins.
- The pericallosal arteries and the corpus callosum are identified. The trajectory through the corpus callosum is defined by the location of the lesion. It is strongly encouraged to proceed with the help of neuronavigation.
- Latex and long cotton sponges should be used to help retract and protect the medial surface of the brain.

Endoscopic Phase

- Proceed using the steps described in the "Endoscopic Phase" of the section on the "Transbasal + Endoscopic Endonasal Approach Technique."

Postoperative Care, Complications, and Special Considerations

- Patients are monitored in the neurological ICU after surgery and should be assessed with a neurological exam every hour for the first 24 to 48 hours.
- Postoperative MRI or CT scans should be performed within 24 hours of surgery to rule out postoperative hematoma, pneumocephalus, or CSF leakage. Patients should be advised to avoid activities that may raise intracranial pressure (e.g., bending over, lifting heavy objects, nose-blowing, and similar types of strain) and to sneeze open-mouthed. Stool-softening medication can also be administered to reduce straining.
- Patients receiving adjuvant radiotherapy have an increased risk of postoperative CSF leakage. These patients should be monitored closely with regular CSF leakage assessment, and

arrangements for appropriate CSF leak management should be in place. These arrangements may include 1 to 2 weeks of bed rest, placement of a lumbar drain, and/or surgical treatment.

- Fluid intake and urine output should be monitored daily alongside fluid and electrolyte management. Administer third-generation cephalosporins to reduce the risk of infection.
- Perform nasal debridement 2 weeks post-operation and then every 1 to 2 weeks following until crusting ceases. Care should be taken to avoid debridement over the nasoseptal flap, as this could cause CSF leakage.
- Patients with unsatisfactory postoperative hormone levels or postoperative diabetes should be placed on appropriate hormone replacement therapy.

Surgical Pearls

- Greater resection can be achieved when a combined transcranial-endoscopic endonasal approach is used for certain large tumors centered around the midline of the anterior and/or central skull base.
- These approaches can be done simultaneously or staged in separate operations. When performing staged operations for large pituitary adenomas, the patient must be observed closely in between the two operations to ensure that the residual tumor does not infarct and swell, causing clinical symptoms.
- It is particularly important to close the endonasal operation securely, ideally using a vascularized nasoseptal flap, to ensure that sinonasal contents do not penetrate the craniotomy site.

References

1. Patel, SG, et al., Craniofacial surgery for malignant skull base tumors: report of an international collaborative study. *Cancer*, 2003. **98**(6): p. 1179–87.
2. Omar, A., TP Andrew, and WB. Gavin, *Basic Principles of Skull Base Surgery*. 2017: p. 955–5.
3. Aryan, HE, et al., Subfrontal transbasal approach and technique for resection of craniopharyngioma. *Neurosurg Focus*, 2005. **18**(6a): p. E10.
4. Feiz-Erfan, I., et al., Proposed classification for the transbasal approach and its modifications. *Skull Base*, 2008. **18**(1): p. 29–47.
5. Michael A. Cohen, Jean A. Eloy, James K. Liu, Midline subfrontal approaches: the transbasal approach and extended modifications to access the clivus, in *Chordomas and Chondrosarcomas of the Skull Base and Spine*. 2017, Elsevier, p. 131–40.
6. Yasargil, MG, and S.I. Abdulrauf, Surgery of intraventricular tumors. *Neurosurgery*, 2008. **62**(6 Suppl 3): p. 1029–40; discussion 1040–1.
7. Delfini, R., and A. Pichierri, Transcallosal approaches to intraventricular tumors, in *Cranial, Craniofacial and Skull Base Surgery*, P. Cappabianca, G. Iaconetta, and L. Califano, eds. 2010, Springer, p. 87–105.
8. Seckin, H., et al., The work horse of skull base surgery: orbitozygomatic approach. Technique, modifications, and applications. *Neurosurg Focus*, 2008. **25**(6): p. E4.
9. L. Fernando Gonzalez, et al., Skull base approaches to the basilar artery. *Neurosurgical Focus*, 2005. **19** (2): p. 1–12.
10. Ciappetta, P., and PI D'Urso, *Subtemporal Approach, in Cranial, Craniofacial and Skull Base Surgery*, P. Cappabianca, G. Iaconetta, and L. Califano, eds. 2010, Springer, p. 107–36.
11. Aziz, KM, et al., The Kawase approach to retrosellar and upper clival basilar aneurysms. *Neurosurgery*, 1999. **44**(6): p. 1225–34; discussion 1234–6.
12. Miller, CG, et al., Transpetrosal approach: surgical anatomy and technique. *Neurosurgery*, 1993. **33** (3): p. 461–9; discussion 469.
13. Solari, D., et al., Anatomy and surgery of the endoscopic endonasal approach to the skull base. *Translational Medicine @ UniSa*, 2012. **2**: p. 36–46.
14. Kassam, AB, et al., Expanded endonasal approach: fully endoscopic, completely transnasal approach to the middle third of the clivus, petrous bone, middle cranial fossa, and infratemporal fossa. *Neurosurg Focus*, 2005. **19**(1): p. E6.
15. Doglietto, F., et al., Brief history of endoscopic transsphenoidal surgery – from Philipp Bozzini to the First World Congress of Endoscopic Skull Base Surgery. *Neurosurg Focus*, 2005. **19**(6): p. E3.
16. Walcott Brian, PB, Chordoma: current concepts, management, and future directions. *Lancet Oncology*. 2012. **13**(2): p. 69–76.
17. Gardner, PA, CH Snyderman, RL Carrau, and DM Prevedello, Endoscopic endonasal approaches to the skull base and paranasal sinuses, in *Otologic Surgery*. 2010, Elsevier, p. 667–80.

18. Li, J., et al., Definition, evaluation, and management of brain relaxation during craniotomy. *British Journal of Anaesthesia*, 2016. **116**(6): p. 759–69.
19. Bander, ED, et al., Endoscopic endonasal versus transcranial approach to tuberculum sellae and planum sphenoidale meningiomas in a similar cohort of patients. *Journal of Neurosurgery*, 2018. **128**(1): p. 40–8.
20. Muskens, IS, et al., The endoscopic endonasal approach is not superior to the microscopic transcranial approach for anterior skull base meningiomas-a meta-analysis. *Acta Neurochir*, 2018. **160**(1): p. 59–75.
21. Clark Aaron, JA, Endoscopic surgery for tuberculum sellae meningiomas: a systematic review and meta-analysis. *Neurosurgical Review*. 2013. **36**(3): p. 349–59.
22. Hayashi, N., et al., A novel graft material for preventing cerebrospinal fluid leakage in skull base reconstruction: technical note of perifascial areolar tissue. *Journal of neurological surgery. Part B. Skull Base*, 2015. **76**(1): p. 7–11.
23. Barger, J., et al., The posterior nasoseptal flap: a novel technique for closure after endoscopic transsphenoidal resection of pituitary adenomas. *Surgical Neurology International*, 2018. **9**: p. 32.
24. Hadad Gustavo, G., A novel reconstructive technique after endoscopic expanded endonasal approaches: vascular pedicle nasoseptal flap. *Laryngoscope*. 2006. **116**(10): p. 1882–6.
25. Yuen, AP, CF Fung, and KN Hung, Endoscopic cranionasal resection of anterior skull base tumor. *Am J Otolaryngol*, 1997. **18**(6): p. 431–3.
26. Yip, J., et al., The inferior turbinate flap in skull base reconstruction. *Journal of Otolaryngology – Head & Neck Surgery*, 2013. **42**(1): p. 6.
27. Alleyne, CH, DL Barrow, and NM Oyesiku, Combined transsphenoidal and pterional craniotomy approach to giant pituitary tumors. *Surgical Neurology*, 2002. **57**(6): p. 380–90.
28. Nicolai, P., et al., Endoscopic surgery for malignant tumors of the sinonasal tract and adjacent skull base: a 10-year experience. *Am J Rhinol*, 2008. **22**(3): p. 308–16.
29. Liu James, KJ, Combined endoscopic and open approaches in the management of sinonasal and ventral skull base malignancies. *Otolaryngologic Clinics of North America*. 2017. **50**(2): p. 331–46.
30. Stamates, MM, et al., Combined open and endoscopic endonasal skull base resection of a rare endometrial carcinoma metastasis. *Journal of Neurological Surgery Reports*, 2018. **79**(1): p. e9–e13.
31. Patel, NJ, and I. Dunn, Resection of a retrochiasmatic craniopharyngioma by combined modified orbital craniotomy and transnasal endoscopic techniques. *J Neurol Surg B*, 2018. **79**(S 03): p. S243–4.
32. Leung, GKK, et al., An endoscopic modification of the simultaneous 'above and below' approach to large pituitary adenomas. *Pituitary*, 2012. **15**(2): p. 237–41.
33. D'Ambrosio, AL, et al., Simultaneous above and below approach to giant pituitary adenomas: surgical strategies and long-term follow-up. *Pituitary*, 2009. **12**(3): p. 217–25.
34. Koechlin, NO, et al., Combined transnasal and transcranial removal of a giant clival chordoma. *Journal of Neurological Surgery Reports*, 2014. **75** (1): p. e98–102.
35. Lombardi, D., et al., Giant hypervascular lesion of the sinonasal tract invading the anterior skull base and orbit: a puzzling case. *Ann Otol Rhinol Laryngol*, 2008. **117**(9): p. 653–8.
36. Leung, GKK, et al., Combined simultaneous transcranial and transsphenoidal resection of large-to-giant pituitary adenomas. *Acta Neurochirurgica*, 2011. **153**(7): p. 1401–8.

Chapter 6

Combined Transcranial Approach for Tumor Resection and Anterior Circulation Vascular Bypass

Kumar Vasudevan, Rima S. Rindler, Andrew M. Erwood, and Gustavo Pradilla

Introduction

The propensity of skull base tumors to encase, parasitize, and occasionally invade critical neurovascular structures is often a barrier to achieving surgical goals. Understanding the relationship between these lesions, their blood supply, and neighboring vascular structures is key for planning safe resection and determining perioperative risk. Cerebral revascularization is an important adjunct in the treatment of skull base tumors. It may maximize tumor resection and prevent cerebral ischemia by allowing a large tumor-feeding vessel to be sacrificed or by allowing the portions of the vessel involved by the tumor to be resected en bloc. Similarly, emergency revascularization may be required in cases of inadvertent vessel injury (1,2). This latter indication is becoming more common in an era when many skull base tumors are resected following radiation therapy or previous operations that might predispose a vessel to injury (3). Open cerebrovascular bypass remains the backbone of the revascularization technique, although some endovascular therapies are emerging as useful supplements or alternatives. In this chapter, we discuss the historical basis for cerebrovascular bypass in skull base tumor surgery, the continued need for bypass in the modern era of tumor treatment, the microanatomy of common bypasses, patient selection, and endovascular options for revascularization.

Historical Perspective

The goal of cerebrovascular bypass surgery is to augment or preserve cerebral blood flow given lost or diminished vessel integrity. Since the conception of the technique by Dr. Yasargil in the 1960s (4), much work has been devoted to studying the anatomy and flow characteristics of various bypass constructs. Direct, flow-augmenting bypass techniques between external carotid arteries (ECA) and internal carotid arteries (ICA), or between ICA and ICA, are well described. "Low-flow" bypasses are typically reserved for flow augmentation in chronic ischemia such as moyamoya disease or chronic vessel occlusion, and they involve anastomosis of a branch of the superficial temporal artery (STA) to a distal branch of an intracranial artery, typically the middle cerebral artery (MCA). "Intermediate-flow" constructs utilize more proximal portions of the external carotid circulation such as the internal maxillary artery or the proximal STA. Radial-artery jump grafts are utilized when anatomically necessary and are usually reserved for failed STA-MCA bypass procedures. "High-flow" bypasses, on the other hand, are usually flow-replacement or flow-preserving procedures used to address pathology at the circle of Willis and its proximal branches (5). Such bypasses require large-caliber graft vessels to anastomose ECA-ICA or ICA-ICA vessels in order to maintain adequate distal blood flow. In the context of tumor resections, bypass constructs should provide appropriate replacement flow for the arterial segment affected by resection (6). The three bypass types should be employed as necessary. Anatomical specifics of high-flow ECA-ICA bypasses, which are most commonly used in skull base tumor resections, are discussed in more detail later in this chapter. Refer to Figure 6.1 for a schematic illustration of bypass types.

Vascular bypass in skull base tumor resection is highly individualized to the patient and is a difficult problem to study, owing to the wide variety of operative indications and techniques published in medical literature. Much of the evidence supporting revascularization techniques hails from flow-augmentation procedures in

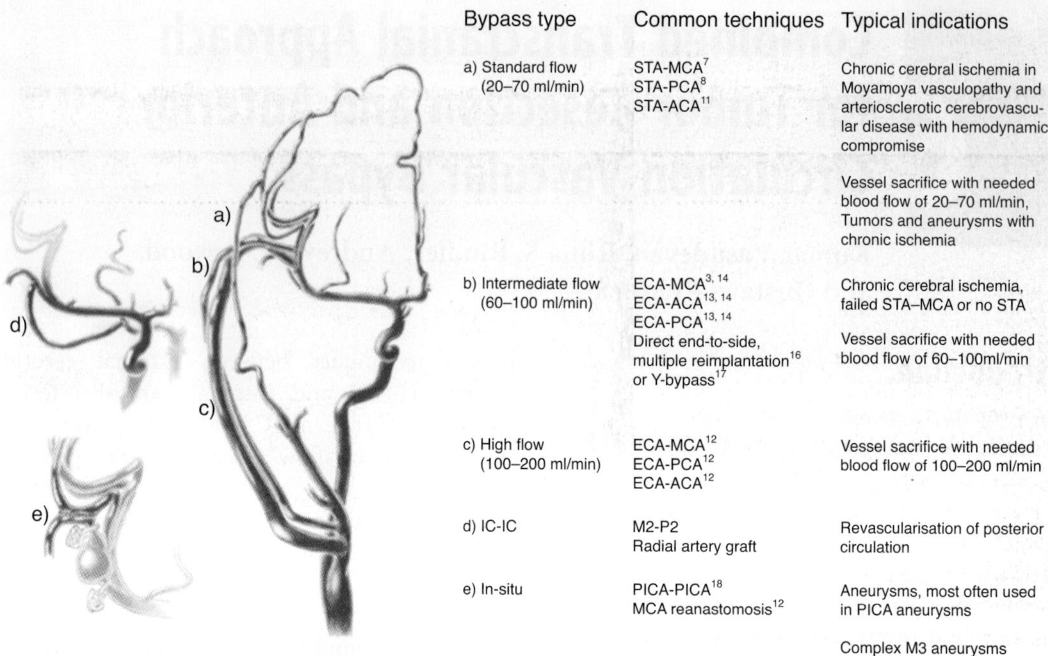

Figure 6.1 A number of intracranial vascular bypass grafts have been described. Rows (a)-(c) describe various EC-IC bypasses and their indications. When successfully anastomosed, the ECA provides a robust source of cerebral blood flow for revascularization, and can supply a range of flow rates depending on the donor vessel selected. Rows (d) and (e) demonstrate revascularization options for posterior circulation lesions, which are not discussed in detail in this chapter. Adapted from Wessels et al. (4), with permission.

patients with chronic ischemia. A 1985 ECA-ICA bypass study demonstrated that despite excellent technical results (95% bypass patency), ECA-ICA bypass failed to reduce stroke rates compared with nonsurgical therapy in patients with ICA occlusion (7). This study prompted a dramatic decrease in the frequency of these operations, despite criticisms regarding its methodology (exclusion of many surgical patients and ineffective preoperative evaluations) (1). Similarly, the 2012 Carotid Occlusion Surgery Study showed no benefit for ECA-ICA bypass in secondary prevention of stroke; in fact, the procedure led to significant rates of postoperative stroke (8). In contrast, the 2014 Japanese Adult Moyamoya trial demonstrated that bilateral ECA-ICA bypass may be protective against rebleeding events in this population (9).

The results of these studies on flow-augmentation bypasses cannot necessarily be extrapolated to flow-preserving bypasses in skull base tumor patients. Specifically, the patient characteristics and outcome measures are not comparable; the vascular anatomy involved is highly variable, and the goals of surgery are quite different. Nevertheless, these trials did demonstrate that cerebrovascular bypass is a safe and replicable procedure when performed by experienced surgeons. Patients across all trials maintained high graft patency rates and a relatively low risk of complications. Furthermore, these studies fostered a new understanding of cerebral perfusion dynamics during brain ischemia, including the physiology related to temporary vessel occlusion during bypass operations. This new understanding helped identify subgroups of patients with oligemia who might benefit from revascularization (10), now more readily identified with modern imaging studies. Postoperatively, magnetic resonance angiography (MRA) and computed tomography angiography (CTA) are able to confirm bypass patency (11). CT perfusion and other dynamic imaging studies have been performed to study changes in revascularized tissue after flow-augmenting bypass, but they have shown variable increases in perfusion or blood flow (12–17). Flow-preserving and non-ECA-ICA bypasses remain understudied in terms of their long-term patency, perioperative morbidity, functional outcomes, and radiographic

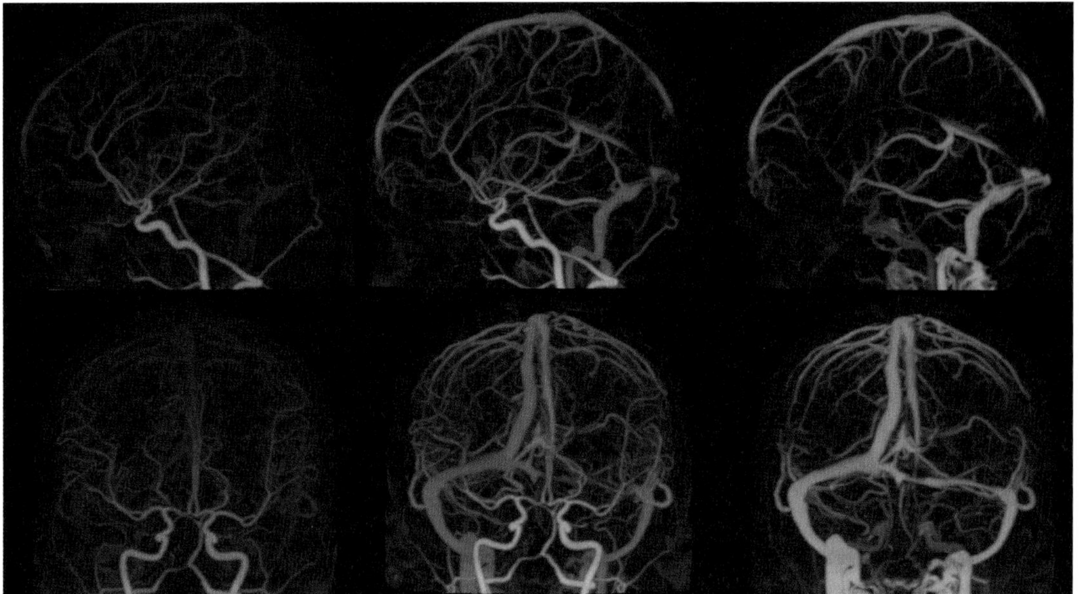

Figure 6.2 Dynamic CT angiography can be used in preoperative planning for skull base tumors, and may be useful for planning vascular bypass. In this modality, a non-contrast CT "template" is subtracted from a contrast-enhanced CT to produce a view of the intracranial vasculature. Staged image acquisition is then used to simulate a dynamic view of blood flow across multiple phases. The above sagittal (top panel) and AP (bottom panel) images simulate, from left to right, the early arterial, late arterial, and venous phases of a standard catheter angiogram.

monitoring on a large scale, but evidence from the ECA-ICA bypass literature may support their use in revascularization for other indications.

Indications for Vascular Bypass in Skull Base Tumor Resection

Modern Management Approaches

The last several decades have witnessed a paradigm shift in the goals and methods for treating both benign and malignant skull base lesions. This shift is due to a combination of advancements in neuroimaging, nonsurgical treatment options, and an improved understanding of tumor behavior and natural history. Aggressive, gross-total resection of tumors involving the skull base and associated vessels was once a common approach, with a sacrifice of involved vasculature and bypass as needed. This approach is now less commonly employed for benign-behaving lesions, for which many surgeons perform maximally safe resection followed by serial imaging and/or radiotherapy for residual and recurrent tumors. This is a commonly utilized approach for most vestibular schwannomas, pituitary adenomas, chordomas, and chondrosarcomas. For meningiomas and recurrent, highly malignant, or locally invasive tumors, management is more variable. In these tumors, ICA narrowing and encasement are often indicative of vessel wall invasion, especially within the cavernous sinus (18). Some surgeons assert that these tumors can be debulked with attempts to peel away tumors from the involved vasculature then observed or irradiated with good long-term control, depending on the pathological diagnosis (1). Other surgeons continue to advocate for a more complete operative resection with vascular sacrifice and bypass (3,6,19–24). This is especially relevant if a recurrent tumor has undergone radiation therapy, as associated radiation vasculopathy could make unprotected dissection around the artery unsafe (1,6).

The decision to perform a vascular bypass procedure for skull base tumors is complex and multifactorial. Vascular bypass should only be considered when there is a reasonable expectation that vessel sacrifice would increase the likelihood of long-term tumor control and overall prognosis without adding significant perioperative morbidity (25). A thorough exploration of all possible alternatives, including observation, planned subtotal resection, staged operations, or adjuvant radiation, is key to ensuring that a bypass is truly necessary. As the field as a whole trends away from aggressive surgical removal in favor of maximal safe resection and adjunctive treatment, the number of bypasses performed by skull base tumor surgeons will likely continue to fall and concentrate within a small number of highly specialized centers. There is evidence that mortality, length of hospital stay, neurological complications, and some medical complications are reduced for patients undergoing flow augmentation for flow-preserving bypasses at these high-volume centers (26). Individual surgeons must therefore weigh the operative risks against their own skill and comfort in performing a technically challenging bypass procedure.

With these considerations in mind, cerebrovascular bypass will likely continue to play a unique role in the treatment of skull base tumors (27). Tumor characteristics, cerebrovascular anatomy and perfusion, and individual patient characteristics are three key factors in deciding the appropriateness and feasibility of a vascular bypass.

Tumor Characteristics

Predicting the "resectability" of skull base tumors requires a high degree of experience and may be difficult to do preoperatively. Imaging factors such as the degree of vascular encasement for particular tumors may be predictive of complications after skull base tumor resection, but these do not necessarily speak to the appropriateness or long-term results of bypass for those lesions (28). For some tumors, vessel sacrifice and bypass are required to prevent a catastrophic hemorrhagic event. This is true for proximal vessels in the cerebral circulation that have clear tumor invasion of the vessel wall and for vessels that are left exposed and at risk of injury due to bony erosion from tumor. For other tumors, the decision to perform a bypass may be less clear. For chordomas, chondrosarcomas, adenoid cystic carcinomas, and other tumors where complete resection offers the best chance for a surgical cure, vascular sacrifice and bypass might be seriously considered. Sometimes these tumors can be easily dissected off of a vessel surface, at which point bypass may no longer be necessary. For head and neck malignancies such as squamous cell carcinomas, vascular bypass could still be performed in order to secure negative margins, as radical resection of these tumors has been shown to improve overall survival.

Characteristics of Cerebral Vasculature and Perfusion

It is imperative to understand the relationship between intracranial vascular anatomy and a skull base tumor prior to considering a bypass during tumor resection. Preoperative evaluation of bypass candidates should focus on the following: (1) radiographic assessment of the need for revascularization, (2) anatomical feasibility of the bypass, (3) planned bypass trajectory and the area requiring revascularization, and (4) potential intraoperative backup or salvage options (3,29–31).

Radiographic evaluation begins with an imaging assessment of the current state of disease and its relationship to vascular structures. Typically, this includes contrast-enhanced MRI and MR angiography (MRA) of the head and neck. Thin-cut CT of the head through the skull base may offer additional information about bony involvement that may put arteries at risk during resection. These modalities are generally sensitive and specific enough to detect carotid artery involvement in head and neck masses, although they are not always predictive of the need for vessel resection. Likewise, although evidence is lacking for specific imaging factors that would predict the need for bypass, some radiographic findings are suggestive of this need, including vessel encasement, vessel stenosis, infarction in an affected vessel territory, and enlarged extracranial or intracranial collaterals. These findings should raise suspicion of clinically relevant vessel involvement, scarring, or invasion (30) and prompt dedicated cerebrovascular imaging to evaluate the course and caliber of parent and target vessels and to determine their candidacy for a possible bypass procedure. Digital subtraction cerebral angiography (DSA) is the gold-standard imaging modality to best assess the circle of Willis and its branches, vessels supplying the tumor, and extracranial arteries that may be utilized for bypass. For flow-augmenting bypasses, DSA allows for a better assessment of distal arteries that may be potential bypass recipients (32). Furthermore,

DSA can assess blood flow dynamics and identify local venous drainage, areas at risk for ischemia, and other factors that influence the decision to perform a bypass. Finally, it allows for test occlusion and endovascular sacrifice, as described later in this chapter.

Some centers are now relying solely on CTA or MRA for preoperative cerebrovascular evaluation (33), citing that these modalities more accurately define vascular anatomy in relation to surrounding structures and provide a three-dimensional reconstruction of extracranial structures. In addition, the procedural risks of DSA (e.g., vascular dissection, stroke, and femoral artery complications) are avoided. Some centers utilize CT perfusion to assess microcirculatory blood flow, but this is of limited value in flow-replacement procedures, as chronic ischemia is not often a primary concern in skull base tumor patients (2). More recently, dynamic CT angiography has been introduced to capture the dynamic element of DSA. In this modality, image processing subtracts a non-contrast, thin-cut CT image from a contrast-enhanced image to create a 3-D view of intracranial vessels (see Figure 6.2). By pulsing image acquisition on and off in 1-second increments, dynamic CTA can obtain a dynamic view of blood flow similar to DSA (34,35). Dynamic CTA has been used successfully in preoperative assessment of arterial anatomy for tumor resection, but whether it provides the visuospatial or time resolution required to plan bypasses remains to be seen (36). Regardless, DSA remains a cornerstone of preoperative workup in most centers due to its superior ability to approximate flow and suggest the type of bypass required.

Revascularization is necessary when vessel sacrifice is anticipated or vessel test occlusion causes a drop in cerebral blood flow (CBF) with associated regional ischemia. Preoperative radiography, as described previously, can suggest the need for a bypass on an anatomical basis, but cannot assess whether hypoperfusion due to planned vessel sacrifice translates to a need for bypass. This is dependent on cerebrovascular reserve and is difficult to assess clinically. As a result, there are two main strategies for preoperative bypass planning based on the perceived utility of preoperative testing (37). Proponents of a *selective approach* perform a bypass when preoperative testing suggests that vessel sacrifice will not be tolerated, whereas those supporting a *universal approach* perform a bypass in all cases where vessel sacrifice is required. Balloon test occlusion (BTO) has historically been used to simulate ICA sacrifice while evaluating vascular collaterals via DSA. During occlusion, a number of tests can evaluate the effectiveness of collaterals, including neurological status, electroencephalography, transcranial doppler ultrasound, xenon-enhanced CT, and single-photon emission computed tomography (SPECT) (38–40,41). Additionally, induced hypotension during BTO may simulate the effects of hypoperfusion on collateral circulation.

Proponents of a universal approach to bypass point to the risk of morbidity during BTO in addition to procedural risks for an overall risk of 3–4%, which increases with prolonged occlusion time (42). Most BTO protocols have been established for anterior circulation only, which is of particular concern for skull base lesions that require posterior circulation revascularization. In addition, the hypervascularity of some skull base tumors may create a "steal phenomenon" during BTO that leads to incorrect estimates of cerebrovascular reserve. Some authors advocate placing the balloon distal to the lesion to avoid steal, but anatomical constraints may make this difficult (43). Finally, the risk of postoperative stroke after passing BTO ("false negative") has been reported to be as high as 22%, although occlusion times and methods of assessment vary considerably among published series (44). In addition to technical inaccuracies during the initial procedure, post-BTO thromboembolism is a proposed mechanism yielding the false-negative rate (45). For these reasons, many surgeons operate under the principle that if the ICA can be bypassed or reconstructed safely, then it is best to avoid carotid sacrifice without revascularization.

Patient Characteristics

A general assessment of patient health and comorbidities is required to determine whether the patient can tolerate a lengthy bypass operation under general anesthesia, changes in blood pressure (e.g., induced hypertension, sometimes utilized to keep bypass grafts patent), and antiplatelet agents and/or anticoagulation agents. A thorough history should include past surgeries, radiotherapy, or traumatic injuries that might make dissection difficult or make vascular bypass graft donors unavailable. A history of transient ischemic attacks or focal neurological symptoms could suggest proximal carotid vascular disease that may compromise a bypass or limit donor vessel candidates. A personal or family history of rheumatological, vasculitic, or coagulation disorders may affect postoperative bypass viability. In all cases, a thorough head, neck, and neurological examination may offer insights into anatomical constraints and identify patients for whom a bypass may be high-risk or unfeasible.

Patients with malignant disease are staged preoperatively in consultation with medical and radiation oncologists. Staging procedures utilize positron emission tomography (PET), SPECT, or other whole-body imaging technologies to determine the extent of disease and patient candidacy. In general, younger patients with higher Karnofsky Performance Status (KPS) scores (70 or higher), in good cardiovascular and respiratory health, and with otherwise long-life expectancies from comorbid diseases are the ideal candidates for vascular bypass and subsequent skull base tumor resections.

Microanatomical Considerations

When planning an intracranial revascularization procedure, it is important to carefully choose the recipient, donor, and graft vessels. At times, this can only be accomplished intraoperatively after direct inspection of the vessels. In addition to general vessel health, cerebral blood flow requirements and size-matching between vessels and the chosen graft are the two main factors that influence the choice of vessels. In most cases, IC sacrifice for skull base tumor resection requires an extracranial-intracranial (EC-IC) high-flow bypass (>50 ml/min) to reconstitute distal blood flow (46). Common bypasses include cervical external carotid artery/internal carotid artery-M2 (ECA/ICA-M2), cervical ECA/ICA-petrous ICA, and petrous ICA-supraclinoid ICA (47). Only anterior circulation bypasses will be considered here.

First, a recipient vessel at least 4 mm in size, of adequate length, and free of perforators must be chosen (47). It is important to understand intracranial vascular anatomy in order to optimize the exposure of the recipient vessel. The primary MCA branches from the ICA terminus and courses anterolaterally toward the Sylvian fissure. It becomes the M2 segment lateral to the limen insulae and turns posteriorly at the genu to travel over the insula within the Sylvian fissure, where it usually bifurcates. The upper and lower trunks continue posteriorly, and the M3 opercular branches turn laterally toward the medial frontal and temporal lobes, respectively. The M4 segments continue over the cerebral convexities of the frontal, parietal, and temporal lobes as terminal MCA branches (47). The primary ACA segment branches from the ICA terminus and courses anteromedially over the optic nerve. It then joins the contralateral ACA over the optic chiasm by the anterior communicating artery. The A2 segment for each vessel continues to course anteriorly in front of the lamina terminalis and into the interhemispheric fissure, then curves posteriorly over the genu of the corpus callosum (A3) as the pericallosal artery, which runs in the callosal sulcus/pericallosal cistern. The callosomarginal artery arises from the A2 or A3 branch and runs over the cingulate gyrus within the cingulate sulcus (47).

First, a recipient vessel is chosen. An M2 branch is usually the desired recipient site; it maintains a relatively large diameter (1.76 +/- 0.36 mm) that can perfuse the MCA and anterior cerebral artery (ACA) territories, and it is easily exposed through a pterional craniotomy and transsylvian approach (47). The ICA terminus or supraclinoid ICA (3.95 +/- 0.56 mm) between the ophthalmic and posterior communicating arteries are also recipient vessel candidates. The supraclinoid ICA is sometimes unsuitable due to atherosclerotic disease. Occasionally, the horizontal petrous carotid (5.42 +/- 0.68 mm) is utilized as a recipient vessel after its extradural exposure in the middle fossa. Rarely, an A2 (2.35 +/- 0.60 mm) or A3 (1.98 +/- 0.35 mm) bypass is required for tumor resection. The M1 is not amenable to bypass because of its fragile lenticulostriate branches that are intolerant of temporary occlusion during anastomosis due to lack of collateral circulation.

Second, the graft vessel is chosen. Saphenous vein (SVG) (46) or radial artery grafts (RAG) (48) are typically used for high-flow bypasses, as either can meet the blood-flow demands to perfuse the territories of the anterior circulation (SVG 100-250 ml/min and RAG 50-100 ml/min). A graft is chosen based on the size of the recipient vessel and the availability of the graft. A RAG should be at least 2.4 mm in diameter (mean diameter 3.55 +/- 0.45 mm) – especially if the anastomosis involves the smaller M2 branch – to be implanted in a vessel at least 2 mm in diameter (1,47). The SVG has a larger diameter of at least 3 mm (mean 4.0 +/- 0.6 mm) and should be implanted in a vessel at least 2.4 mm in diameter, which is suitable for a supraclinoid ICA recipient. In general, the RAG is the preferred graft. It is easier to harvest, lacks valves, and is less prone to intimal denudation and subsequent thrombosis compared with an SVG. SVG also carries a higher risk of vessel size mismatch than RAG. RAGs, however, are plagued by vasospasm, which can be effectively managed with the pressure distension technique as described in the following section. If uncertainty exists, choose the graft with the higher flow capacity (1). The vessels can be evaluated preoperatively either with ultrasonography or brachial arteriogram for the RAG or with duplex ultrasonography for the SVG. If an RAG is used, an Allen test should confirm adequate collateral flow from the ulnar artery to the hand through the palmar branch.

Third, a donor vessel must be chosen. Blood is best supplied by an extracranial carotid artery donor vessel such as the cervical ICA (8.57 +/- 1.34 mm) or ECA (5.75 +/-0.94 mm) after exposure within the anterior triangle of the neck. The appropriate vessel should be free from branches or atherosclerotic disease and is in relatively close proximity to the recipient vessel. An ECA donor is chosen if there is poor intracranial collateral circulation that would preclude prolonged temporary ICA occlusion during the bypass procedure. The use of ECA branches (e.g., the superficial temporal artery or maxillary artery) as donors is reserved for low-flow bypasses. Anastomosis at the distal common carotid artery has been described (29). A bypass from the petrous portion of the internal carotid artery to the supraclinoid ICA or M2 vessel can also be considered, as first described by Sekhar (19) and Spetzler (45) using an SVG.

Surgical Technique

The patient should first be intubated under general anesthesia. Trace and mark the course of the graft vessel on the arm or leg using Doppler ultrasonography. Avoid placing arterial lines on the side of a RAG. Place a femoral sheath if intraoperative angiography is planned. Administer perioperative antibiotics within 1 hour of the incision. Perform neuromonitoring that at least consists of somatosensory evoked potentials and motor evoked potentials, the latter of which requires total intravenous anesthesia. Prior to temporary vessel occlusion, burst-suppress the patient with propofol to decrease cerebral metabolic demand, and elevate the blood pressure to ensure adequate collateral perfusion. Administer intravenous heparin (4,000–5,000 U) and aspirin (325 mg) at the start of the operation or at the time of the first anastomosis.

If bypass and tumor resection are performed sequentially in a single session, the positioning of the patient and head is determined by the necessary approach to the primary pathology being addressed. Otherwise, the patient is positioned supine on the operating room table in a three-point fixation device for stabilization, with the head turned about 45 degrees to the contralateral side. The recipient artery is exposed after a pterional or fronto-temporal craniotomy with cranial base approaches to provide adequate exposure and control. A proximal M2 branch is easily exposed after wide dissection of the Sylvian fissure. If using the supraclinoid ICA, flatten the sphenoid ridge, remove the anterior clinoid, expose the proximal optic canal, and cut the distal dural ring in order to accommodate a temporary clip proximal to the ophthalmic artery. If using the horizontal petrous ICA, expose it extradurally under the temporal lobe dura by drilling the petrous ridge between V3 and the foramen spinosum, so that the opening is about 1 cm in length.

The ICA or ECA donor vessel is then exposed in the neck through the anterior carotid triangle. Expose the ICA from the bifurcation to beyond the digastric muscle (which should be divided) to maximize graft length. Expose the ECA at least 2 cm distal to the bifurcation to the superficial temporal artery and internal maxillary artery branches.

Dissect the chosen graft during the preparation of the recipient vessel, but do not harvest it until ready to perform the anastomosis. Harvest the saphenous vein from the upper leg/lower thigh, as it has a uniform caliber in this location (1). It can be harvested with an open technique or endoscopically, depending on the surgeon's experience. Remove the adventitia about 1 cm from each end, and flush the lumen with heparinized saline. The direction of the graft is not reversed while it is relocated to the anastomotic site to allow blood to flow along the direction of the valves. Harvest the RAG from the wrist to just below the elbow. Flush the vessels with heparinized saline. To prevent vasospasm in the RAG, use the pressure distension technique to expand the artery and improve elasticity (3,19,49). In this maneuver, the end of the artery is pinched around a blunt-tip needle attached to a syringe of heparin. The artery is sequentially squeezed proximally to distally as heparin is infused to distend the walls of the artery. The artery diameter will not change much, but the artery will be more elastic. Some surgeons have applied botulinum toxin to the ex-vivo graft with good results (50). The adventitia is then removed about 1 cm from either end of the artery. The ends of the RAG are cut sharply at a diagonal and fish-mouthed at the distal end.

Vessel anastomoses are usually performed end-to-end or end-to-side. Perform the intracranial anastomosis first. Apply temporary clips to the recipient artery. The recipient artery is then ligated (for an end-to-end anastomosis), or a 3- to 5-mm arteriotomy is made on the side of the recipient artery (for an end-to-side anastomosis). Perform the anastomosis with a 10-0, 9-0, or 8-0 nylon suture in either a running or interrupted fashion. Flush both vessels with saline, and back-bleed the anastomosis to ensure patency. Place a temporary clip 1 cm proximal to the anastomosis on the graft. Next, tunnel the graft to the neck either through an open incision or through a chest tube in the post-auricular (for either the SVG or RAG) or preauricular (for the RAG) subcutaneous space. It is critical to prevent graft torsion. Create a 6- to 8-mm arteriotomy in the ICA or ECA, and perform an end-to-side anastomosis with an 8-0 or 7-0 nylon suture. Back-bleed the RAG, and flush the SVG with saline to remove bubbles before removing the temporary clips. If an end-to-side anastomosis to the petrous carotid is created, use 8-0 or 6-0 nylon sutures (47).

Graft patency should then be assessed. There are many methods for accomplishing this, including the use of indocyanine green (ICG) and qualitative or quantitative Doppler ultrasonography. DSA can confirm patency if other methods are equivocal. Ultrasonic micro-flow probes can be used to approximate flow volume in-situ. Both proximal and distal anastomoses should be evaluated for stenosis. Evaluate the brain for adequate perfusion by ensuring that blood flow through the graft is faster than flow through the extracranial circulation (19). Assessing graft patency intraoperatively alerts the surgeon to any acute problems and allows him or her to promptly address the issue. Non-patency of the graft intraoperatively is most often caused by stenosis at the suture line, intraluminal thrombosis, or vessel kinking and should be immediately evaluated and corrected. Redose heparin during graft re-exploration. Place temporary clips on the recipient vessel, donor vessel, and distal graft. Create an arteriotomy 1 cm from the distal end of the graft. Remove the temporary clips from the recipient vessel to evaluate for backflow; if there is none, explore this end. Next, remove the temporary clips from the graft and donor vessel; if there is no flow, explore this end. If both ends lead to good back-flow within the graft, this indicates dynamic kinking of the graft or recipient vessel when there is full flow. Tack the graft to the dura to prevent this. Once patency has been confirmed, close the dura and craniotomy in the usual fashion, leaving ample room for the graft to pass through. Do not reverse heparin.

The patient should be monitored in the intensive care unit setting postoperatively. Assess graft patency frequently using a Doppler probe for the first 48 hours, with daily transcranial Doppler ultrasonography. If an intraoperative DSA was not performed, perform a CTA immediately postoperatively. Otherwise, perform DSA within 12 hours of the procedure.

If a RAG was used, vascular checks of the hand should continue for 24 hours postoperatively. If an SVG was used, start the patient on aspirin (81 mg daily) and a statin, and continue to administer subcutaneous heparin (5,000 U) three times daily. Blood pressure should be maintained at least less than 140 mmHg for 1 week to prevent hyperemia and perfusion-related hemorrhage. Allow the patient to recover for up to a week before tumor resection to allow the effects of anticoagulation to dissipate.

Bypass Outcomes for Skull Base Tumors

The selection of SVG versus RAG as the graft for high-flow EC-IC bypass varies considerably (30). Unfortunately, many published patient series assessing bypass graft outcomes do not distinguish between graft types or among indications for bypass; therefore, outcomes are pooled for aneurysms, tumors, cerebral ischemia, and emergency revascularization (30). In general, perioperative graft failure rates are as low as 0.6% in some series but as high as 7% for SVG (compared with 2% for RAG) in other series, and failure usually occurs within the first week (45, 51). Early failure is typically caused by delayed thrombosis from mechanical trauma to the endothelium or vasospasm. Acute stroke risk for revascularization procedures is 7–11% (19,45). If thrombosis occurs within 12 hours of surgery without associated cerebral infarction, endovascular thrombolysis can be attempted; otherwise, open surgical revision of the anastomosis with a new graft is indicated. Angioplasty or administration of intra-arterial vasodilators may be used to treat vasospasm (49). The use of the pressure-distension technique, as described previously, is a reliable way to reduce the frequency of vasospasm in RAG.

Delayed graft failure for intracranial bypasses has been studied most extensively for intracranial aneurysms (6). The failure rate for intracranial SVG is estimated to be 1–1.5% higher in the first year (52). For perioperative failures, some authors have reported long-term failure rates for SVG compared with RAG (1), although other series report equivalent long-term failure rates (6,51). Long-term occlusion rates of SVG and RAG range from 0–27% (1–8.3% in recent series) (1,6,38,45,53) and occur at a median of 6 months. Occlusion is associated with a relatively low stroke risk of 0–0.3% per year, likely due to the development of collateral vessels (45). This is in comparison to a much higher 1.9% annual stroke risk for carotid sacrifice without revascularization despite a normal BTO (45). Remote occlusion of SVGs is thought to be a result of delayed atherosclerosis (54,55). Rarely, grafts can occlude and spontaneously reopen at a later date, although it is unclear whether this is due to relief of vasospasm, resolution of a luminal thrombus, or changes in flow dynamics related to flow through collateral vessels (6). Once graft occlusion is identified, primary operative repair is recommended.

In-graft stenosis occurs at a rate of 12.5% at a median of 8 months (6). Graft stenosis is often due to intimal hyperplasia from turbulent flow and can lead to transient ischemic attacks, possibly due to changes in flow dynamics as collateral vessels are being established. Graft stenosis can be observed if it is minimal and asymptomatic. For more severe or symptomatic stenosis, endovascular balloon angioplasty or intraluminal stenting can be considered for extracranial pathology. Longer stenotic segments or intracranial stenosis should be repaired surgically with excision and primary reanastomosis, interposition graft, or Y-construct to bypass the stenosis (6).

Due to the risk of remote graft failure, maintain patients on aspirin and statins for at least 1 year. Graft patency is monitored with CTA or MRA at 3 months, then yearly.

Clinical Outcomes for Skull Base Tumors

A number of published series have described institutional experiences of EC-IC bypass for resection of skull base tumors. In total, these series include tumors of all types, various bypass techniques and graft choices, and variable rates of postoperative radiation therapy. Thus, it remains difficult to draw conclusions regarding the safety and efficacy of bypass for skull base tumors. In general, bypass for radical resection of skull base tumors can have a high success rate for disease control with low procedural complication rates in experienced hands. A recent systematic review evaluated the outcomes of EC-IC bypass for resection of skull base tumors of all types in the literature (30). Most resections were performed for meningiomas (61%). Overall gross total resection rates range from 63% to 73%, with residual disease left for benign lesions involving cranial nerves or critical perforating arteries, followed by radiotherapy (1,6,56–58). Perioperative morbidity from tumor resection ranges from 7–33% and includes extra-axial hematoma, infection, cerebrospinal fluid leak, hydrocephalus, and seizures (53,59). Perioperative mortality rates range from 0% to 9.1% from either medical or bypass-related stroke complications (1,6,53). Recurrence rates depend entirely on tumor pathology. Despite aggressive resection, long-term mortality rates are high and often occur due to tumor progression or surgery-related disability (3.9–36.3%) (1,6,38,51).

Meningiomas

Skull base meningiomas are the most common indication for vascular bypass and radical resection. The natural history of skull base meningiomas is largely uncharacterized, but several series suggest most progress over time (60–76% of petroclival meningiomas, as an example) (60,61). Skull base meningiomas are mostly benign (WHO I). Atypical and malignant grades are exceedingly rare at the skull base in comparison to other locations (WHO II, 4.2–5.9% versus 35.5%, and WHO III, 0% versus 1.2%) (62). Resection of all skull base meningiomas is associated with a 17.9% morbidity and low mortality rate (0.9%) (31). For these reasons, some surgeons argue that maximal resection at initial operation for most skull base meningiomas is indicated to reduce recurrence risk (31).

Even still, gross total resection rates of skull base meningiomas without vascular bypass are lower (41–53%) than for non-skull base cranial tumors (78%) (31,63). The overall 5-year recurrence-free survival (RFS) rate for grossly resected meningiomas is higher for non-skull base locations (76%) than for skull base locations (67%). Similarly, when comparing Grade I meningiomas alone (including all extents of resection, with or without radiation), non-skull base locations had a higher RFS (69%) than skull base locations (56%) in one series, although another series cited a much higher RFS rate for Grade I skull base meningiomas of 88% (31). Interestingly, although subtotal resection of all meningioma grades without adjuvant radiation produced similar 5-year RFS rates for skull base and non-skull base locations (37%), the RFS was much improved for radiated residual skull base tumors (89%) than for radiated residual non-skull base tumors (50%) (63). Other series confirm the importance of postoperative radiation of low-grade residual skull base (cavernous sinus) disease, resulting in 82.3–94.7% (up to 100% in one series) 5-year progression-free survival (PFS) rates, good functional status, and 0–9% tumor-related long-term mortality (31,64,65).

Vascular bypass with resection of a benign skull base meningioma increases gross total resection rates to upward of 70%, maintains low mortality rates (6.8% at 4 years), and high PFS (88% at 4 years) (19). These outcomes are comparable to subtotal resection with adjuvant radiation; therefore, the added benefit of vascular bypass to achieve gross total resection of these primary tumors may be very low. Bypass should be reserved for recurrent and/or progressive tumors.

Five-year RFS rates for atypical (0–59%) or malignant (8.4–50%) meningiomas are much lower at all cranial locations than for WHO Grade I tumors (31,63,66). Some series demonstrate improved RFS following adjuvant radiosurgery for WHO Grade II tumors (100%) (66). Most recurrent tumors return within the first 5 years with or without radiosurgery and with high mortality rates at 10 years (46.7% for WHO Grade II and 85.8% for WHO Grade III tumors) (67). For this reason, some surgeons advocate aggressive resection of recurrent, irradiated, or primary WHO Grade II/III skull base meningiomas with vascular bypass, if needed. In one small series of four patients with near-total or gross total resection of atypical meningioma or solitary fibrous tumor, all maintained a KPS greater than 70 up to 3.5 years from surgery without tumor recurrence (69). Unfortunately, the impact of radical resection with vascular bypass on long-term outcomes in these patients is largely uncharacterized, as the cases in larger series cannot be extracted from other tumor types.

Chordomas and Chondrosarcomas

Other rare skull base tumors such as chordoma and chondrosarcoma have been treated with radical resection and vascular bypass. Gross total resection with postoperative radiation at primary presentation is the current standard treatment. Current series endorse a 62–74% gross total resection rate, at least 52–56% 5-year RFS, and 76.6–93% overall survival for standard resection with or without radiation (23,70,71). Resection alone is associated with an 18–26% complication rate and 0–7.8% perioperative death rate, which is highest for patients with previously resected/irradiated or recurrent disease and is associated with vascular injury (23,70-72). KPS scores at 6 months or at last follow-up remain greater than 70 for the vast majority of patients (23,71,72). The addition of vascular bypass for resection is typically reserved for advanced or recurrent disease or to repair inadvertent intraoperative vascular injuries. This is associated with a lower gross total resection rate (42.8–67%), a slightly lower recurrence rate (42.8%), and lower survival rate at 2 years (71.4%) (19). Perioperative stroke with or without revascularization has been reported at 0–1.3% (23,71). It is unclear whether it is the bypass and resection technique alone or the advanced stage of disease or tumor aggressiveness that is responsible for poorer outcomes.

Head and Neck Malignancies

Advanced head and neck malignancies that extend to the skull base are another unique entity that may require arterial sacrifice for oncological control (6,73). Such malignancies, which include squamous cell carcinomas, osteogenic sarcoma, and adenoid cystic carcinomas (ACCs), were historically considered inoperable. Several international collaborative studies have reported results for radical craniofacial resection of malignant skull base tumors and include high 5-year overall (up to 62%) and recurrence-free (55–57%) survival rates, but also relatively high surgical complication rates (up to 36.3%) (73,74). Perioperative mortality rates range from 1.4% to 4.8%. However, these resections do not include revascularization procedures for carotid artery involvement at the skull base. In such cases, some groups have attempted gross total resection with revascularization followed by chemotherapy and radiation. These cases appear to have higher surgery-related death rates, ranging from 11% to 20%, and much lower survival rates than patients without ICA involvement or sacrifice (2-year survival rate 11–43%, mean 14–31 months) (59,75,76). Furthermore, survival after resection and revascularization is likely dependent upon the histology, with ACC associated with improved survival rates after aggressive resection with or without revascularization procedures compared with other carcinomas or sarcomas (59,77). For these reasons, some authors argue that radical resection should be reserved for these tumors alone (59).

Future Directions

As neurosurgery moves toward minimally invasive, technology-intensive techniques, cerebrovascular bypass "stands against these trends by requiring a few simple instruments, steady hands, and meticulous technique" (78). Still, the pre- and postoperative evaluation of bypass patients, and the necessity of bypass itself, is very susceptible to the changing technological standard. This is especially true in skull base tumor resections.

Several techniques have been employed to make vascular bypass safer. The excimer laser-assisted nonocclusive anastomosis (ELANA) technique avoids temporary arterial occlusion and has shown promising results. ELANA allows the surgeon to suture a small metal ring onto the recipient artery to which the SVG is then attached (56–58). Through a side branch, the laser is introduced into the SVG lumen, and an arteriotomy is made through the metal ring. This technique precludes the need for temporary occlusion of cerebral arteries and may open up the option of using vessels with poor collateral circulation. However, the use of this technique is not yet widespread, due to the high cost of the laser and its limited application to SVGs only. Some groups have described successfully performing awake craniotomies for EC-IC bypasses to ensure the adequacy of cerebral perfusion during and after the anastomosis (79).

Advancements in endovascular therapies have broadened the treatment repertoire for intracranial vascular disease, including applications for skull base tumors involving cerebral vasculature. The endovascular armamentarium includes balloon angioplasty, bare metal balloon-mounted stents, and self-expanding intracranial stents, as well as flow-diverting stents such as the Pipeline NED stent (1). In cases where a tumor encases the ICA, preoperative stenting can allow for safer radical resection while avoiding bypass. This method has been applied to malignant, extracranial tumors of the head and neck, wherein the deepest resection margins are taken to the mesh interstices of the stent. Neointima that has formed within the stent is relied upon to provide vessel continuity. To our knowledge, this technique has not been applied to skull base tumors, but it may present a future alternative to vascular bypass for at-risk vessels. Endovascular techniques, such as balloon angioplasty or stenting, may address perioperative ischemia caused by graft stenosis or vasospasm (1). Cases of delayed graft stenosis can also be treated with percutaneous transluminal angioplasty as a salvage method for high-flow arterial grafts (80). Finally, endovascular therapies can effectively treat iatrogenic vascular injuries that occur during resection of skull base tumors, such as occlusions, stenosis, dissections, or vessel wall injury that leads to pseudoaneurysms, fistula formation, or actual vascular rupture. Endovascular management varies, from parent artery occlusion, pseudoaneurysm coil embolization, or covered stent or flow diversion (81). Endovascular applications for skull base tumors will only increase in the coming years as new techniques and indications are evaluated.

New non-invasive imaging methods will reduce the likelihood of stroke after bypass operations. Improvements in imaging modalities will allow for more accurate preoperative evaluation of cerebrovascular reserve; hypercapnic blood oxygen level–dependent MRI and MRA-based fractional flow measurements have already shown promise in patients with chronic ischemia and could be employed for tumor patients to avoid DSA (83,82). MRI with higher magnetic flux density (3 T and 7 T) may more clearly define neurovascular relationships and help anticipate surgical events.

The future of revascularization for skull base tumor resection is inextricably linked to advances in oncological treatment. The last two decades have seen rapid growth in the genetic characterization of meningiomas, chordomas, schwannomas, and other skull base lesions. This has helped redraw their classifications, enhance the understanding of their natural histories, and refine treatment algorithms. The field of targeted and gene-based therapies for the lesions has exploded and is likely to soon yield new adjuvant therapies that will improve tumor control rates. These advances, together with new radiation technologies, are making the strategy of "planned subtotal resection" more prevalent. Although it is unclear whether this strategy will result in better long-term outcomes, it is inevitable that newer, safer adjunctive tumor control strategies will emerge. With these strategies, we expect that the indications for bypass will shrink unless new techniques or teaching methods can make the procedure safer and technically easier.

Conclusions

Skull base tumors pose a unique challenge in their intimate relationship to neurovascular structures, and a number of them will require the resection of major cerebral vessels for definitive control. Cerebrovascular bypass is a well-established method for revascularizing the territory supplied by these vessels. These "flow replacement" bypasses are rare and highly individualized, and they require an intricate understanding of the patient's cerebral hemodynamics and vascular anatomy. Although multidisciplinary management of skull base tumors continues to evolve with technology, bypass techniques remain indispensable for the comprehensive skull base surgeon. The ability to perform a successful bypass ensures that vessel involvement is not a barrier to maximal tumor resection, and it is essentially a "backup plan" in the event of unanticipated vessel injury. Bypass techniques should continue to evolve in tandem with tumor control modalities.

Key Points

- There has been a paradigm shift in the management of skull base tumors in recent years from the goal of maximal primary resection to the goal of maximally safe resection with adjuvant therapy
- Radical resection of skull base tumors with high-flow vascular bypass of the anterior circulation remains an important tool for addressing recurrent or malignant tumors
- As skull base tumor management evolves with advancements in oncological, radiation, and endovascular therapies, vascular bypass techniques for tumor resection will likely be concentrated in specialized centers of excellence

References

1. Sekhar LN, Natarajan SK, Ellenbogen RG, Ghodke B. Cerebral revascularization for ischemia, aneurysms, and cranial base tumors. *Neurosurgery*. 2008;**62**(6 Suppl 3):1373–408; discussion 408–10.
2. Walker M, Acharya J, Bird CR, Partovi S. Evaluation of EC-IC bypass grafts using CT angiography. *Barrow Quarterly*. 2001;**17**(3).
3. Mohit AA, Sekhar LN, Natarajan SK, Britz GW, Ghodke B. High-flow bypass grafts in the management of complex intracranial aneurysms. *Neurosurgery*. 2007;**60**(2 Suppl 1):ONS105–22; discussion ONS22–3.
4. Wessels L, Hecht N, Vajkoczy P. Bypass in neurosurgery-indications and techniques. *Neurosurg Rev*. 2019;**42**(2):389–93.
5. Tayebi Meybodi A, Huang W, Benet A, Kola O, Lawton MT. Bypass surgery for complex middle cerebral artery aneurysms: an algorithmic approach to revascularization. *J Neurosurg*. 2017;**127**(3):463–79.
6. Ramanathan D, Temkin N, Kim LJ, Ghodke B, Sekhar LN. Cerebral bypasses for complex aneurysms and tumors: long-term results and graft management strategies. *Neurosurgery*. 2012;**70**(6):1442–57; discussion 57.

7. Group EIBS. Failure of extracranial-intracranial arterial bypass to reduce the risk of ischemic stroke. Results of an international randomized trial.*New England Journal of Medicine*. 1985;**313**(19):1191–200.
8. Grubb RL Jr., Powers WJ, Clarke WR, Videen TO, Adams HP Jr., Derdeyn CP, et al. Surgical results of the Carotid Occlusion Surgery Study. *J Neurosurg*. 2013;**118**(1):25–33.
9. Miyamoto S, Yoshimoto T, Hashimoto N, Okada Y, Tsuji I, Tominaga T, et al. Effects of extracranial-intracranial bypass for patients with hemorrhagic moyamoya disease: results of the Japan Adult Moyamoya Trial. *Stroke*. 2014;**45**(5):1415–21.
10. Esposito G, Amin-Hanjani S, Regli L. Role of and Indications for Bypass Surgery After Carotid Occlusion Surgery Study (COSS)? *Stroke*. 2016;**47**(1):282–90.
11. Ginat DT, Smith ER, Robertson RL, Scott RM, Schaefer PW. Imaging after direct and indirect extracranial-intracranial bypass surgery. *AJR Am J Roentgenol*. 2013;**201**(1):W124–32.
12. Langner S, Fleck S, Seipel R, Schroeder HW, Hosten N, Kirsch M. Perfusion CT scanning and CT angiography in the evaluation of extracranial-intracranial bypass grafts. *J Neurosurg*. 2011;**114**(4):978–83.
13. Teng MM, Jen SL, Chiu FY, Kao YH, Lin CJ, Chang FC. Change in brain perfusion after extracranial-intracranial bypass surgery detected using the mean transit time of computed tomography perfusion. *J Chin Med Assoc*. 2012;**75**(12):649–53.
14. Low SW, Teo K, Lwin S, Yeo LL, Paliwal PR, Ahmad A, et al. Improvement in cerebral hemodynamic parameters and outcomes after superficial temporal artery-middle cerebral artery bypass in patients with severe stenoocclusive disease of the intracranial internal carotid or middle cerebral arteries. *J Neurosurg*. 2015;**123**(3):662–9.
15. Serrone JC, Jimenez L, Hanseman DJ, Carroll CP, Grossman AW, Wang L, et al. Changes in computed tomography perfusion parameters after superficial temporal artery to middle cerebral artery bypass: an analysis of 29 cases. *Journal of Neurological Surgery Part B, Skull Base*. 2014;**75**(6):371–7.
16. Kwon WK, Kwon TH, Park DH, Kim JH, Ha SK. Efficacy of superficial temporal artery-middle cerebral artery bypass in cerebrovascular steno-occlusive diseases: Hemodynamics assessed by perfusion computed tomography. *Asian Journal of Neurosurgery*. 2017;**12**(3):519–24.
17. Vos PC, Riordan AJ, Smit EJ, de Jong HW, van der Zwan A, Velthuis BK, et al. Computed tomography perfusion evaluation after extracranial-intracranial bypass surgery. *Clinical Neurology and Neurosurgery*. 2015;**136**:139–46.
18. Kotapka MJ, Kalia KK, Martinez AJ, Sekhar LN. Infiltration of the carotid artery by cavernous sinus meningioma. *J Neurosurg*. 1994;**81**(2):252–5.
19. Sekhar LN, Bucur SD, Bank WO, Wright DC. Venous and arterial bypass grafts for difficult tumors, aneurysms, and occlusive vascular lesions: evolution of surgical treatment and improved graft results. *Neurosurgery*. 1999;**44**(6):1207–23; discussion 23–4.
20. Natarajan SK, Sekhar LN, Schessel D, Morita A. Petroclival meningiomas: multimodality treatment and outcomes at long-term follow-up. *Neurosurgery*. 2007;**60**(6):965–79; discussion 79–81.
21. Sekhar LN, Kalavakonda C. Cerebral revascularization for aneurysms and tumors. *Neurosurgery*. 2002;**50**(2):321–31.
22. Sekhar LN, Tzortzidis FN, Bejjani GK, Schessel DA. Saphenous vein graft bypass of the sigmoid sinus and jugular bulb during the removal of glomus jugulare tumors. Report of two cases. *J Neurosurg*. 1997;**86**(6):1036–41.
23. Tzortzidis F, Elahi F, Wright D, Natarajan SK, Sekhar LN. Patient outcome at long-term follow-up after aggressive microsurgical resection of cranial base chordomas. *Neurosurgery*. 2006;**59**(2):230–7; discussion 207.
24. Tzortzidis F, Elahi F, Wright DC, Temkin N, Natarajan SK, Sekhar LN. Patient outcome at long-term follow-up after aggressive microsurgical resection of cranial base chondrosarcomas. *Neurosurgery*. 2006;**58**(6):1090–8; discussion 1098.
25. Kalavakonda C, Sekhar LN. Cerebral revascularization in cranial base tumors. *Neurosurgery clinics of North America*. 2001;**12**(3):557–74, viii–ix.
26. Akbarian-Tefaghi H, Kalakoti P, Sun H, Sharma K, Thakur JD, Patra DP, et al. Impact of hospital caseload and elective admission on outcomes after extracranial-intracranial bypass surgery. *World Neurosurgery*. 2017;**108**:716–28.
27. Yang T, Tariq F, Chabot J, Madhok R, Sekhar LN. Cerebral revascularization for difficult skull base tumors: a contemporary series of 18 patients. *World Neurosurgery*. 2014;**82**(5):660–71.
28. McCracken DJ, Higginbotham RA, Boulter JH, Liu Y, Wells JA, Halani SH, et al. Degree of vascular encasement in sphenoid wing meningiomas predicts postoperative ischemic complications. *Neurosurgery*. 2017;**80**(6):957–66.

29. Wolfe SQ, Tummala RP, Morcos JJ. Cerebral revascularization in skull base tumors. *Skull Base*. 2005;**15**(1):71–82.

30. Wolfswinkel EM, Landau MJ, Ravina K, Kokot NC, Russin JJ, Carey JN. EC-IC bypass for cerebral revascularization following skull base tumor resection: current practices and innovations. *J Surg Oncol*. 2018;**118**(5):815–25.

31. Di Maio S, Ramanathan D, Garcia-Lopez R, Rocha MH, Guerrero FP, Ferreira M Jr., et al. Evolution and future of skull base surgery: the paradigm of skull base meningiomas. *World Neurosurgery*. 2012;**78**(3–4):260–75.

32. Farsad K, Hayek RA, Mamourian AC, Friedman JA. Computerized tomographic angiography for preoperative assessment of the superficial temporal artery for external carotid artery to internal carotid artery bypass: Case illustration. *Cases J*. 2008;**1**(1):119.

33. Kramer M, Vairaktaris E, Nkenke E, Schlegel KA, Neukam FW, Lell M. Vascular mapping of head and neck: computed tomography angiography versus digital subtraction angiography. *Journal of Oral and Maxillofacial Surgery*. 2008;**66**(2):302–7.

34. Bi WL, Brown PA, Abolfotoh M, Al-Mefty O, Mukundan S Jr., Dunn IF. Utility of dynamic computed tomography angiography in the preoperative evaluation of skull base tumors. *J Neurosurg*. 2015;**123**(1):1–8.

35. Matsumoto M, Kodama N, Endo Y, Sakuma J, Suzuki K, Sasaki T, et al. Dynamic 3D-CT *Angiography*. 2007;**28**(2):299–304.

36. Gupta S, Bi WL, Mukundan S, Al-Mefty O, Dunn IF. Clinical applications of dynamic CT angiography for intracranial lesions. *Acta Neurochirurgica*. 2018;**160**(4):675–80.

37. Ramina R, de Aguiar PHP, Tatagiba M. *Samii's Essentials in Neurosurgery*. Springer Berlin Heidelberg; 2014.

38. Sia SF, Morgan MK. High flow extracranial-to-intracranial brain bypass surgery. *J Clin Neurosci*. 2013;**20**(1):1–5.

39. Leech PJ, Miller JD, Fitch W, Barker J. Cerebral blood flow, internal carotid artery pressure, and the EEG as a guide to the safety of carotid ligation. *J Neurol Neurosurg Psychiatry*. 1974;**37**(7):854–62.

40. Sorteberg A, Bakke SJ, Boysen M, Sorteberg W. Angiographic balloon test occlusion and therapeutic sacrifice of major arteries to the brain. *Neurosurgery*. 2008;**63**(4):651–60; discussion 60–1.

41. Barr JD, Lemley TJ, McCann RM. Carotid artery balloon test occlusion: combined clinical evaluation and xenon-enhanced computed tomographic cerebral blood flow evaluation without patient transfer or balloon reinflation: technical note. *Neurosurgery*. 1998;**43**(3):634–7; discussion 7–8.

42. Sorteberg A. Balloon occlusion tests and therapeutic vessel occlusions revisited: when, when not, and how. *AJNR American Journal of Neuroradiology*. 2014;**35**(5):862–5.

43. Sorteberg A, Sorteberg W, Bakke SJ, Lindegaard KF, Boysen M, Nornes H. Varying impact of common carotid artery digital compression and internal carotid artery balloon test occlusion on cerebral hemodynamics. *Head & Neck*. 1998;**20**(8):687–94.

44. Origitano TC, al-Mefty O, Leonetti JP, DeMonte F, Reichman OH. Vascular considerations and complications in cranial base surgery. *Neurosurgery*. 1994;**35**(3):351–62; discussion 62–3.

45. Lawton MT, Hamilton MG, Morcos JJ, Spetzler RF. Revascularization and aneurysm surgery: current techniques, indications, and outcome. *Neurosurgery*. 1996;**38**(1):83–92; discussion 94.

46. Lougheed WM, Marshall BM, Hunter M, Michel ER, Sandwith-Smyth H. Common carotid to intracranial internal carotid bypass venous graft. Technical note. *J Neurosurg*. 1971;**34**(1):114–18.

47. Kawashima M, Rhoton AL Jr., Tanriover N, Ulm AJ, Yasuda A, Fujii K. Microsurgical anatomy of cerebral revascularization. Part I: Anterior circulation. *J Neurosurg*. 2005;**102**(1):116–31.

48. Ausman JI, Nicoloff DM, Chou SN. Posterior fossa revascularization: anastomosis of vertebral artery to PICA with interposed radial artery graft. *Surgical Neurology*. 1978;**9**(5):281–6.

49. Evans JJ, Sekhar LN, Rak R, Stimac D. Bypass grafting and revascularization in the management of posterior circulation aneurysms. *Neurosurgery*. 2004;**55**(5):1036–49.

50. Strickland BA, Rennert RC, Bakhsheshian J, Bulic S, Correa AJ, Amar A, et al. Botulinum toxin to improve vessel graft patency in cerebral revascularization surgery: report of 3 cases. *J Neurosurg*. 2018;130:1–7.

51. Sia SF, Davidson AS, Assaad NN, Stoodley M, Morgan MK. Comparative patency between intracranial arterial pedicle and vein bypass surgery. *Neurosurgery*. 2011;**69**(2):308–14.

52. Regli L, Piepgras DG, Hansen KK. Late patency of long saphenous vein bypass grafts to the anterior and posterior cerebral circulation. *J Neurosurg*. 1995;**83**(5):806–11.

53. Bulsara KR, Patel T, Fukushima T. Cerebral bypass surgery for skull base lesions: technical notes incorporating lessons learned over two decades. *Neurosurgical Focus*. 2008;**24**(2):E11.

54. Nwasokwa ON. Coronary artery bypass graft disease. *Annals of Internal Medicine*. 1995;**123** (7):528–45.

55. Shuhaiber JH, Evans AN, Massad MG, Geha AS. Mechanisms and future directions for prevention of vein graft failure in coronary bypass surgery. *European Journal of Cardio-Thoracic Surgery*. 2002;**22**(3):387–96.

56. Streefkerk HJ, Bremmer JP, Tulleken CA. The ELANA technique: high flow revascularization of the brain. *Acta Neurochirurgica Supplement*. 2005;**94**:143–8.

57. Streefkerk HJ, Bremmer JP, van Weelden M, van Dijk RR, de Winter E, Beck RJ, et al. The excimer laser-assisted nonocclusive anastomosis practice model: development and application of a tool for practicing microvascular anastomosis techniques. *Neurosurgery*. 2006;**58**(1 Suppl):ONS148–56; discussion ONS56.

58. Streefkerk HJ, Wolfs JF, Sorteberg W, Sorteberg AG, Tulleken CA. The ELANA technique: constructing a high flow bypass using a non-occlusive anastomosis on the ICA and a conventional anastomosis on the SCA in the treatment of a fusiform giant basilar trunk aneurysm. *Acta Neurochirurgica*. 2004;**146** (9):1009–19; discussion 1019.

59. Kalani MY, Kalb S, Martirosyan NL, Lettieri SC, Spetzler RF, Porter RW, et al. Cerebral revascularization and carotid artery resection at the skull base for treatment of advanced head and neck malignancies. *J Neurosurg*. 2013;**118**(3):637–42.

60. Terasaka S, Asaoka K, Kobayashi H, Yamaguchi S, Sawamura Y. Natural history and surgical results of petroclival meningiomas. *No Shinkei Geka. Neurological Surgery*. 2010;**38**(9):817–24.

61. Van Havenbergh T, Carvalho G, Tatagiba M, Plets C, Samii M. Natural history of petroclival meningiomas. *Neurosurgery*. 2003;**52**(1):55–62; discussion 64.

62. Pearson BE, Markert JM, Fisher WS, Guthrie BL, Fiveash JB, Palmer CA, et al. Hitting a moving target: evolution of a treatment paradigm for atypical meningiomas amid changing diagnostic criteria. *Neurosurgical Focus*. 2008;**24**(5):E3.

63. Kshettry VR, Ostrom QT, Kruchko C, Al-Mefty O, Barnett GH, Barnholtz-Sloan JS. Descriptive epidemiology of World Health Organization grades II and III intracranial meningiomas in the United States. *Neuro-oncology*. 2015;**17** (8):1166–73.

64. McGovern SL, Aldape KD, Munsell MF, Mahajan A, DeMonte F, Woo SY. A comparison of World Health Organization tumor grades at recurrence in patients with non-skull base and skull base meningiomas. *J Neurosurg*. 2010;**112** (5):925–33.

65. Litre CF, Colin P, Noudel R, Peruzzi P, Bazin A, Sherpereel B, et al. Fractionated stereotactic radiotherapy treatment of cavernous sinus meningiomas: a study of 100 cases. *International Journal of Radiation Oncology, Biology, Physics*. 2009;**74**(4):1012–17.

66. Skeie BS, Enger PO, Skeie GO, Thorsen F, Pedersen PH. Gamma knife surgery of meningiomas involving the cavernous sinus: long-term follow-up of 100 patients. *Neurosurgery*. 2010;**66**(4):661–8; discussion 8–9.

67. Aghi MK, Carter BS, Cosgrove GR, Ojemann RG, Amin-Hanjani S, Martuza RL, et al. Long-term recurrence rates of atypical meningiomas after gross total resection with or without postoperative adjuvant radiation. *Neurosurgery*. 2009;**64** (1):56–60.

68. Durand A, Labrousse F, Jouvet A, Bauchet L, Kalamarides M, Menei P, et al. WHO grade II and III meningiomas: a study of prognostic factors. *Journal of Neuro-oncology*. 2009;**95**(3):367–75.

69. Wanibuchi M, Akiyama Y, Mikami T, Iihoshi S, Miyata K, Horita Y, et al. Radical removal of recurrent malignant meningeal tumors of the cavernous sinus in combination with high-flow bypass. *World Neurosurgery*. 2015;**83**(4):424–30.

70. Di Maio S, Rostomily R, Sekhar LN. Current surgical outcomes for cranial base chordomas: cohort study of 95 patients. *Neurosurgery*. 2011;**70** (6):1355–60.

71. Tzortzidis F, Elahi F, Wright DC, Temkin N, Natarajan SK, Sekhar LN. Patient outcome at long-term follow-up after aggressive microsurgical resection of cranial base chondrosarcomas. *Neurosurgery*. 2006;**58** (6):1090–8.

72. Sekhar LN, Pranatartiharan R, Chanda A, Wright DC. Chordomas and chondrosarcomas of the skull base: results and complications of surgical management. *Neurosurgical Focus*. 2001;**10**(3):1–4.

73. Gil Z, Patel SG, Singh B, Cantu G, Fliss DM, Kowalski LP, et al. Analysis of prognostic factors in 146 patients with anterior skull base sarcoma: an international collaborative study. *Cancer*. 2007;**110**(5):1033–41.

74. Ganly I, Patel SG, Singh B, Kraus DH, Bridger PG, Cantu G, et al. Complications of craniofacial

resection for malignant tumors of the skull base: report of an International Collaborative Study. *Head & Neck*. 2005;**27**(6):445–51.

75. Feiz-Erfan I, Han PP, Spetzler RF, Lanzino G, Ferreira MA, Gonzalez LF, et al. Salvage of advanced squamous cell carcinomas of the head and neck: internal carotid artery sacrifice and extracranial-intracranial revascularization. *Neurosurgical Focus*. 2003;**14**(3):e6.

76. Chazono H, Okamoto Y, Matsuzaki Z, Ogino J, Endo S, Matsuoka T, et al. Extracranial-intracranial bypass for reconstruction of internal carotid artery in the management of head and neck cancer. *Annals of Vascular Surgery*. 2003;**17** (3):260–5.

77. Gormley WB, Sekhar LN, Wright DC, Olding M, Janecka IP, Snyderman CH, et al. Management and long-term outcome of adenoid cystic carcinoma with intracranial extension: a neurosurgical perspective. *Neurosurgery*. 1996;**38** (6):1105–12; discussion 12–13.

78. Lawton MT, Lang MJ. The future of open vascular neurosurgery: perspectives on cavernous malformations, AVMs, and bypasses for complex aneurysms. *J Neurosurg*. 2019;**130**(5):1409–25.

79. Abdulrauf SI. Awake craniotomies for aneurysms, arteriovenous malformations, skull base tumors, high flow bypass, and brain stem lesions. *Journal of Craniovertebral Junction & Spine*. 2015;**6**(1):8–9.

80. Chen C, Yang Y, Ling C, He H, Luo L, Wang H. Percutaneous transluminal angioplasty for radial artery graft stenosis after high-flow superficial temporal artery trunk to middle cerebral artery interposition bypass. *British Journal of Neurosurgery*. 2019:1–4.

81. Aydin E, Gok M, Esenkaya A, Cinar C, Oran I. Endovascular management of iatrogenic vascular injury in the craniocervical region. *Turk Neurosurg*. 2018;**28**(1):72–8.

82. Dlamini N, Shah-Basak P, Leung J, Kirkham F, Shroff M, Kassner A, et al. Breath-hold blood oxygen level–dependent MRI: a tool for the assessment of cerebrovascular reserve in children with Moyamoya disease. *AJNR Am J Neuroradiol*. 2018;**39**(9):1717–23.

83. Ge X, Zhao H, Zhou Z, Li X, Sun B, Wu H, et al. Association of fractional flow on 3D-TOF-MRA with cerebral perfusion in patients with MCA stenosis. *AJNR Am J Neuroradiol*. 2019;**40** (7):1124–31.

Chapter 7

Hybrid/Combined Strategies for Vestibular Schwannomas

Philip V. Theodosopoulos

Introduction

Traditional treatment algorithms for vestibular schwannomas have heavily favored gross total tumor resection, allowing for less-than-complete resections only under extraordinary circumstances. For large tumors, surgical treatment strategies focused on complete tumor resections were, in general, associated with good postoperative facial nerve function at rates varying between 30% and 80%, mostly centered around 50%. With the development and advancement of radiosurgery over the past two decades, non-microsurgical treatment of vestibular schwannomas has expanded significantly (1,2,3,4,5). Several recent natural history studies have also brought into question the premise that the majority of schwannomas grow, advocating for a wait-and-see strategy using serial scans (6,7). As a consequence, today the average patient with a vestibular schwannoma is given a choice between three reasonable options: observation with interval imaging, radiotherapy, and surgical resection.

Microsurgical resection has been shown to have the worst facial nerve and general wellness outcome when compared with the other two options, both prospectively and retrospectively (8). In an effort to improve the outcomes of microsurgical resection, the treatment algorithm and goals of treatment have been redefined. This careful reconsideration has resulted in the development of hybrid strategies for the treatment of vestibular schwannomas.

The case for hybrid treatment strategies is most applicable to large tumors. Microsurgical resection remains, in general, the only viable primary treatment option. However, because of the high rates of poor facial nerve function associated with microsurgical resection, lesions addressed with this technique often receive subtotal resections, even when total resection is the goal. The development of hybrid treatments has helped advance treatment in this regard. In an attempt to improve facial nerve outcomes, Raftopoulos et al. initially suggested intentional subtotal resection of large acoustic neuromas in a 2005 publication in which they reported their preliminary experience with 15 patients with HB 1 or 2 (9).

These preliminary results gave rise to several studies evaluating less-than-complete microsurgical resections of larger tumors. Premier among them was the ANSRS (Acoustic Neuroma Subtotal Resection Study), a prospective trial of intentional subtotal resections of tumors larger than 2.5 cm in maximal diameter with close follow-up observation of residual tumor and radiosurgical treatment for any radiographic or clinical evidence of progression. The first publication of this multicenter trial included data from at least one year of follow-up (10). Sixty-six patients were included in the study. Ten patients underwent gross total resection (GTR), 20 underwent near-total resection (NTR; leaving residuals less than 5 mm thick), and 36 underwent subtotal resection (STR). Long-term facial nerve outcomes were optimal in the near-total resection group and were statistically significantly better in both STR and NTR groups compared with the GTR group. Tumor regrowth was three times more likely in the STR group compared with the GTR and the NTR groups. The authors concluded that, based on their findings, an NTR provides the optimal combination of tumor control and functional outcome. The late results of this study are expected to be published soon and will shed more light on the long-term benefits of planned subtotal resections.

Reviewing all the intentional subtotal resections that we performed during the period of the trial, but outside the trial given logistic and patient choice reasons, we reported on 52 patients with large acoustic neuromas (Koos grade 3 and 4) who were treated with the same decision-making algorithm intraoperatively as the patients in the prospective trial (11). Although all three groups – gross total, near-total, and subtotal resection – had good long-term facial nerve outcome (HB 1 and 2 in more than 91% in all groups) the rate of tumor progression/recurrence was 0% in the GTR group, 8% for the NTR group, and 17% for the STR group. Long-term tumor control was 90% in one NTR and nine STR patients requiring postoperative radiation treatment. Similarly to the ANSRS trial, we concluded that a near-total resection appears to be the optimal extent of resection.

Several other studies have shown similar results, proving that subtotal resections followed by radiosurgery to the residual are a feasible and safe approach (4,12,13,14). A Dutch study of 50 patients with large vestibular schwannomas (average maximal diameter 3.5 cm) undergoing intentional subtotal resection followed by radiosurgery to any progressing residual reported 90% tumor control at 34 months of median follow-up with 94% good (HB 1 and 2) facial nerve function (12).

Indications for This Combined Approach

Combined approaches with subtotal resection followed by radiosurgery are optimally suited to large tumors. Koos grade 3 and 4 vestibular schwannomas are good examples of cases that often involve areas of the tumor that are densely adherent to neurovascular structures. In particular, the interface of a large tumor with the facial nerve along the distal cisternal segment toward the porus of the IAC, as well as along the surface of the ventral brainstem, are areas that can be difficult to dissect without injuring the neural tissue. Violation of the pial surface near the brainstem can have critical consequences; aggressive dissection near the facial nerve can easily, inadvertently cause permanent loss of function. A similar combined strategy can be employed for smaller tumors, however. Based on all the data available, the durability of a gross total resection is preferred whenever possible, and smaller tumors rarely have dense adhesions to neural tissue that significantly limit the safety of dissection.

Patient selection for combined approaches has not been well defined. Multiple factors contribute to the decision-making for such a treatment strategy. Even when a combined approach is indicated and planned, if intraoperative findings prove favorable, a complete resection is preferable in most circumstances. One should be adept at the various techniques of microsurgical dissection of tumor from the facial nerve and the brainstem. Should the tumor easily peel away from the surrounding structures, removal of the entirety of the tumor is always indicated.

A large tumor in a mostly-asymptomatic patient, significant medical comorbidities, advanced age, or no prior treatment are all circumstances that favor a combined approach. Although no absolute contraindications exist, the younger the age of the patient, the more important it becomes to attempt complete resection. Prior radiosurgical treatment should also prompt the surgeon to attempt a complete resection. Our data indicate that complete resection with a good facial nerve outcome is possible – and, in fact, likely – in the case of post-radiosurgery growth (15). However, the thickening of the surrounding arachnoid plane associated with radiation therapy can limit the ability to achieve safe aggressive complete resection (16,17). It should be noted that if there is intervening growth of the tumor after radiosurgical treatment, whatever residual is left following microsurgical resection can likely be safely "re-treated" with radiosurgery, as it may not have received much or any radiation during the first radiosurgical procedure (Figure 7.1).

Radiosurgery has been well established as an alternative to microsurgery for vestibular schwannomas (18–23). For large tumors, alternative approaches to combined treatment include aggressive microsurgical resection and radiation therapy (fully fractionated, hypofractionated, or even as a single fraction) (24). Recurrent tumors following either prior microsurgical or radiosurgical treatment pose a unique challenge. Often large and extensive, they can have dense adhesions as a result of the primary treatment. Surgery following prior microsurgery has proven to be the most difficult, and if also combined with any form of radiation therapy, the chances of a complete resection diminish significantly. In such instances, one should be very careful to avoid neurovascular injury, which can be catastrophic. Interestingly, the literature indicates that tumors that fail microsurgery are also frequently resistant to radiosurgery, possibly indicative of a more aggressive tumor phenotype (24). In

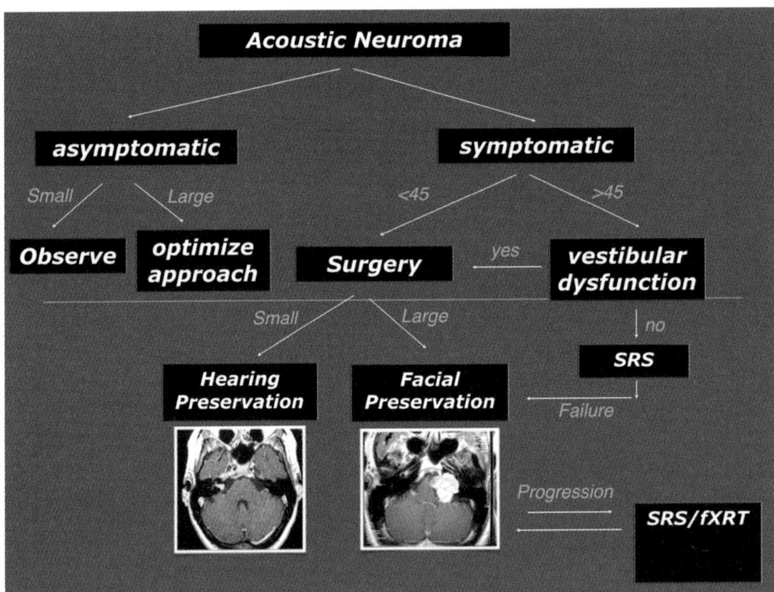

Figure 7.1 Treatment algorithm for acoustic neuroma

summary, when treating recurrent tumors, particularly multiply-recurrent ones, enthusiasm for a complete resection should be carefully tempered by the increased risks. Such tumors are best treated by expert microsurgeons and should not be taken lightly.

The recent development and refinement of hypofractionated radiosurgery platforms have introduced three- or five-fraction radiosurgery as a viable treatment paradigm, even for large tumors (25–27). The data are limited, and the long-term viability of such treatments is still unknown. There is a real risk of symptom-worsening secondary to perilesional edema development. Steroids and, in cases of refractory edema-related symptoms, bevacizumab can be used to improve edema and resolve symptoms with good results. However, the mass effect is rarely improved with such medical treatments, making any symptomatic improvement possibly short-lived and often requiring cytoreductive treatments.

Preoperative Planning

A complete hearing evaluation is imperative. It should be noted that microsurgery affords a disappointingly low rate of serviceable hearing preservation. On average, most modern studies suggest 10–15% serviceable hearing preservation, despite intraoperative monitoring and careful microsurgical dissection of tumor away from the audiovestibular nerve. As the vascular supply to the cochlea is often shared with the tumor, interruption of the tumor blood supply can inadvertently cause cochlear ischemia, resulting in abrupt hearing loss. Aside from traction-related, auditory brainstem-evoked potential hearing loss, most other intraoperative causes of hearing loss are sudden and irreversible. As such, patients should be advised that little can be done during microsurgical resection to preserve hearing, especially when operating on large tumors.

In cases where there is no serviceable hearing on preoperative testing, the 8th cranial nerve can be sectioned to obtain better exposure to the facial nerve at the root entry zone and to minimize the chances of postoperative development or worsening of tinnitus, particularly given the high chance of complete loss of hearing.

Standard preoperative imaging in our practice involves thin-cut MRI of the brain through the IAC with FIESTA sequence to attempt to identify the course of the facial and audiovestibular nerves. A stereotactic scan is used in conjunction with an intraoperative guidance system as an additional method of estimating residual tumor, enhancing the chances of an optimal subtotal resection. The location of the tumor and its tethering by the cranial nerves make significant intraoperative registration inaccuracies due to CSF drainage rare, with frequent accurate volumetric localization along the cerebellopontine angle.

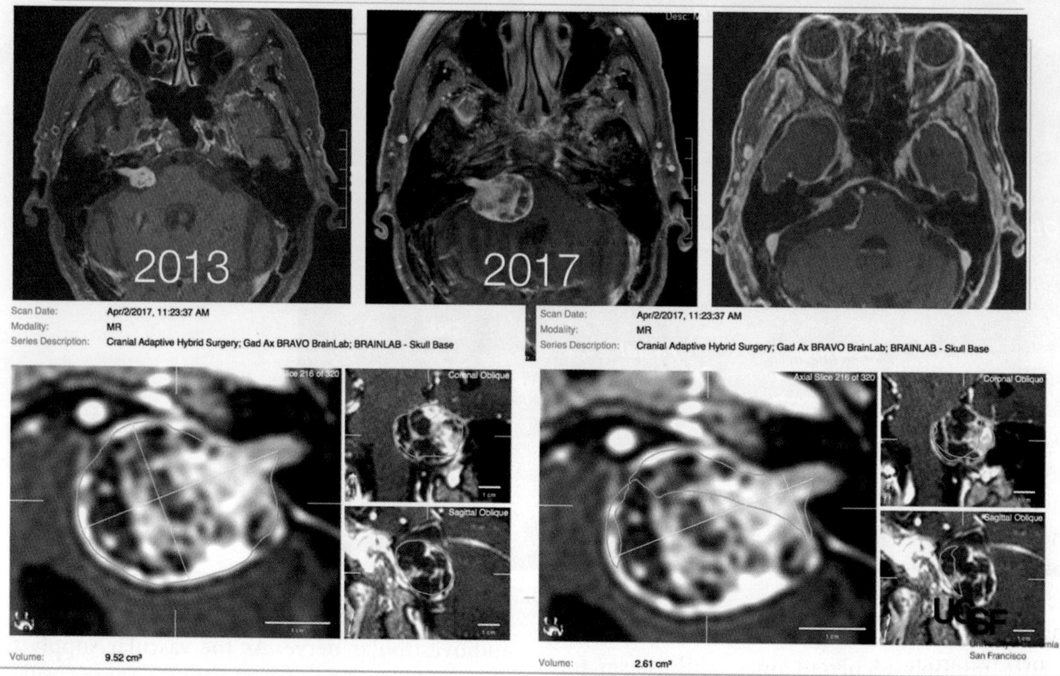

Figure 7.2 Case of an 83-year-old woman with a rapidly enlarging acoustic neuroma. The third panel on the top right is the postoperative MRI. The bottom panels show the various tumor dimensions.

Intraoperative navigation software currently exists that allows for a preoperative determination of the intended residual. The Brainlab ASC software provides intraoperative updates of the extent of resection based on offline preoperative evaluation of the optimal potential radiosurgical volume. Although the accuracy of such systems remains to be determined, such software provides another tool for attempting an optimal subtotal resection (Figure 7.2).

Operative Technique

Any microsurgical approach to a vestibular schwannoma is absolutely dependent on a detailed knowledge of the anatomy of the cerebellopontine angle. The retrosigmoid approach is most commonly used in our practice. The most important anatomical nuances with which one should become familiar include the relevant bony landmarks, the required exposure of the craniectomy, the relationship of the tumor, the approach angle to the cranial nerves, and the limitations of visualization.

I do not find the asterion a dependable marker for the necessary exposure. Instead, I prefer the line joining the root of the zygoma to the inion as an accurate surrogate for the position of the transverse sinus. On average, this line crosses the pinna toward its upper third portion.

Once the CPA is exposed one can appreciate the depths of the three sets of cranial nerves, with the lower cranial nerves most superficial at the jugular foramen; the facial and audiovestibular nerves, a bit deeper; and, finally, the trigeminal nerve, the deepest (this is a key anatomic fact). The relationship of the tumor, particularly a large tumor, to the petrosal vein is important to appreciate. Safe division of the vein is almost always necessary for maximal exposure and mobilization of the superior aspect of the tumor. The trigeminal nerve is almost always displaced anteriorly and is located along the most superior aspect of the ventral tumor capsule. The facial nerve course is variable, with the ventral location most common, followed by the superior, and, less frequently, the dorsal location along the capsule of the tumor first encountered during CPA dissection. The nerve root entry zone, in general, is identified along the most medial and inferior portion of the tumor. However, the facial nerve course distal to its origin is highly variable. Even when it remains along the ventral surface of the tumor it can cross the CPA along the most inferior aspect of the tumor capsule, turn abruptly superiorly, and join the trigeminal nerve – crossing over the trigeminal nerve or following any course in-between. Within the IAC, the facial nerve again returns to a relatively reproducible location along the ventral superior aspect.

The optimal retrosigmoid approach involves positioning the patient in the lateral decubitus position, taking care to place an axillary roll and to pad all pressure points. Except for cases of obstructive hydrocephalus, prior to the final positioning, a lumbar puncture is performed and 30 cc of CSF removed to relax the posterior fossa. If there is ventriculomegaly, a right frontal EVD insertion may be performed. The neck can be flexed and turned; however, the optimal positioning of the petrous face is perpendicular to the floor. Over-rotation makes adequate exposure difficult. Two fingerbreadths of space between the contralateral mandible and clavicle is recommended to prevent venous hypertension by jugular compression. A curvilinear incision is made with the apex below the line joining the zygoma and the inion and three fingerbreadths behind the pinna. An inferiorly-based curvilinear incision – first popularized by Dandy – is preferable to prevent postoperative headaches, as it allows for limited dissection around the greater occipital nerve.

It is strongly recommended to perform a craniectomy rather than a craniotomy in order to minimize the chances of venous sinus injury. Even in the case of a craniotomy, further drilling along the ventral and superior aspects of the bone flap is almost always necessary, making the bone flap mostly inadequate during the closure. The craniectomy is performed, and the bone dust is collected and saved for the closure. The drilling starts laterally and inferiorly and proceeds anteriorly and superiorly. Dissection is frequently performed anteriorly and superiorly epidurally to localize the sinuses. Once the sigmoid sinus is localized with careful epidural dissection, a coarse diamond burr is used to continue drilling anteriorly to allow for maximal exposure. The transverse sigmoid junction is exposed. The bone along the convexity of the posterior fossa, in general, involves an angle change of the rostrocaudal axis with respect to the transverse as the bone courses toward the foramen magnum. The caudal extent of the craniectomy needs to come to the point of maximal change in orientation of the bone but no further, as removal of the bone as it veers toward the foramen magnum provides little to no additional exposure. In cases where the size of the tumor requires opening of the foramen magnum, a "hockey-stick" incision is preferable, as it allows for safe dissection and wide exposure of the foramen.

The dura is opened along the transverse sigmoid angle, leaving at least 5 mm of dural margin to the sinuses. The operative microscope is brought into the field. Careful dissection perpendicular to the orientation of the folia leads to the cisterna magna and allows for the safe release of CSF. Dissection along the orientation of the folia leads to the CPA. Care should be taken to ensure that there are no superficial bridging veins along the most superior aspect of the cerebellar hemisphere, and, if identified, that they are carefully coagulated and divided.

Under high microscopic magnification, the CPA is exposed and the arachnoid layers surrounding the tumor are carefully identified and preserved. In general, an acoustic neuroma is enveloped medially by two layers of arachnoid. Dividing the superficial layer and preserving the deeper layer allows for safe mesial dissection. Extensive stimulation of the facial nerve along the dorsal capsule is imperative prior to any coagulation and dissection. In the absence of any positive responses, the capsule is coagulated and incised, and tumor cytoreduction commences with an ultrasonic aspirator.

Capsular dissection away from the cerebellum, and eventually the brainstem, can proceed inferiorly with constant facial nerve stimulation to identify the facial nerve root entry zone (28). The audiovestibular nerve root is often found superficial to the facial nerve root, and in the absence of an auditory brainstem response (ABR) or serviceable hearing, it can be divided to allow for improved visualization. Dissection then is performed superiorly and the trigeminal nerve and, often, the distal part of the facial nerve identified anteriorly. Exposure of the origin of any of the nerves requires enough cytoreduction to allow for medial capsule mobilization. In cases of uniquely vascular tumors, it is helpful to interrupt the blood supply by coagulating intratumorally along a line parallel to the petrous face.

Early identification of the facial nerve root entry zone is critical. However, in large tumors, particularly in those with a firm consistency or vascular lesion, it may be difficult to debulk the tumor at its ventral depth without extensive capsule coagulation in the area; this is contraindicated before the facial nerve is identified. Lateral dissection can be performed following drilling of the IAC and identification of the distal facial nerve. Dissection of the tumor away from the nerve can be performed. One should be careful, however, as distal-to-proximal tumor dissection along the interface with the facial nerve can injure the nerve by avulsing it from its lateral insertion into the labyrinthine canal. It is crucial to remember that the facial nerve is quite mobile in the CPA; it has already been stretched and is relatively laterally immobile, as it is tethered at its bony insertion.

A residual tumor is often left behind proximal to the course of the facial nerve and along areas of the capsule that are adherent to the brainstem pia. Lack of clear visualization of the capsule along the ventral aspect of such residuals makes it difficult to maximally reduce their bulk, but this can be carefully attempted with the ultrasonic aspirator. Along the lateral aspect of the tumor, careful stimulation of the capsule both inferiorly and superiorly just proximal to the porus can help identify the relative course of the facial nerve, allowing for minimal residual tumor.

It is recommended that any residual tumor be observed expectantly with serial MRI scans or treated with radiosurgery. The usual regimen of follow-up MRI involves an immediate postoperative study performed within 48 hours followed by 6 months postop, a year postop, and then yearly thereafter. Evaluating for residual tumor growth can be challenging, as the residual tumor almost always changes configuration within the first 3 months as the brainstem re-expands to its more native position. Residual tumor configuration often starts as a concave shell along the brainstem and along the course of the facial nerve in the CPA. With brainstem re-expansion following tumor resection, it ends up collapsing to form a more compact shape. Postoperative enhancement on early imaging is difficult to distinguish from true tumor enhancement. In general, if expectant management is performed, it should be done with the understanding that an accurate assessment of any true tumor size change, indicating growth may not be reliably made until close to a year postoperation. Any time such a determination of growth is made on any postoperative imaging, it is strongly recommended to proceed with salvage radiosurgical treatment. Postoperative determination of residual tumor growth is always associated with persistent and, on occasion, more rapid growth than anticipated, and timely treatment is important.

Adjuvant radiosurgery has become an increasingly preferred treatment strategy for both primary and recurrent disease. Early data from the prospective ANSRS trial and data from other subtotal resection trials have identified a small subset of tumor remnants that recur relatively rapidly and are especially difficult to manage. Up-front radiosurgery may provide the optimal treatment strategy for this minority set of tumors, although no clear data confirming this exist in the literature.

No matter the timing, for adjuvant or salvage disease, radiosurgery has been shown to be effective in the treatment of tumor residual following microsurgical resection (29–34).

Most studies report tumor control rates of 94% or better (Figure 7.3). However, there is some indirect evidence in the literature suggesting that radiosurgical control of residuals may be inferior to control of untreated tumors. This

Study	Number of patients	Tumor volume (cm^3)	Median dose (Gy)	SRS control rate (%)
Pollock 1998	78	2.8	12	94
Unger 2002	50	3.4	13	96
Pollock 2008	55	3	14	94
Huang 2017	173	2.7	13	94
UCSF 2017	11	1.2	12.5	100

Figure 7.3 Summary of radiosurgery outcomes for acoustic neuromas

mostly relates to large or rapidly-growing residuals, potentially indicating that tumors that progress rapidly despite microsurgical resection may also progress through salvage radiosurgical treatment (12,24).

The majority of radiosurgical data is derived from the gamma knife literature and relates to single-fraction treatments at a 12–13 Gy marginal dose. Several linear accelerator (linac) platforms have been used in both a single-fraction and hypofractionated regimen for the treatment of residual; however, these studies are small, and it is difficult to draw robust conclusions from them (25,26).

Based on the published data, it appears that any modality of radiation treatment as primary treatment for vestibular schwannomas is highly effective in controlling tumor growth. Three different prospective trials comparing single-fraction radiosurgery and fully-fractionated treatment have shown no difference in yielding high rates of tumor control (35,36). Available published studies on radiosurgical treatment by linear accelerator platforms have, in general, reproduced the outcomes of much larger data sets reported on single-fraction gamma knife treatments. In our practice, although we have both the gamma knife and two linear accelerator-based radiosurgery platforms, we prefer single-fraction gamma knife treatment whenever possible, as it is the modality with most proven success to date. Although it is difficult to assess, dose heterogeneity afforded by the gamma knife with "multiple hotspots" receiving more than 20 Gy, while the marginal dose remains 12.5 Gy, may be a contributor to the high rate of tumor control. This assumption is further corroborated by published data that show decreased control rates with increased plan uniformity (32).

Our institutional data indicate that radiosurgery to residual tumor is highly effective in tumor control whether used as adjuvant or salvage treatment (34). Given the relatively slow growth rate of such tumor residuals, it is unlikely that we will soon know the optimal timing of such treatment following radiosurgery. In our practice, given the small but currently unpredictable minority of cases that exhibit rapid growth following subtotal microsurgical resection, we gravitate toward treating every residual in the adjuvant setting.

Residual tumor morphology tends to change in its geometry between the immediate postoperative period and follow-up. Due to this, we wait at least three months before treating with radiosurgery to allow the tumor capsule remnant to collapse on itself as the brainstem re-expands. In general, this results in a more compact volume for radiosurgery. As there is never a conclusive reason for immediate postoperative radiosurgery for residual tumor, we recommend adjuvant radiosurgery be completed between three and six months from microsurgery.

Complications

It is important to remember that subtotal microsurgical resection carries the same neurovascular risks as any other microsurgical approach to such lesions, as the majority of the procedure remains the same. Limiting the facial nerve dissection may be beneficial to preserving nerve function, as limiting aggressive dissection along the brainstem surface can limit pial transgressions. However, facial nerve dysfunction still occurs in a fair number of patients undergoing subtotal resections. This is often due to injury caused to the facial nerve during attempts to determine the degree of tumor-nerve adhesion, and subtotal resection tends to be the approach for tumors with a high degree of adhesion. Minimizing the dissection along the nerve while accurately determining the degree of adhesion is difficult but extremely important.

Tumor remnants that fail hybrid treatment strategies pose a unique challenge. Further treatment, either microsurgical or radiosurgical, is often required. The risks of such treatments are higher than with primary treatment. Repeat microsurgery carries an increased risk of ischemic events and facial nerve injury, as well as the likelihood of another incomplete resection. Given all this, it is our recommendation that repeat microsurgery be used in cases where there is bulky residual growth, particularly in close proximity to the brainstem, or rapid recurrence. When undertaken, it should be understood that, in general, repeat microsurgery will likely be followed by another round of radiation therapy. As such, if there is no significant mass effect or rapid growth, another round of radiosurgery may be the preferable salvage treatment. There is adequate evidence of the effectiveness and safety of repeat radiosurgery for the treatment of vestibular schwannomas that have progressed through primary radiosurgery. The safety of such treatments stands to reason; often, large parts of the tumor at the time of radiosurgical retreatment have never received any prior radiation, as those parts of the tumor may not have been present during the primary treatment. The effectiveness, however, of treatments such as salvage radiosurgery following multiple therapies remains largely unproven.

Salvage microsurgical treatment of acoustic neuromas has been shown to be safe and effective following primary radiosurgery (15,37,38). Following prior microsurgery, however, our experience indicates that a significant increase in the number of adhesions along the area of the prior dissection tends to result. Arachnoid planes, which are of paramount importance for safe dissection of the tumor capsule away from normal neurovascular structures, are thickened and, in many cases, become opaque, making safe dissection more difficult. Sharp dissection is imperative for safe resection, and small portions of a tumor should be left on neurovascular structures if they are found to be too densely adherent.

It should be noted, however, that dissection is often most difficult along the brainstem surface or along the interface with the facial nerve. These areas may well be free of abnormal adhesions if dissection was never carried out along those planes. Tumors that have previously undergone a suboptimal subtotal resection and present with large bulky residuals are easier to resect during the second microsurgical resection compared with tumors that were optimally treated with an aggressive subtotal or near-total resection and have now progressed with significant regrowth. This is because, in the latter case, all of the dissection planes are often affected by adhesions. In choosing the optimal salvage therapy, it is of paramount importance to first verify the extent of dissection previously performed by evaluating the postoperative imaging obtained immediately following the first microsurgical resection.

When considering microsurgery as salvage therapy, the surgical approach should be carefully considered. In our practice, barring no limiting factors, a different surgical approach corridor is preferred to the primary one as it often results in fewer adhesions. In general, a retrosigmoid approach is preferable following primary treatment via a translabyrinthine approach, and vice versa. Even in rare instances where the repeat microsurgical approach follows the same trajectory as the primary approach, it is important to modify the trajectory at least enough to allow for dissection along arachnoid planes that have not already been extensively dissected and scarred. In the case of repeat retrosigmoid approaches, a much wider bony removal is preferred, especially inferiorly, as well as an early opening into the foramen magnum. For repeat translabyrinthine approaches, a good option is an extended translabyrinthine approach with sectioning of the tentorium. This allows for a panoramic view of the superolateral brainstem and superior cerebellopontine angle resulting in a significantly increased field of view.

The efficacy of medical therapies at salvage has not been proven extensively. Yet, there are a number of small-molecule inhibitors that have shown promise in the treatment of sporadic acoustic neuromas. Among them, bevacizumab remains the most effective (39). Dosing is standard, but duration of treatment is unknown, and there are no data reported on its use in the salvage setting. In the few recurrent cases, bevacizumab has been used in our practice, the chosen duration was six months. Phase I studies of other small-molecule inhibitors have not yet been reported, although studies have been open for years now. This may be due to the slow-accrual, long-term follow-up necessary to determine treatment effect or negative results.

Follow-Up

Our suggested follow-up for all treated acoustic neuromas includes an immediate follow-up MRI with contrast within 48 hours of surgical resection, a repeat scan at 3 months (to determine whether the residual has collapsed to a more compact target in order to guide the timing of adjuvant radiosurgery), a repeat scan at 6 months if no adjuvant treatment has yet been undertaken, and yearly scans for the first 5 years. Following this, we typically obtain a 7- and a 10-year scan, provided there is no evidence of radiographic or clinical progression. After 10 years, there is no set follow-up recommendation, yet most patients prefer to continue with occasional repeat radiological imaging.

Recent data on the timing of response to primary radiosurgical treatment would suggest that there are late responses often missed by the yearly scans over the first 5 years post-treatment (34). This would suggest that longer-term follow-up is important. Yet, in our experience, tumor progression is generally evident over the first 3 years following primary treatment; late significant tumor progression cases are rare.

The most recent published data on long-term follow-up of subtotally resected acoustic neuromas seem to indicate that tumor-remnant progression is correlated to the length of follow-up (40). If that indeed is the case, then one would expect the majority, if not all, of the subtotally resected tumors to progress given enough time. As such, long-term follow-up remains very important, even in given early radiographic stability.

Clinical Pearls

Hybrid treatment strategies for acoustic neuromas are increasingly popular. Early data from both prospective and retrospective trials suggest high percentages of good facial nerve function even for large tumors, a subset of vestibular schwannomas that, under the old paradigm of complete tumor resection, were associated with up to 50% poor facial nerve function. The more experience we collectively acquire with such treatment strategies, the more pitfalls and limitations we identify.

The indications for hybrid treatment should be carefully evaluated in every case. Subtotal resection should not be a replacement for meticulous, expert tumor resection and should never be preferred to a complete resection if at all possible with acceptable risk. This is likely the most important point, as some advocate subtotal resection for any acoustic neuroma, a strategy that is not supported by existing data or even common sense. To the best of our analysis of present data, there is no question that any amount of residual tumor has a significant risk of further growth and, likely, need for further treatment. Tumors smaller than 2.5 cm should rarely, if ever, qualify for anything but an attempted gross total resection. Maintenance of technical excellence and expertise in the surgical resection of acoustic neuromas is founded on the ability to safely dissect tumor away from the facial nerve and brainstem for a complete tumor resection. This remains the definition of optimal treatment of acoustic neuromas.

Optimizing the residual tumor size is a difficult process to master. Although the initial theoretical intent of such resections was to create a safe radiosurgical target, continued, subsequent resection should be attempted to minimize the size of the remnant as much as possible. The perfect balance between limiting the risk to the facial nerve and the size of the residual is often elusive. Meticulous and systematic debulking of the tumor is imperative in this process.

Younger patients, particularly those younger than 30 years of age with large tumors, pose a special conundrum to the surgeon. Complete resection is preferable for such patients, but permanent facial nerve dysfunction can be a significant and limiting lifelong morbidity. In such cases, if residual tumor remains, it is strongly recommended to treat the residual with adjuvant radiosurgery early on.

Rarely, in cases of multiple prior treatments, surgical re-operation needs to proceed in a lateral-to-medial fashion in order to interrupt all the blood supply to the lesion and allow for safe visualization. This approach often results in severing the facial and audiovestibular nerves at the porus acusticus and should only be used in cases where the facial nerve is already non-functional. It allows, however, for effective devascularization of the tumor from its predominant blood supply around the IAC and can be beneficial in the safe resection of such formidable lesions.

The most critical part of the decision-making process for a subtotal resection involves a good appreciation of the degree of adhesion between the facial nerve/brainstem and the capsule of the tumor. With increased experience, the surgeon can identify tumors that pose a high risk of facial nerve injury earlier in the dissection. This may result in lower rates of facial dysfunction but has yet to be proven in the literature.

Close follow-up of any residual tumor is imperative. Whenever there is evidence of tumor progression, further treatment is important as, in general, such growth in the absence of radiation therapy is often linear. Our practice has mostly shifted to early adjuvant radiosurgery to the residual tumor in order to avoid the well-defined minority of tumor remnants that exhibit aggressive regrowth.

Limitations

Despite extensive research on hybrid treatment therapies and subtotal microsurgical resections of acoustic neuromas, there remain several unanswered questions. The predictors of tumor remnant progression are unknown. The size of the residual seems to be the factor identified in most studies as the greatest predictor of progression; however, there are published studies that find residual size not to be a predictor of progression. Outside of residual size, there are no well-defined predictors of growth. Additionally, it remains unknown whether progression depends on some inherent tumor characteristic or is a result of the effect of treatment on the genetics of the tumor.

Possibly the biggest limitation of combination treatments is the fact that the size of tumor residual and postoperative facial nerve function are not linearly related. As a result, in utilizing such strategies, one could end up with a suboptimal, bulky residual tumor and also poor facial nerve function. Although there is yet no clear understanding of how to avoid this, meticulous microsurgical technique and early identification of the facial nerve are critical in predicting good outcomes.

Key Points

- Combination treatment of vestibular schwannomas is effective and safe for reducing facial nerve morbidity.
- The optimal size of tumor residual remains unknown.
- The optimal timing of radiosurgical treatment is unknown, although early adjuvant treatment may prevent the rare development of rapid tumor regrowth.

References

1. Samii M, Gerganov V, Samii A. Improved preservation of hearing and facial nerve function in vestibular schwannoma surgery via the retrosigmoid approach in a series of 200 patients. *Journal of Neurosurgery*. 2006 Oct 1;**105**(4):527–35.
2. Raftopoulos C, Serieh BA, Duprez T, Docquier MA, Guerit JM. Microsurgical results with large vestibular schwannomas with preservation of facial and cochlear nerve function as the primary aim. *Acta Neurochirurgica*. 2005 Jul 1;**147**(7):697–706.
3. Sughrue ME, Kaur R, Rutkowski MJ, Kane AJ, Kaur G, Yang I, Pitts LH, Parsa AT. Extent of resection and the long-term durability of vestibular schwannoma surgery. *Journal of Neurosurgery*. 2011 May 1;**114**(5):1218–23.
4. Haque R, Wojtasiewicz TJ, Gigante PR, Attiah MA, Huang B, Isaacson SR, Sisti MB. Efficacy of facial nerve-sparing approach in patients with vestibular schwannomas. *Journal of Neurosurgery*. 2011 Nov 1;**115**(5):917–23.
5. Falcioni M, Fois P, Taibah A, Sanna M. Facial nerve function after vestibular schwannoma surgery. *Journal of Neurosurgery*. 2011 Oct 1;**115** (4):820–6.
6. El Bakkouri W, Kania RE, Guichard JP, Lot G, Herman P, Huy PT. Conservative management of 386 cases of unilateral vestibular schwannoma: tumor growth and consequences for treatment. *Journal of Neurosurgery*. 2009 Apr 1;**110**(4):662–9.
7. Stangerup SE, Caye-Thomasen P, Tos M, Thomsen J. The natural history of vestibular schwannoma. *Otology & Neurotology*. 2006 Jun 1;**27**(4):547–52.
8. Pollock BE, Driscoll CL, Foote RL, Link MJ, Gorman DA, Bauch CD, Mandrekar JN, Krecke KN, Johnson CH. Patient outcomes after vestibular schwannoma management: a prospective comparison of microsurgical resection and stereotactic radiosurgery. *Neurosurgery*. 2006 Jul 1;**59**(1):77–85.
9. Raftopoulos C, Serieh BA, Duprez T, Docquier MA, Guerit JM. Microsurgical results with large vestibular schwannomas with preservation of facial and cochlear nerve function as the primary aim. *Acta Neurochirurgica*. 2005 Jul 1;**147**(7):697–706.
10. Monfared A, Corrales CE, Theodosopoulos PV, Blevins NH, Oghalai JS, Selesnick SH, Lee H, Gurgel RK, Hansen MR, Nelson RF, Gantz BJ. Facial nerve outcome and tumor control rate as a function of degree of resection in treatment of large acoustic neuromas: preliminary report of the Acoustic Neuroma Subtotal Resection Study (ANSRS). *Neurosurgery*. 2016 Aug 1;**79** (2):194–203.
11. Anaizi AN, Gantwerker E, Pensak M, Theodosopoulos PV. Facial nerve preservation surgery for Koos stage 3 and 4 vestibular schwannomas. *Journal of Neurological Surgery, Part B: Skull Base*. 2014 Feb;**75**(S 01):A131.
12. van de Langenberg R, Hanssens PE, van Overbeeke JJ, Verheul JB, Nelemans PJ, de Bondt BJ, Stokroos RJ. Management of large vestibular schwannoma. Part I. Planned subtotal resection followed by Gamma Knife surgery: radiological and clinical aspects. *Journal of Neurosurgery*. 2011A Nov 1;**115**(5):875–84.
13. Theodosopoulos PV, Pensak ML. Contemporary management of acoustic neuromas. *The Laryngoscope*. 2011 Jun;**121**(6):1133–7.
14. Gurgel RK, Theodosopoulos PV, Jackler RK. Subtotal/near-total treatment of vestibular

schwannomas. *Current Opinion in Otolaryngology & Head and Neck Surgery*. 2012 Oct 1;**20**(5):380–4.

15. Breshears JD, Osorio JA, Cheung SW, Barani IJ, Theodosopoulos PV. Surgery after primary radiation treatment for sporadic vestibular schwannomas: case series. *Operative Neurosurgery*. 2017 Aug 1;**13**(4):441–7.
16. Roche PH, Khalil M, Thomassin JM, Delsanti C, Régis J. Surgical removal of vestibular schwannoma after failed gamma knife radiosurgery. In *Modern Management of Acoustic Neuroma* 2008 (Vol. **21**, pp. 152–7). Karger Publishers.
17. Wise SC, Carlson ML, Tveiten ØV, Driscoll CL, Myrseth E, Lund-Johansen M, Link MJ. Surgical salvage of recurrent vestibular schwannoma following prior stereotactic radiosurgery. *The Laryngoscope*. 2016 Nov;**126**(11):2580–6.
18. Flickinger JC, Kondziolka D, Niranjan A, Maitz A, Voynov G, Lunsford LD. Acoustic neuroma radiosurgery with marginal tumor doses of 12 to 13 Gy. *International Journal of Radiation Oncology, Biology, Physics*. 2004 Sep 1;**60** (1):225–30.
19. Lunsford LD, Niranjan A, Kano H, Kondziolka D. The technical evolution of gamma knife radiosurgery for arteriovenous malformations. In *Gamma Knife Radiosurgery for Brain Vascular Malformations* 2013 (Vol. **27**, pp. 22–34). Karger Publishers.
20. Foote RL, Coffey RJ, Swanson JW, Harner SG, Beatty CW, Kline RW, Stevens LN, Hu TC. Stereotactic radiosurgery using the gamma knife for acoustic neuromas. *International Journal of Radiation Oncology, Biology, Physics*. 1995 Jul 15;**32**(4):1153–60.
21. Yang I, Aranda D, Han SJ, Chennupati S, Sughrue ME, Cheung SW, Pitts LH, Parsa AT. Hearing preservation after stereotactic radiosurgery for vestibular schwannoma: a systematic review. *Journal of Clinical Neuroscience*. 2009 Jun 1;**16**(6):742–7.
22. Murphy ES, Suh JH. Radiotherapy for vestibular schwannomas: a critical review. *International Journal of Radiation Oncology, Biology, Physics*. 2011A Mar 15;**79**(4):985–97.
23. Murphy ES, Barnett GH, Vogelbaum MA, Neyman G, Stevens GH, Cohen BH, Elson P, Vassil AD, Suh JH. Long-term outcomes of Gamma Knife radiosurgery in patients with vestibular schwannomas. *Journal of Neurosurgery*. 2011B Feb 1;**114**(2):432–40.
24. Yang HC, Kano H, Awan NR, Lunsford LD, Niranjan A, Flickinger JC, Novotny J, Bhatnagar JP, Kondziolka D. Gamma Knife radiosurgery for larger-volume vestibular schwannomas. *Journal of Neurosurgery*. 2011 Mar 1;**114**(3):801–7.
25. Kim HJ, Roh KJ, Oh HS, Chang WS, Moon IS. Quality of life in patients with vestibular schwannomas according to management strategy. *Otology & Neurotology*. 2015 Dec 1;**36**(10):1725–9.
26. Lo WL, Yang KY, Huang YJ, Chen WF, Liao CC, Huang YH. Experience with Novalis stereotactic radiosurgery for vestibular schwannomas. *Clinical Neurology and Neurosurgery*. 2014 Jun **1**;121:30–4.
27. van de Langenberg R, de Bondt BJ, Nelemans PJ, Dohmen AJ, Baumert BG, Stokroos RJ. Predictors of volumetric growth and auditory deterioration in vestibular schwannomas followed in a wait and scan policy. *Otology & Neurotology*. 2011B Feb 1;**32**(2):338–44.
28. Bozorg Grayeli A, Kalamarides M, Fraysse B, Deguine O, Favre G, Martin C, Mom T, Sterkers O. Comparison between intraoperative observations and electromyographic monitoring data for facial nerve outcome after vestibular schwannoma surgery. *Acta oto-laryngologica*. 2005 Jan 1;**125**(10):1069–74.
29. Brokinkel B, Sauerland C, Holling M, Ewelt C, Horstmann G, van Eck AT, Stummer W. Gamma Knife radiosurgery following subtotal resection of vestibular schwannoma. *Journal of Clinical Neuroscience*. 2014 Dec 1;**21**(12):2077–82.
30. Huang MJ, Kano H, Mousavi SH, Niranjan A, Monaco EA, Arai Y, Flickinger JC, Lunsford LD. Stereotactic radiosurgery for recurrent vestibular schwannoma after previous resection. *Journal of Neurosurgery*. 2017 May 1;**126**(5):1506–13.
31. Iwai Y, Ishibashi K, Watanabe Y, Uemura G, Yamanaka K. Functional preservation after planned partial resection followed by gamma knife radiosurgery for large vestibular schwannomas. *World Neurosurgery*. 2015 Aug 1;**84**(2):292–300.
32. Pollock BE, Link MJ, Foote RL. Failure rate of contemporary low-dose radiosurgical technique for vestibular schwannoma clinical article. *Journal of Neurosurgery*. 2009 Oct 1;**111**(4):840–4.
33. Pollock BE, Lunsford LD, Flickinger JC, Clyde BL, Kondziolka D. Vestibular schwannoma management: Part I. Failed microsurgery and the role of delayed stereotactic radiosurgery. *Journal of Neurosurgery*. 1998 Dec 1;**89**(6):944–8.
34. Breshears JD, Chang J, Molinaro A, Sneed P, Mcdermott MW, Tward A, Theodosopoulos PV. Duration and timing of transient tumor enlargement after gamma knife radiosurgery for vestibular schwannomas. *Journal of Neurological Surgery, Part B: Skull Base*. 2018 Feb;**79**(S 01): A086.

35. Andrews DW, Suarez O, Goldman HW, Downes MB, Bednarz G, Corn BW, Werner-Wasik M, Rosenstock J, Curran Jr WJ. Stereotactic radiosurgery and fractionated stereotactic radiotherapy for the treatment of acoustic schwannomas: comparative observations of 125 patients treated at one institution. *International Journal of Radiation Oncology, Biology, Physics*. 2001 Aug 1;**50**(5):1265–78.

36. Combs SE, Welzel T, Schulz-Ertner D, Huber PE, Debus J. Differences in clinical results after LINAC-based single-dose radiosurgery versus fractionated stereotactic radiotherapy for patients with vestibular schwannomas. *International Journal of Radiation Oncology, Biology, Physics*. 2010 Jan 1;**76**(1):193–200.

37. Friedman RA, Brackmann DE, Hitselberger WE, Schwartz MS, Iqbal Z, Berliner KI. Surgical salvage after failed irradiation for vestibular schwannoma. *The Laryngoscope*. 2005 Oct;**115**(10):1827–32.

38. Iwai Y, Yamanaka K, Yamagata K, Yasui T. Surgery after radiosurgery for acoustic neuromas: surgical strategy and histological findings. *Operative Neurosurgery*. 2007 Feb 1;60(suppl 2): ONS-75.

39. Plotkin SR, Stemmer-Rachamimov AO, Barker FG, Halpin C, Padera TP, Tyrrell A, Sorensen AG, Jain RK, di Tomaso E. Hearing improvement after bevacizumab in patients with neurofibromatosis type 2. *New England Journal of Medicine*. 2009 Jul 23;**361**(4):358–67.

40. Nakatomi H, Jacob JT, Carlson ML, Tanaka S, Tanaka M, Saito N, Lohse CM, Driscoll CL, Link MJ. Long-term risk of recurrence and regrowth after gross-total and subtotal resection of sporadic vestibular schwannoma. *Journal of Neurosurgery*. 2017 May 1;**1**(aop):1–7.

Transchoroidal, Subchoroidal, and Combined Approaches to the Third Ventricle

Zaid Aljuboori, Hayder R. Salih, Brian J. Williams, and Dale Ding

Introduction

Ventricular lesions are considered some of the most challenging pathologies in neurosurgery. They were first described in the mid-nineteenth century; Walter Dandy is generally considered to have the greatest role in advancing our understanding of the diagnosis and treatment of ventricular lesions, culminating in a book he published on the topic in 1933 (1). Since then, there have been significant advances in the management of these lesions. Surgical access to the lateral and third ventricles can be attained by a variety of approaches, which can be generally categorized as either open or endoscopic. Transventricular approaches can also be classified as anterior, lateral, or posterior. All of these approaches inevitably entail traversing unaffected neural tissues. Therefore, judicial selection of the surgical approach is important to optimizing both intraoperative visualization of the pathology and neurological preservation (2). Most open and endoscopic approaches involve entering the third ventricle through the lateral ventricle using the interhemispheric anterior transcallosal, frontal transsulcal, or frontal transcortical approach. In choosing among these approaches, one must consider the site of the pathology, size, and consistency of the lesion; anatomical considerations of the patient; and individual preferences and experience of the neurosurgeon.

Operative corridors to the third ventricle include either working solely through the foramen of Monro (transforaminal approach), which is typically employed for small lesions located in the anterior superior part of the third ventricle, or through the choroidal fissure (transchoroidal or subchoroidal). The foramen of Monro, which can be conceptualized as the dilated end of the choroidal fissure, can be enlarged posteriorly by opening the choroidal fissure in order to expand the surgical field for access to lesions located in, or extending into, the middle or posterior parts of the roof of the third ventricle. Access to the third ventricle through the choroidal fissure requires either opening the taenia fornicis medial to the choroid plexus (transchoroidal approach) or opening the taenia thalami lateral to the choroid plexus (subchoroidal approach).

In this chapter, we will focus on the transchoroidal, subchoroidal, and combined transchoroidal and subchoroidal approaches to the third ventricle, with an exploration of the indications, limitations, and technical nuances of each approach.

Pathology of the Third Ventricle

Several classifications have been applied to ventricular lesions. Broadly speaking, these include primary intraventricular (originating from within the ventricle) or secondary (extending into the ventricle from extraventricular origin or from the wall) pathologies. More specific classifications describe third-ventricular lesions according to their location within the third ventricle (anterior versus posterior), according to their incidence (common versus rare pathologies), or according to the age of the patient at the time of diagnosis.

Intraventricular lesions include both neoplastic and non-neoplastic lesions. The former comprises primary and metastatic tumors, whereas the latter comprises cysts, vascular malformations, infectious foci, and inflammatory lesions (Table 8.1).

Open Surgical Approaches to the Third Ventricle

The surgical treatment of third-ventricular lesions remains challenging to neurosurgeons in the modern era, in spite of advances in tools and techniques. Thus the selection of the surgical

Table 8.1 Differential diagnosis of third-ventricular lesion

Intraventricular tumors:	• Astrocytoma (all grades) • Choroid papilloma and carcinoma • Subependymal giant cell astrocytoma • Central neurocytoma • Ependymoma • Optic-hypothalamic pathway glioma • Meningioma • Chordoid glioma of the third ventricle • Metastatic tumors
Extension of suprasellar tumors	• Craniopharyngioma • Germinomas • Pituitary tumors
Extension of pineal tumors:	• Thalamic astrocytomas (grade 2–4) • Germ cell tumors (germinoma, embryonal cell carcinoma, endodermal sinus tumor), choriocarcinoma and teratoma, and mixed tumors • Pineal parenchymal tumors (pineocytoma, pineoblastoma, and mixed tumors) • Metastasis
Cystic lesions:	• Colloid cysts • Epidermoid and dermoid cysts • Arachnoid cyst • Ependymal cysts and large choroid plexus cysts
Infectious/inflammatory lesions:	• Pyogenic abscess • Neurocysticercosis • Tuberculosis, fungal infection • Sarcoidosis • Langerhans cell histiocytosis • Choroid plexus xanthogranuloma
Vascular lesions:	• Arteriovenous malformations, cavernomas, and vein of Galen malformations
Other very rare lesions:	• Primary lymphoma • Medulloblastoma • Hemangioblastoma • Atypical teratoid / rhabdoid tumor

approach is not uniform across all lesions and practitioners; the approach should be individualized according to the lesion type, location, and predicted consistency, the patient's specific anatomy, and the aim of surgery.

Open approaches to the third ventricle can be categorized according to the trajectory through which the surgeon approaches the ventricle or according to the location of the lesion within the third ventricle (Figure 8.1). Depending on the location, the open approach to the third ventricle will take one of three trajectories: anterior, lateral, or posterior (3).

Anterior Trajectory to the Third Ventricle

The anterior trajectory to the third ventricle comprises the following approaches, each with its related corridors or modifications.

Anterior Interhemispheric Transcallosal Approach

This approach is generally preferred, since it affords the shortest working distance to the third ventricle. After performing the callosotomy and entering the lateral ventricle, use one or a combination of the following four corridors.

1. The transforaminal corridor, which uses the foramen of Monro.
    - The foramen of Monroe can be pathologically enlarged by superior extensions of third-ventricular lesions.
    - It represents a normal anatomical aperture into the third ventricle.
    - It can be traversed with minimal violation of surrounding critical structures.
    - This corridor only provides access to the anterior superior part of the third ventricle.
2. The transchoroidal corridor, a posterior extension of the transforaminal corridor, in which the choroidal fissure is opened medial to the choroid plexus.
3. The subchoroidal corridor, also a posterior extension of the transforaminal corridor, in

which the choroidal fissure is opened lateral to the choroid plexus.

4. The interforniceal corridor, which is attained by dividing the fornices. Note that this approach provides limited working space laterally and presents a considerable risk of bilateral forniceal injury (4).

The Frontal Transcortical Approach

This approach is more suitable for large third-ventricular lesions with dilated lateral ventricles and provides wider operative exposure than the interhemispheric approach, with more flexibility in the working angles. Upon entering the lateral ventricle, the transcortical approach shares corridors into the third ventricle with the interhemispheric transcallosal approach, including the transforaminal, transchoroidal, and subchoroidal corridors.

The Subfrontal Approach

This approach is favored for small lesions localized to the anterior inferior part of the third ventricle. Three corridors can be used to access the third ventricle from the subfrontal approach: the translamina terminalis, opticocarotid, and subchiasmatic corridors.

The Transsphenoidal Approach

This approach – which can be performed endoscopically or microscopically from an endonasal approach or microscopically from a sublabial approach – is usually reserved for suprasellar pathologies that extend superiorly and posteriorly into the lower part of the third ventricle (e.g., craniopharyngiomas). Although the details of this approach are beyond the scope of the present chapter, one must take precautions to minimize the risk of postoperative CSF leak and meningitis (e.g., using a pedicled nasoseptal flap or placing a lumbar drain) when targeting intradural lesions from a transsphenoidal approach.

Lateral Trajectory to the Third Ventricle

The lateral trajectory to the third ventricle comprises two approaches: the subtemporal approach and the pterional approach. The subtemporal approach represents the primary lateral access to the third ventricle, and it can be applied to lesions extending inferolaterally to the middle cranial fossa. The pterional approach requires a wide Sylvian fissure dissection, but it provides a relatively narrow operative corridor into the third ventricle through the lamina terminalis. Therefore, the pterional approach is a reasonable option for multi-compartmental lesions requiring combined operative corridors. Specifically, the pterional approach can be combined with an interhemispheric transcallosal or transcortical transfrontal approach. Similarly to the aforementioned transsphenoidal approach, the pterional approach can be used alone for suprasellar lesions extending into the anterior inferior third ventricle. The suprasellar cistern is encountered at the depth of the anterior Sylvian fissure dissection. From there, opening the lamina terminus allows access to the anterior inferior third ventricle. Additionally, it is relatively easier to ensure a watertight dural closure to prevent CSF leaks from a transcranial compared with a transsphenoidal approach.

Posterior Trajectory to the Third Ventricle

The posterior trajectory to the third ventricle comprises multiple approaches that are usually reserved for the resection of pineal lesions that extend into the posterior third ventricle or, in rare instances, for small lesions that reside solely in the posterior third ventricle. This can be achieved through the supracerebellar infratentorial, posterior interhemispheric transcallosal, or occipital transtentorial approaches. The relative use of these approaches depends on the relationship of the lesion to the Galenic venous complex and on the lesion's lateral extension (Figure 8.1).

Indications of the Combined Transcortical, Transchoroidal, and Subchoroidal Approach

Lesions of the third ventricle can be challenging, and they may drive surgeons to design innovative approaches that provide better exposure with less transgression of critical anatomical structures. Both the transchoroidal and subchoroidal approaches are methods to enlarge the foramen of Monro during resection of third-ventricular lesions. Either the transcallosal or transcortical routes can be used to enter the lateral ventricle, after which the neurosurgeon can use either the transchoroidal or subchoroidal approach to

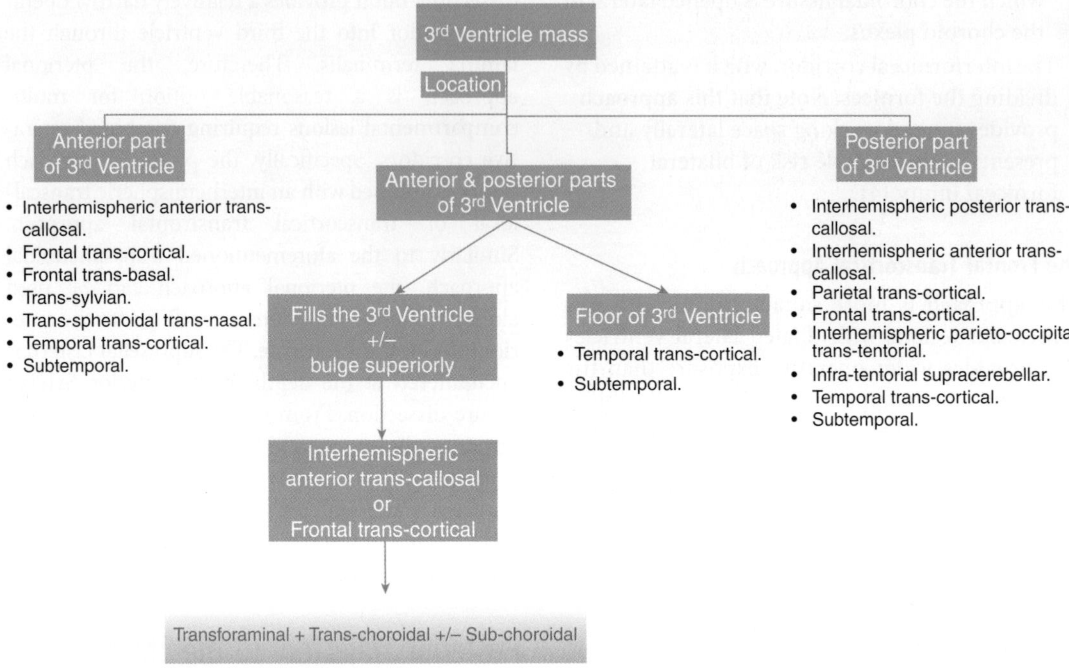

Figure 8.1 Open approaches to the third ventricle according to the location of the lesion

access the third ventricle. In general, the transcallosal route is preferred for small or medium-sized lesions, whereas the transcortical route provides a wider operative corridor for access to larger lesions (diameter >3 cm) (5,6).

In this chapter, we introduce and explore the combined transchoroidal and subchoroidal approach. Surgical access to the third ventricle can be substantially increased by combining the transchoroidal and subchoroidal approaches, ligating the septal vein, and skeletonizing and laterally mobilizing the internal cerebral vein while preserving the thalamostriate vein, thereby minimizing the risk of postoperative venous infarction. This combined approach provides adequate exposure of the middle and posterior regions of the third ventricle (Figure 8.2). The combined transchoroidal and subchoroidal approach is typically applied to large third-ventricular lesions extending into the posterior part of third ventricle. This approach is particularly useful for lesions that do not readily collapse with internal debulking (7).

Alternative Approaches

The primary alternative routes to the combined transchoroidal and subchoroidal approach are the interforniceal and transforniceal approaches. The interforniceal approach requires division along the midline between the two fornices that form the roof of the third ventricle. It is limited by the junction of the anterior commissure and the fornices; thus, this approach is preferable for anteriorly located third-ventricular lesions. The interforniceal approach carries a profound risk of patient memory loss, as injury to both fornices is common during the attempt to split them. The transforniceal approach is also generally not favored by surgeons, as it involves transgression of the body of fornix and resultant patient memory deficits (8).

Pertinent Microanatomy

A safe and precise neurosurgical procedure to resect a third-ventricular mass requires detailed knowledge of the microsurgical anatomy of the lateral and third ventricles, choroidal fissure, and foramen of Monro. The preoperative planning process focuses on the relevant neurovascular anatomy, with particular attention paid to venous circulation, which is of paramount importance during third-ventricular surgery. Additionally, considering the potential distortion of normal anatomy by the lesion itself or by the associated hydrocephalus is a critical factor in avoiding complications.

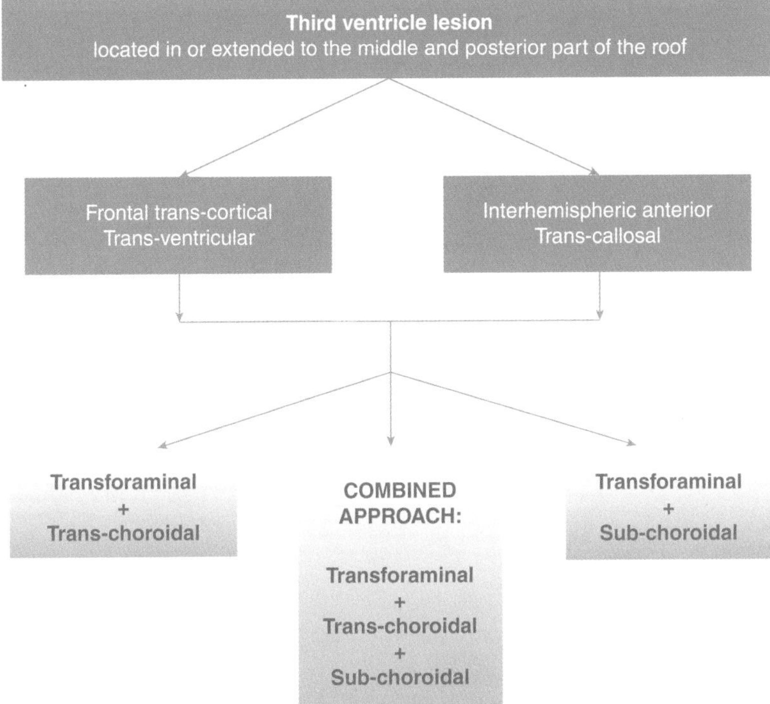

Figure 8.2 Decision-making scheme for a large lesion located in the roof of the third ventricle.

Through the interventricular foramen of Monro, the choroid plexus of the lateral and third ventricles is continuous. The choroid plexus arises from a membranous structure called the tela choroidea. The tela choroidea is attached to the ventricular wall via the tenia. The tenia on the medial side of the choroidal fissure (attached to the fornix) is called the *tenia fornicis*, whereas the tenia on the lateral side of the choroidal fissure (attached to the thalamus) is called the *tenia choroidea* or *tenia thalami*.

The foramen of Monro is an elliptical space between the columns of the fornix (anteriorly), the thalamus (posteriorly), and the genu of the internal capsule (laterally). Its diameter is around 0.5 cm in normal individuals. The foramen of Monro can be conceptualized as the dilated terminus of the choroidal fissure. While it is continuous with the choroidal fissure posteriorly, it is anatomically divided from the choroidal fissure by the junction of the septal and thalamostriate veins at the venous angle.

The third ventricle is a slit-like midline CSF cavity with a roof, floor, and anterior, posterior, and lateral walls. The roof of the third ventricle is comprised of five layers. The first layer (upper or neural) includes the fornices. The superior and inferior layers of the tela choroidea form the second and fourth layers of the roof of the third ventricle. The superior and inferior layers of the tela choroidea have a space in between them called the *velum interpositum*, which represents the third layer. The velum interpositum contains the medial posterior choroidal arteries, which are branches of the proximal posterior cerebral artery (P2 segment), and the internal cerebral veins, which join the bilateral basal veins of Rosenthal posteriorly to form the vein of Galen. The fifth (lower) layer is formed by the choroid plexus. The choroidal fissure is located in the lateral margin of the roof of the third ventricle.

The anterior wall of the third ventricle is formed, from top to bottom, by the lamina terminalis, suprachiasmatic recess, and optic chiasm.

The floor is formed, from anterior to posterior, by the pituitary infundibulum, tuber cinereum, mammillary bodies, and posterior perforated substance.

The lateral walls are formed by the thalamus and hypothalamus on each side.

Finally, the posterior wall is formed by the posterior commissure, pineal body, and habenular commissure (Figure 8.3).

The medial posterior choroidal arteries most frequently arise from the P2 segment of the posterior

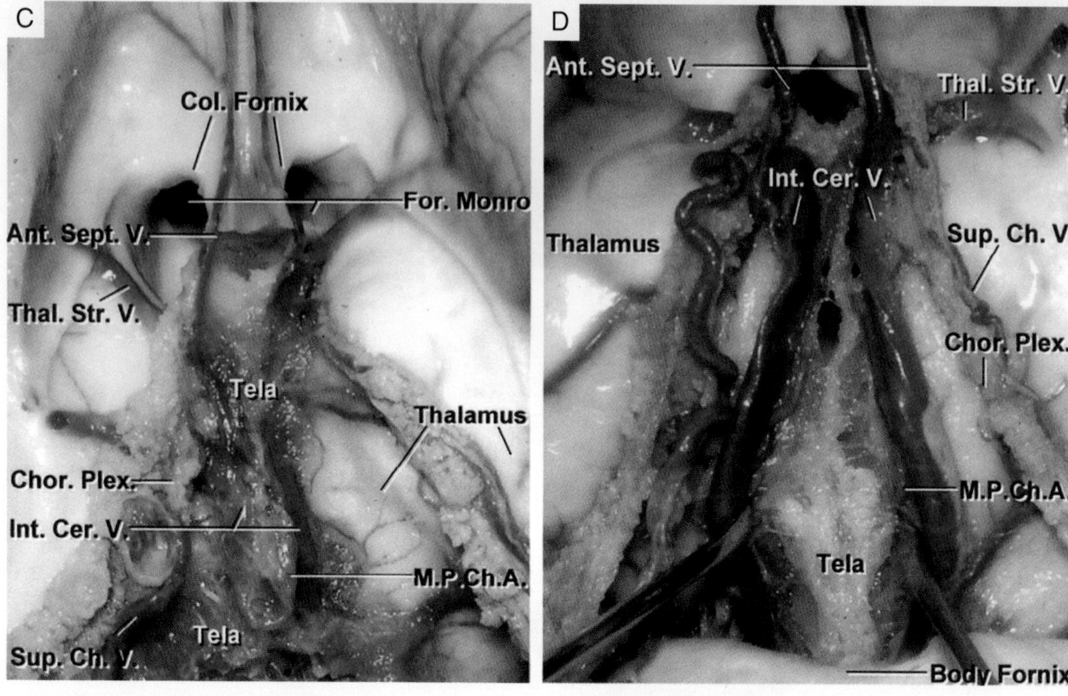

Figure 8.3 Roof of the third ventricle. Superior views. C, the tela is a thin, arachnoid-like membrane, through which the internal cerebral veins and the medial posterior choroidal arteries can be seen. The anterior septal veins pass above the foramen of Monro. D, the upper layer of tela has been removed to expose the internal cerebral veins and medial posterior choroidal arteries. The internal cerebral veins have been retracted laterally. The anterior septal veins course along the septum and join the internal cerebral veins near the foramen of Monro. Ant., anterior; Cer., cerebral; Ch., choroidal; Chor., choroid; Col., column; For., foramen; M.P.Ch.A., medial posterior choroidal artery; Plex., plexus; Sept., septal; Sup., superior; Thal.Str., thalamostriate; V., vein. (Rhoton AL Jr. The lateral and third ventricles. Neurosurgery. 2002;51(4) (Suppl): S1-228). Courtesy of the Rhoton Collection, American Association of Neurological Surgeons [AANS]/Neurosurgical Research and Education Foundation [NREF].

cerebral artery in the interpeduncular and crural cisterns. They then turn forward on each side of the pineal gland to enter the roof of the third ventricle and course from posterior to anterior within the velum interpositum adjacent to the internal cerebral veins. These arteries supply the choroid plexus in the roof of the third ventricle.

The internal cerebral veins are formed primarily by the convergence of the anterior septal and thalamostriate veins near the foramen of Monro (this angiographic landmark is known as the venous angle) in the anterior part of the velum interpositum, and they exit the velum interpositum above the pineal body to enter the quadrigeminal cistern. There, they join the bilateral basal veins of Rosenthal to form the vein of Galen. The anterior septal vein courses medially from the tip of the frontal horn, curves posteriorly along the septum pellucidum and over the column of the fornix, and passes above the foramen of Monro to join the thalamostriate vein to form the internal cerebral vein (2,8,9–13).

The anatomy of the lateral ventricles is also important to note, and especially the relationship among the anterior septal vein, thalamostriate vein, and choroidal fissure. Identification of the venous angle will further help the surgeon safely enter the third ventricle. The venous angle is composed of the juncture of the anterior septal and the thalamostriate veins, and it is located along the posterior edge of the foramen of Monro. In some patients, it extends 3–7 mm beyond the posterior margin of the foramen of Monro; this anatomic configuration can facilitate transforaminal access to the third ventricle.

Interhemispheric Anterior Transcallosal versus Frontal Transcortical Approach to the Third Ventricle

The transcortical approach is most notably limited by its preference for a dilated lateral ventricle to facilitate transventricular access, but its advantages include the relative technical ease of the approach compared with the transcallosal approach, the lack of bridging veins at risk for injury, avoidance of an incision in the corpus callosum, and a more lateral-to-medial trajectory to access the ventricular system. Since the size of the frontal corticotomy or corticectomy can be adjusted to the size of the tumor, the transcortical approach is generally preferred for larger tumors. On the other hand, the transcallosal approach is limited by the significant risk it poses to the bridging veins, fornices, and corpus callosum, but it has the advantages of an easier approach given normal ventricular size and a shorter working distance. Both approaches can cause seizures, hemiparesis, memory loss, confusion, and mutism, as well as disconnection syndromes at variable incidences (14–17).

Although it is extremely rare, the senior author encountered a case during his training in which an adult patient with a third-ventricular epidermoid cyst had agenesis of the anterior portion of the falx cerebri in the presence of a normal superior sagittal sinus (SSS) (18). Since the anterior and posterior portions of the falx cerebri have distinct embryological origins, one can have an absent anterior falx but present posterior falx. However, since the falx cerebri develops in conjunction with the overlying SSS, it was very unusual in this particular case for the patient to have a normally developed SSS but an absent anterior falx cerebri. This anomaly was not noted preoperatively and, therefore, the planned approach was an anterior interhemispheric transcallosal approach to the third ventricle. However, when the dura was opened, the absent falx was noted and the medial surfaces of the two cerebral hemispheres were noted to be densely adherent with traversing veins. Since this precluded an anterior interhemispheric corridor, a frontal transcortical approach was performed to resect the lesion. Due to the rarity of this abnormality, we cannot recommend screening every patient for absence of a falx cerebri. Rather, this example serves to underscore the importance of a thorough evaluation of preoperative neuroimaging.

Transchoroidal, Subchoroidal, and Combined Approaches

Preoperative Planning

The following are of the utmost importance for the success of third-ventricular surgery:

- Obtaining good quality neuroimaging studies (e.g., brain MRI with and without contrast with neuronavigation protocol; MR venography)
- Careful evaluation of the origin, location, size, and imaging characteristics of the tumor
- Careful evaluation of the age and medical comorbidities of the patient

In addition, a clear understanding of vascular (particularly venous) anatomy is critical to the success of this operation. MR venography (MRV) is crucial to understanding the venous anatomy around the lesion, particularly, the subependymal veins (anterior septal and thalamostriate veins) of the lateral ventricle and their relationships to the foramen of Monro. Notably, a duplication of venous drainage can be helpful during the procedure, as it will allow the sacrifice of specific vein(s) with minimal risk of venous infarct. Additionally, the location of the venous angle can be determined from the MRV. MRV is particularly important for the anterior interhemispheric approach, as it identifies the major cortical veins draining into the superior sagittal sinus. The parasagittal craniotomy for the interhemispheric approach must be tailored to the anatomy of the draining veins. A large draining vein that bisects the dural opening effectively halves the size of the craniotomy for this approach. Furthermore, locating the medial posterior choroidal arteries can help to characterize blood supply to the tumor. Computed tomography angiography, MR angiography, or digital subtraction angiography can provide a more comprehensive picture of the arterial anatomy(8).

Operative Procedure

General Positioning Principles

- Affix the head in a Mayfield skull clamp.
- Use frameless stereotactic neuronavigation if helpful, but this is not necessary.
- Mark the incision and shave hair as needed.
- Prep and drape the incision.
- Use a Budde halo or Greenberg retractor system if needed.
- A variety of head positions have been proposed for approaches to the third ventricle. Conventionally, the head is positioned straightforward in the neutral position with

the head anteriorly translated and the neck extended to facilitate venous outflow through the internal jugular veins. The straightforward neutral head position keeps the surgeon oriented toward the surface and deep anatomy. This position can be utilized for the transcortical approach as well. Alternatively, the head can be rotated approximately 20–30 degrees to the left for a right-frontal transcortical approach so that the operative corridor is perpendicular to the floor.

- Proponents of retractor less surgery will perform the anterior hemispheric approach with the patient in a supine position with the shoulders rotated 30–45 degrees toward the side of the approach and the head rotated 90 degrees toward the side of the approach so that the patient's nose is parallel to the floor. This positions the contralateral side up and the ipsilateral side down, which allows gravity to retract the ipsilateral cerebral hemisphere (i.e., the side of the approach) downward, thereby obviating the need for a fixed retractor. This approach also allows the surgeon's hands to operate side-by-side along the long axis of the ventricle rather than front-to-back, as is necessary with the conventional head position.

Frontal Transcortical Approach

The incision is usually a curvilinear or reverse "question mark" shape, starting at the zygomatic process of the temporal bone, extending upward toward the superior temporal line, then curving toward the widow's peak. A subgaleal scalp flap that preserves the temporal fascia is typically sufficient, since the superior temporal line to which the temporalis muscle attaches approximates the inferior frontal sulcus.

After the scalp flap is elevated, a right frontoparietal craniotomy is performed. Before opening the dura, use neuronavigation if available to confirm that the exposure from the craniotomy is sufficient. The dural opening can be C-shaped with the pedicle toward the SSS, or it can be made in a cruciate fashion.

A corticectomy is made through the middle frontal gyrus to create a corridor into the right lateral ventricle. This is most easily performed by first establishing a tract from the cortical surface to the lateral ventricle using either a brain cannula or an external ventricular drain. After the initial tract has been made and the CSF flow confirmed, the transcortical corridor can be expanded to the appropriate width for the size of the lesion.

At this point, a brain retractor system is placed to maintain the transcortical corridor into the ventricle. Typically, multiple retractor blades are necessary to prevent herniation of adjacent parenchyma into the operative field.

Interhemispheric Anterior Transcallosal Approach

The incision is typically a two-thirds or three-quarters bicoronal incision biased toward the side of the approach or a U-shaped incision with two-thirds on one side of the SSS and one-third on the other side. After opening the incision and exposing the periosteum, use retractors to maintain the bony exposure. Neuronavigation can be used to plan the craniotomy flap over the body of the corpus callosum, but in general, a parasagittal craniotomy two-thirds anterior and one-third posterior to the coronal suture will provide sufficient exposure. Patients with one or more large bridging veins as identified on preoperative MRV may require a larger craniotomy in the anteroposterior dimension in order to provide a sufficiently wide interhemispheric operative corridor.

The craniotomy flap should measure 3-by-3 inches, although this may vary based on the venous anatomy. The flap will include the SSS, which should be carefully dissected off of the overlying periosteum, particularly in older patients, in order to avoid sinus injury and postoperative thrombosis, air embolism, and significant intraoperative blood loss. The dural opening is typically made in a C-shape with the pedicle toward the SSS, although one must take great care to preserve any large draining veins entering the dura up to 1 cm lateral to the margin of the SSS. If the dural opening traverses a bridging vein, the opening must be modified to go around, rather than through, the vein to minimize the risk of postoperative venous infarction.

Microsurgical dissection is performed to access the interhemispheric fissure. It may be necessary to sacrifice a bridging vein from the medial cerebral hemisphere to the falx in order to adequately open the interhemispheric fissure; however, carefully consider the attendant risk of venous infarction before taking this approach.

While attempting to reach the corpus callosum, one must take care not to mistake the cingulate gyrus for the corpus callosum, particularly in patients with interdigitating and/or adherent medial hemispheres. The corpus callosum has a distinctive, bright white appearance, but the surgeon should not rule out the possibility of inadvertent entrance into the cingulate gyrus until the ventricle is entered.

Once the corpus callosum is properly identified, attention must be paid to preserving the callosomarginal and pericallosal arteries, the latter of which runs on the surface of the corpus callosum. Once the corpus callosum is adequately exposed, perform the callosotomy, which is generally 2–3 cm in length, to access the ipsilateral lateral ventricle. Ensure, either by visual inspection or using neuronavigation, that the opening in the body of the corpus callosum is made at least 2 cm posterior to the genu. A callosotomy that begins too anteriorly, or one with an anterior rather than perpendicular trajectory, will cross the genu of the corpus callosum without ever encountering the ventricle. Typically, there is enough space between the two pericallosal arteries to perform the callosotomy in between them. However, in cases where the pericallosal arteries run closely side-by-side and/or are eccentric to one side, perform a callosotomy to the side of the vessels. The callosotomy can be enlarged for larger lesions, but note that the risk of a disconnection syndrome is greater for longer callosotomies.

For both the transcortical and interhemispheric approaches, it is important to identify the normal anatomical landmarks after entering the lateral ventricle so as to determine the ventricle's laterality. Visually identify the choroid plexus, the foramen of Monro, the thalamostriate vein, and the septal vein. Sometimes, the lesion can be seen through the foramen of Monro.

Transchoroidal Approach

The transchoroidal approach is based on the dissection of the choroidal fissure to gain access to the roof and middle and posterior portions of the third ventricle. One typically begins the dissection by gently lifting the choroid plexus and then coagulating it. In many cases, bipolar electrocauterization of the choroid plexus alone will sufficiently shrink it to allow for visualization of the choroidal fissure with gentle mobilization of the fornix to the contralateral side. For patients with particularly large choroid plexuses, this approach may require partial resection.

Next, an opening is made in the tenia fornicis from the foramen of Monro to the atrium of the lateral ventricle. This will allow the choroid plexus to be retracted laterally. The superior membrane of the tela choroidea is divided, and the internal cerebral veins and branches of the medial posterior choroidal arteries are exposed. Further dissection is performed between the two internal cerebral veins, since there are typically no bridging vein connections between them. Finally, the last two layers of the roof of the third ventricle, namely the inferior membrane of the tela choroidea and the choroid plexus of the third ventricle, are opened.

The entirety of the transchoroidal approach should be accomplished without sacrificing any neural or vascular structures except the anterior septal vein, which should be ligated to connect the choroidal fissure anteriorly to the foramen of Monro and provide additional working space. Ligation of the septal vein allows lateral mobilization of the ipsilateral thalamostriate and internal cerebral vein complex, which expands the operative corridor (Figure 8.4) (5,19,20).

Subchoroidal Approach

The subchoroidal approach was first described by Hirsch and colleagues (10). In this approach, the roof of the third ventricle is entered between the thalamus and the lateral aspect of the choroid plexus of the lateral ventricle by opening the tenia thalami. The velum interpositum is exposed below the choroid plexus approximately 5–10 mm dorsal to the thalamostriate vein. As a general rule, the surgeon should stay close to the thalamus with minimal elevation of the choroid plexus.

When opening the velum interpositum, one should avoid the internal cerebral vein, which can be identified by its continuity with the thalamostriate vein. After opening the velum, gently retract the choroid plexus of the lateral ventricle medially; the superior choroidal vein will follow the displacement of the choroid plexus medially.

Next, perform microsurgical dissection to open the plane between the thalamus and the ipsilateral internal cerebral vein; open the tela choroidea and the choroid plexus of the third ventricle to enter the ventricle. This opening corresponds to the entire length of the superior portion of the third ventricle between the pineal body and the foramen of Monro.

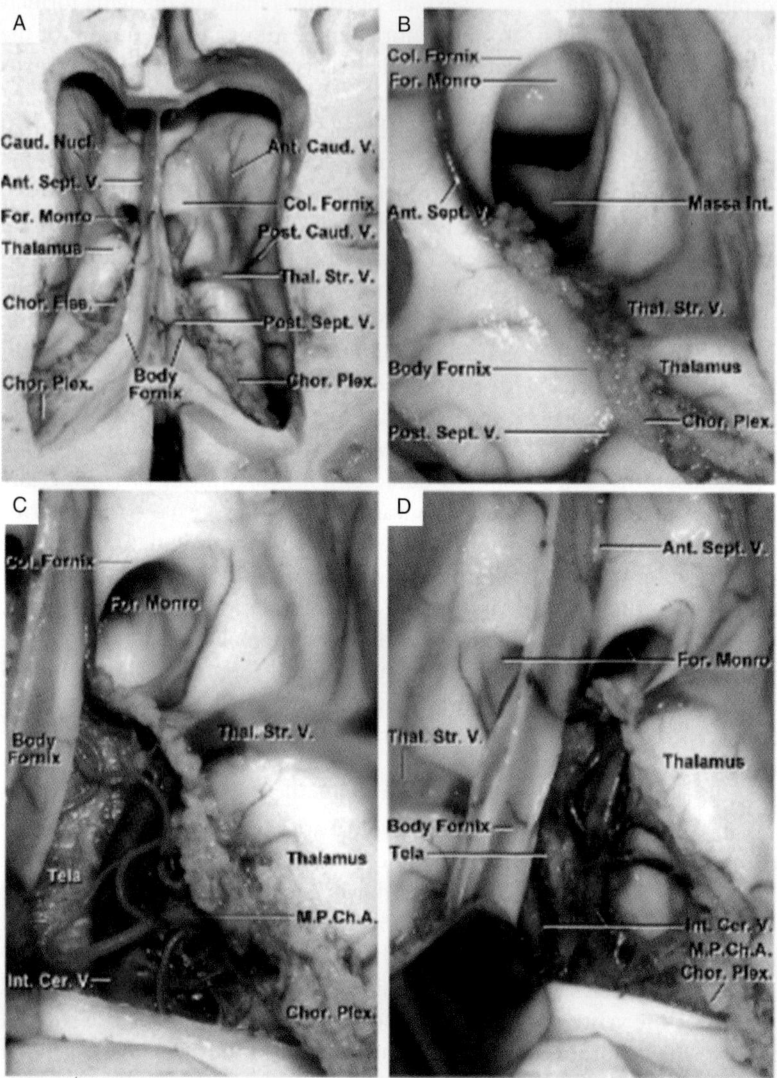

Figure 8.4 Transchoroidal approach to the third ventricle directed along the fornicial side of the choroidal fissure. A, superior view of the frontal horn and body of the lateral ventricle. The left thalamostriate vein passes through the posterior margin of the foramen of Monro, and the right thalamostriate vein passes through the choroidal fissure a few millimeters behind the foramen. The choroidal fissure, located between the thalamus and fornix, is opened by dividing the tenia fornix, which attaches the choroid plexus to the lateral edge of the fornix, leaving the attachment of the choroid plexus to the thalamus undisturbed. B, enlarged view. C, the tenia fornix, which attaches the choroid plexus to the fornix, has been divided and the body of the fornix retracted medially to expose the internal cerebral vein and medial posterior choroidal arteries. The lower layer of tela, which attaches to the striae medullaris thalami and forms the floor of the velum interpositum, is intact. D, the separation of the fornix and choroid plexus has been extended posteriorly to the junction of the atrium and body of the ventricle. The lower layer of tela remains intact. (From Rhoton AL Jr. The supratentorial cranial space: Microsurgical anatomy and surgical approaches. Neurosurgery 51[Suppl 1]: S207–S272, 2002 [9]). Courtesy of the Rhoton Collection, American Association of Neurological Surgeons [AANS]/Neurosurgical Research and Education Foundation [NREF].

The subchoroidal approach is considered safer with respect to the fornix because it is farther away, but it carries a greater risk of injury to the thalamostriate vein (3,5,8,21–24). Notably, some proponents of this approach advocate for routine ligation of the thalamostriate vein at its junction with the internal cerebral vein. While this may be well tolerated in most patients due to the presence of collateral drainage pathways in the deep venous system, the sacrifice of the thalamostriate vein is also associated with potentially devastating thalamic venous infarct. Ligating the thalamostriate vein in the subchoroidal approach is equivalent to ligature of the septal vein in the transchoroidal approach; that is, dividing the thalamostriate vein connects the choroidal fissure anteriorly to the foramen of Monro, and medial mobilization of the ipsilateral septal and internal cerebral vein complex expands the operative corridor of this approach.

Combined Transchoroidal and Subchoroidal Approach

Combining the transchoroidal and subchoroidal approaches has not been adequately described in the literature. This combined approach entails carefully and sequentially performing both the transchoroidal and subchoroidal dissections, aiming to skeletonize the critical structures located in the roof of the third ventricle, with special attention given to preserving the internal cerebral veins (Figure 8.5). This dissection results in wide exposure of the full length of the superior aspect of the third ventricle with access to most of the third ventricle compartments. Furthermore, this exposure excludes inferior angles, but provides feasible negotiation of the target lesion excluding the inferior angles, but allowing feasible negotiation of the target lesion, whether the lesion is located below or between the cerebral veins or around the massa intermedia.

The two critical steps to joining the transchoroidal and subchoroidal approaches are (1) ligation of the septal vein, which allows lateral mobilization of the thalamostriate vein as it drains into the internal cerebral vein (think of the septal vein as a medial tether in this approach), and (2) skeletonizing the ipsilateral internal cerebral vein within the velum interpositum. The combination of these two steps allows lateral transposition of the internal cerebral vein without requiring ligation of the thalamostriate vein and risking venous infarction of the thalamus. The combined approach results in a complete opening of the choroidal fissure from the foramen of Monro to the posterior roof of the third ventricle. As in the transchoroidal approach, the choroid plexus is retracted laterally, although in the combined approach the tenia on both sides of the choroid plexus has been divided. Thus the choroid plexus can be mobilized further laterally to expose the entirety of the choroidal fissure, or it can be resected.

Patients who undergo the combined approach remain at risk of retraction injury to the ipsilateral fornix, since it is not protected by the choroid

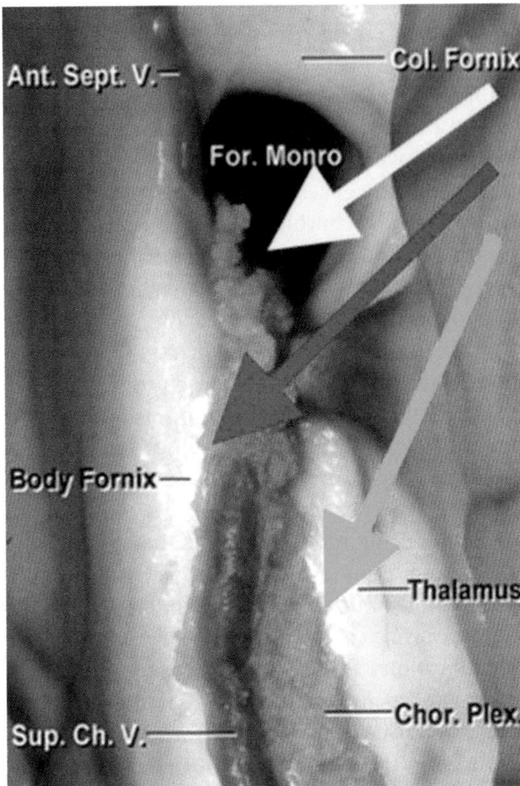

Figure 8.5 Superior view to the foramen of Monro region (Enlarged) shows the combined suprachoroidal and subchoroidal approach. Yellow arrow: pure trans-foraminal approach, Red arrow: supra-choroidal approach: usually called trans-choroidal approach, Green arrow: sub-choroidal approach. Ant., anterior; Ch., choroidal; Chiasm., chiasmatic; Chor., choroid; Col., column; For., foramen; Plex., plexus; Sept., septal; V., vein. (Rhoton AL Jr. The lateral and third ventricles. Neurosurgery. 2002;51(4) (Suppl): 51–219). Courtesy of the Rhoton Collection, American Association of Neurological Surgeons [AANS]/Neurosurgical Research and Education Foundation [NREF].

plexus as in the subchoroidal approach. Therefore, one should conceptualize the combined transchoroidal and subchoroidal approach as a lateral extension of the transchoroidal approach, not as a medial extension of the subchoroidal approach.

Lesion Resection

After the inferior membrane of the tela choroidea and the choroid plexus of the third ventricle have been opened in the midline, the cavity of the third ventricle can be completely visualized. The posterior margin of the foramen of Monro is then dissected from the choroidal fissure while preserving surrounding critical structures. Preserving the thalamostriate and internal cerebral veins bilaterally is crucial for avoiding complications.

A septostomy is usually performed to prevent trapping the ipsilateral ventricle postoperatively; this also allows one to perform a contralateral approach when necessary. In general, lesions within the third ventricle receive blood supply either from the choroidal vessels (e.g., in choroid plexus papillomas and meningiomas) or from the ependymal surface and septum pellucidum (e.g., in gliomas).

Due to the spatial confinements of the anatomically restricted third ventricle, most lesions will be resected in a piecemeal fashion using standard microsurgical techniques. Lesion resection is facilitated by maintaining the dissection plane between the ependyma and the lesion. It is not uncommon for intraventricular tumors to grow slowly and become quite large, in which case the tumor must first be internally debulked. Then the tumor capsule can be inwardly collapsed to allow identification of the interface between the tumor edge and ependyma. The massa intermedia, if present, is usually stretched by the existing hydrocephalus or the tumor. Since the massa intermedia has no reliably demonstrable function, it can be divided if necessary to facilitate resection of the lesion.

After the tumor is resected, it is important to ensure complete hemostasis. Irrigate the ventricles to prevent postoperative hydrocephalus. Leave a ventricular catheter in place for 24 to 48 hours postoperatively to measure ventricular pressure and to demonstrate patency of CSF circulation. Obtain an MRI on the first postoperative day to assess the extent of resection and identify trapped or obstructed ventricles (7,12,19).

Postoperative Considerations

The specific postoperative concerns depend on the pathology of the lesion, but in general, immediately postoperation, the patient should be admitted to an intensive care unit and given frequent neurological assessments. The duration of external ventricular drainage and the need for a permanent CSF shunt depends on the presence of hydrocephalus at presentation, the nature of the causative lesion, the extent of resection, and the absence of postoperative complications (such as intraventricular hemorrhage or ventriculitis). Patients with extensive intraoperative bleeding may require temporary CSF drainage for a longer period postoperatively; these patients are also more likely to require a CSF shunt prior to hospital discharge.

In addition to the routine postoperative brain MRI with and without contrast – which is necessary to assess for immediate postoperative complications and the presence of residual lesion – additional neuroimaging should be performed, as necessary, for new or worsening neurological symptoms. The initial outpatient follow-up usually takes place 10–14 days after surgery to perform suture or staple removal and to assess for any early signs of pseudomeningocele formation. Patients who did not require a CSF shunt during the initial hospitalization should be counseled regarding the signs and symptoms of delayed hydrocephalus, which remains a concern for the first 2–3 months after third-ventricular surgery.

Additionally, a brain MRI with and without contrast should be performed 3 months after surgery to assess for residual or recurrent lesion and to establish a baseline for future follow-up, particularly if there was a known residual tumor or if the pathology is such that eventual tumor recurrence is expected.

Limitations and Complications

Postoperative complications are a consequence of the tumor's location and the surgical approach. Limitations to this approach include a relatively narrow working corridor; the risk of injuring critical neurovascular structures, which limits the amount of retraction; and a limited viewing angle while inside the ventricle.

The main disadvantage of this approach is its proximity to the thalamus, stria medullaris thalami, fornices, and the thalamic vessels. Injury to or division of the thalamostriate vein may result in a venous infarct of the thalamus or basal ganglia and even death.

Possible complications of this approach include the following (3,8,25):

- Stroke (ischemic or hemorrhagic)
- Infection, including superficial wound infection, cerebral abscess, and ventriculitis
- CSF leak manifesting primarily as a pseudomeningocele
- Memory problems due to forniceal injury
- Arousal problems due to thalamic injury

– Hydrocephalus

Illustrative Case

The following case was previously published by the senior author in the *Journal of Neurosciences in Rural Practice* (15).

A 53-year-old male presented with signs of increased intracranial pressure (headache, nausea, vomiting, and seizure). Neuroimaging showed a peripherally enhancing, hemorrhagic lesion attached to the superior aspect of the third ventricle and the septum pellucidum. The decision was made to resect the lesion using a frontal transcortical combined transchoroidal-subchoroidal approach. After performing the transcortical approach to the right lateral ventricle, the anterior portion of the lesion protruding through the foramen of Monro was dissected off of the fornix medially and off of the caudate laterally. The ipsilateral choroidal fissure was then opened widely, cutting both the taenia fornicis medial to the choroid plexus and the taenia thalami lateral to the choroid plexus. The right internal cerebral vein was skeletonized and the anterior septal vein was divided, which allowed lateral transposition of the right internal cerebral vein. This completed the combined transchoroidal and subchoroidal approach to the third ventricle (Figure 8.6). A septostomy was performed, and a contralateral transchoroidal approach was performed to further increase visualization and facilitate dissection of the lesion off of the neurovascular structures on the left side. The lesion was removed in a piecemeal fashion using standard microsurgical techniques, and gross total resection was achieved. The thalamostriate and internal cerebral veins were preserved bilaterally.

Postoperative MRI showed no evidence of residual enhancing tumor (Figure 8.7). The patient had an uncomplicated postoperative course. Histopathological analysis of the lesion revealed a hemorrhagic epithelial cyst (7).

Key Points

- Understanding the surgical anatomy of the lateral and third ventricles is crucial to readily accessing and successfully resecting lesions of the third ventricle.
- For large lesions located in the middle and posterior parts of the third ventricle, the transcortical combined transchoroidal and subchoroidal approach can be used to provide maximum exposure of the third ventricle while preserving the critical thalamostriate and internal cerebral veins.
- The two critical steps in the combined transchoroidal-subchoroidal approach are (1) ligation of the septal vein and (2) skeletonizing the ipsilateral internal cerebral vein. Together, these two maneuvers allow mobilization and lateral transposition of the ipsilateral internal cerebral vein, which allows the widest possible opening of the choroidal fissure after the tenia fornicis and thalami have been divided.
- Meticulous preoperative planning, especially regarding patient-specific anatomy, can significantly improve the safety of this procedure.

References

1. Horwitz NH. Walter Edward Dandy (1886–1946). *Neurosurgery*. 1997 Jan 1;**40**(1):211–15.
2. Yamamoto I, Rhoton Jr AL, Peace DA. Microsurgery of the third ventricle, Part 1: Microsurgical anatomy. *Neurosurgery*. 1981 Mar 1;**8** (3):334–56.
3. Wen HT, Rhoton AL, de Oliveira E Jr. Transchoroidal approach to the third ventricle: an anatomic study of the choroidal fissure and its clinical application. *Neurosurgery*. 1998 Jun 1;**42**(6):1205–17.
4. Carota A, Rizzo E, Broways P, Calabrese P. Pure anterograde memory deficit due to secondary lymphoma of the fornix. *European Neurology*. 2013;**70**(3–4):242.
5. Pendl G, Öztürk E, Haselsberger K. Surgery of tumours of the lateral ventricle. *Acta Neurochirurgica*. 1992 Jun 1;**116**(2–4):128–36.
6. Kasowski HJ, Nahed BV, Piepmeier JM. Transcallosal transchoroidal approach to tumors of the third ventricle. *Operative Neurosurgery*. 2005 Oct **1**;57(suppl 4):ONS-361.
7. Fonseca RB, Black PM, Azevedo Filho H. Approaches to the third ventricle. *Arquivos Brasileiros de Neurocirurgia: Brazilian Neurosurgery*. 2012 Mar;**31**(01):3–9.
8. Fujii K, Lenkey C, Rhoton Jr AL. Microsurgical anatomy of the choroidal arteries: Lateral and third ventricles. *Journal of Neurosurgery*. 1980 Feb;**52** (2):165–88.

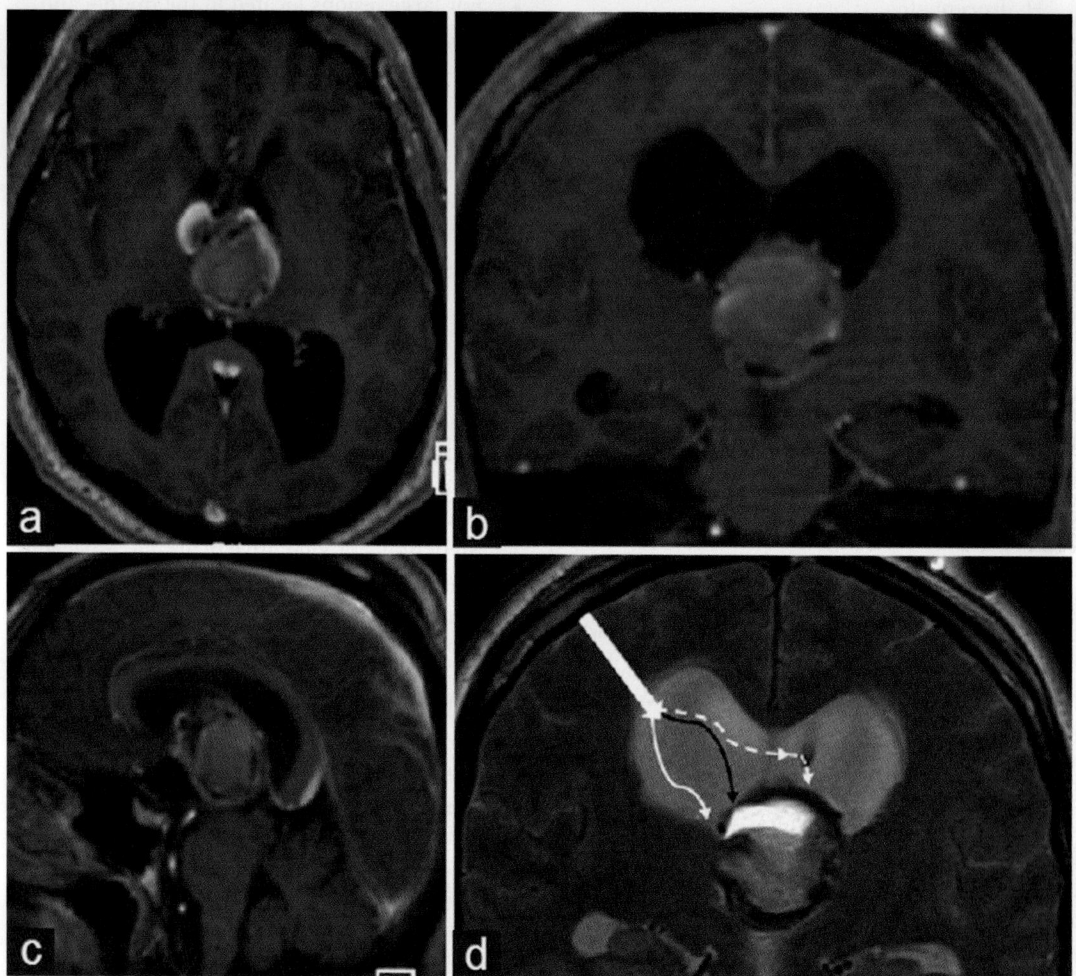

Figure 8.6 Preoperative brain MRI, T1-weighted sequence with gadolinium contrast, (a) axial, (b) coronal, and (c) sagittal views, shows a 3.7 × 3.6 × 3.5 cm, hemorrhagic mass with heterogeneous peripheral enhancement, (d) T2-weighted sequence, coronal view, shows the surgical approach; after a frontal transcortical approach to the right lateral ventricle, (blocked white arrow) an ipsilateral combined transchoroidal (solid black arrow) and subchoroidal (solid white arrow) approach to the third ventricle is performed, and further exposure of the lesion is done by septostomy and contralateral transchoroidal approach (dashed white arrow). Note: This figure was previously published in the *Journal of Neurosciences in Rural Practice.* (15)

9. Villani RM, Tomei G. Approach to tumors of the third ventricle. In Schmidek HH, Roberts DW, eds., *Schmidek and Sweet's Operative Neurosurgical Techniques: Indications, Methods, and Results*, 5th ed. Philadelphia: Saunders Elsevier; 2006:772–85.
10. Hirsch JF, Zouaoui A, Renier D, Pierre-Kahn A. A new surgical approach to the third ventricle with interruption of the striothalamic vein. *Acta Neurochirurgica*. 1979 Sep 1;**47**(3–4):135–47.
11. Rhoton AL Jr. The lateral and third ventricles. *Neurosurgery*. 2002;**51**(4 Suppl): S207–71.
12. Viale GL, Turtas S. The sub choroid approach to the third ventricle. *Surgical Neurology*. 1980 Jul;**14** (1):71–4.
13. Cikla U, Swanson KI, Tumturk A, Keser N, Uluc K, Cohen-Gadol A, Baskaya MK. Microsurgical resection of tumors of the lateral and third ventricles: operative corridors for difficult-to-reach lesions. *Journal of Neuro-oncology*. 2016 Nov 1;**130**(2):331–40.
14. Ito Y, Inoue T, Tamura A, Tsutsumi K. Interhemispheric transchoroidal approach to resect third ventricular teratoma. Neurosurgical focus. 2016 Jan;40(Video Suppl 1):1.
15. Ding D, Furneaux CE. Combined transchoroidal and subchoroidal approach for resection of a large hemorrhagic epithelial cyst: Expanding the operative corridor to the third ventricle. *Journal of Neurosciences in Rural Practice*. 2017 Jan;**8**(1):145.

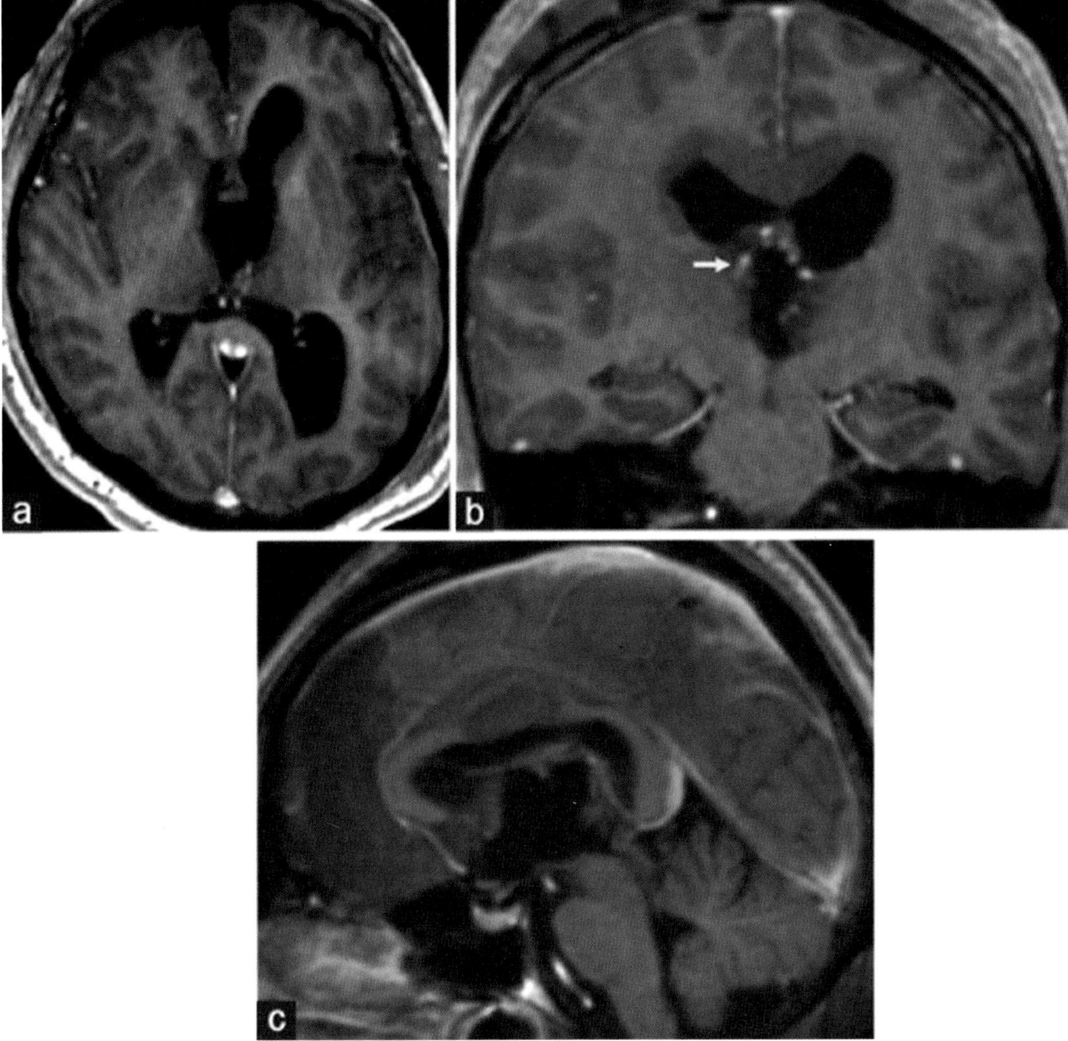

Figure 8.7 Postoperative magnetic resonance imaging brain, T1-weighted sequence with gadolinium contrast, (a) axial, (b) coronal, and (c) sagittal views, no residual tumor is found, (b) the coronal view shows an intact right thalamostriate vein (arrow). Note: This figure was previously published in the *Journal of Neurosciences in Rural Practice*. (15)

16. Anderson RC, Ghatan S, Feldstein NA. Surgical approaches to tumors of the lateral ventricle. *Neurosurgery Clinics*. 2003 Oct 1;**14**(4):509–25.

17. Yasargil MG, Abdulrauf SI. Surgery of intraventricular tumors. *Neurosurgery*. 2008;**62**(6 Suppl 3):1029–40.

18. Finch NW, Ding D, Oldfield EH, Druzgal J. Agenesis of anterior falx cerebri in patient with planned interhemispheric approach to third ventricle mass. *World Neurosurgery*. 2018 Jan 1;**109**:162–4.

19. Petridis, Athanasios K. Commentary. *Journal of Neurosciences in Rural Practice* 2017; **8**(1):147.

20. Türe U, Yaşargil MG, Al-Mefty O. The transcallosal–transforaminal approach to the third ventricle with regard to the venous variations in this region. *Journal of Neurosurgery*. 1997 Nov;**87**(5):706–15.

21. Lang J. Topographic anatomy of preformed intracranial spaces. In *Minimally Invasive Neurosurgery I*. Vienna: Springer; 1992: 1–10.

22. Tubbs RS, Oakes P, Maran IS, Salib C, Loukas M. The foramen of Monro: a review of its anatomy, history, pathology, and surgery. *Child's Nervous System*. 2014 Oct 1;**30**(10):1645–9.

23. Cai Q, Wang J, Wang L, Deng G, Chen Q, Chen Z. A classification of lesions around interventricular foramen and its clinical value. *International Journal of Clinical and Experimental Pathology*. 2015;**8**(9):9950.

24. Taghva A, Liu CY, Apuzzo ML. Transcallosal surgery of lesions affecting the third ventricle: basic principles. In *Schmidek and Sweet Operative Neurosurgical Techniques*. 6th ed. Amsterdam: Elsevier; 2012: 339–50.

25. Patel P, Cohen-Gadol AA, Boop F, Klimo Jr P. Technical strategies for the transcallosal transforaminal approach to third ventricle tumors: expanding the operative corridor. *Journal of Neurosurgery: Pediatrics*. 2014 Oct;**14**(4):365–71.

Combined Orbitofrontal Craniotomy and Direct Orbital Decompression

Viraj J. Mehta, Lain Hermes Gonzalez Quarante, James A. Garrity, and Pradeep Mettu

Introduction

The orbitofrontal craniotomy combined with a direct orbitotomy allows for broad surgical access to the anterior cranial fossa and orbit. This combined approach may be beneficial for pathologies ranging from severe Graves' orbitopathy to various orbital tumors to lesions affecting the skull base, such as sphenoid wing meningioma. Various techniques in orbitofrontal craniotomies have been described by clinicians, with more modern approaches utilizing an endoscopic approach. Jane et al. first described a supraorbital modification to the frontal craniotomy in 1982 (1). This technique allowed for exposure not only to intracranial lesions but also to nearly the entire orbit except the floor. Delashaw et al. further developed this technique to include a frontal bone flap that incorporated the supraorbital rim (2). Many techniques for orbitofrontal craniotomy have been modified and have evolved from these previous descriptions. Advantages of an orbitofrontal approach may include more direct access to structures in the anterior cranial fossa and parasellar region, often with less brain retraction (1,3). The orbitofrontal approach can be especially beneficial when combined with one of the myriad techniques for an orbitotomy to access nearly the entire orbit (4–6).

Indications

Indications for a combined orbitofrontal craniotomy with direct orbitotomy are truly varied and largely dependent on the exact location, size, and nature of the lesion. The surgeon should adhere to a guiding principle for the safest, most direct route to the pathology, which may require a multidisciplinary approach to access large, complex, or deep orbital lesions. Jane et al. described their supraorbital modification to the frontal craniotomy to approach intracranial lesions such as anterior communicating artery aneurysms, pituitary tumors, and other parasellar lesions, as well as orbital tumors (1). Paluzzi et al. described an algorithm for surgical access to the globe and generally reserved a craniotomy and/or lateral orbitotomy for lesions lateral to the supraorbital notch (4). Anterior orbital lesions may best be accessed through a transorbital approach, while posterior orbital lesions may be more amenable to a neurosurgical approach, although the distinction is rather fluid. Examples of such orbital lesions that may benefit from a combined approach include optic nerve gliomas and meningiomas, sphenoid wing meningiomas, hemangiomas, and neurofibromas (7,8).

Orbital decompression in patients with active Graves' orbitopathy is generally reserved for patients with severe proptosis resulting in corneal decompensation or optic neuropathy (Figure 9.1 and 9.3) (9). The goal of surgery in these patients is to increase the effective volume of the orbit, and many patients achieve significant proptosis reduction and improvement of optic neuropathy from two- or three-wall decompressions with or without orbital fat removal (5). In very severe cases with optic neuropathy resistant to other treatments, a combined approach to decompress the orbital roof and lateral wall may be beneficial (Figure 9.2). A neurosurgical approach to the orbital roof decompression in severe Graves' orbitopathy was first described by Howard C. Naffziger in 1932 and has since been modified and adapted (10). One case series described 11 patients who had all failed medical therapy and underwent four-wall decompression with a transcranial approach for the orbital roof. An average reduction of 7 mm in proptosis was noted, along with significant improvements in vision (11,12). Comparatively, a large series by

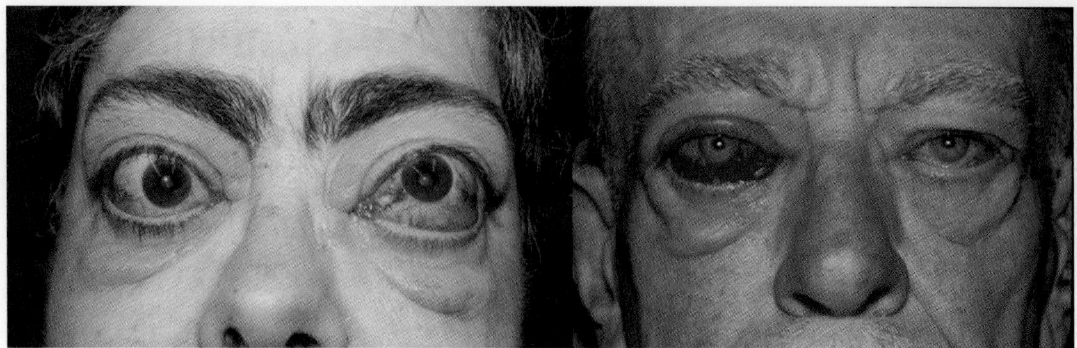

Figure 9.1 Both left and right photographs show patients who presented with active Graves' orbitopathy, proptosis, and severe optic neuropathy which persisted after transantral orbital decompression. In addition, note significant periocular edema and conjunctival injection (present in both patients), as well as severe conjunctival chemosis (present in the patient on the right). Patients presenting with such severe disease are candidates for combined orbito-frontal craniotomy for aggressive decompression to preserve vision.

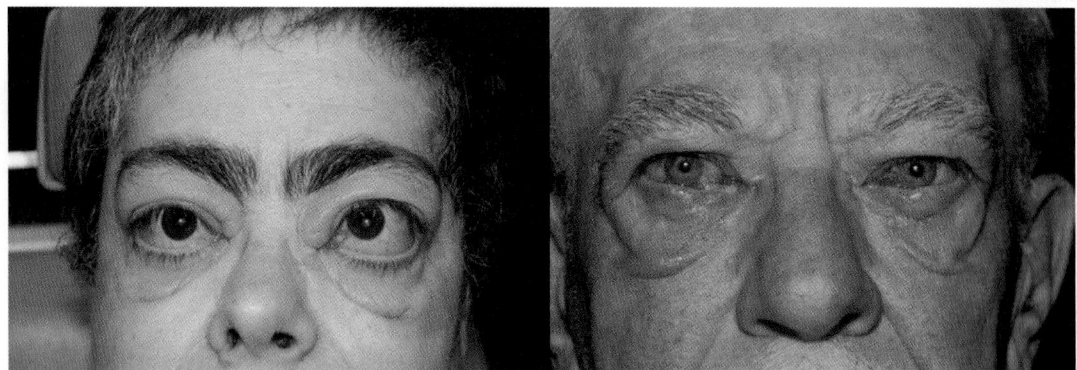

Figure 9.2 Post-operative (combined transfrontal and orbital decompression) photographs of both patients presented in Figure 9.1. Both patients had initially underdone a transantral decompression, but remained symptomatic and proptotic. The patient on the right then underwent bilateral orbito-frontal decompressions, while the patient on the left underwent unilateral orbito-frontal decompression. Both had a significant reduction in proptosis, improvement in corneal exposure, and improvement in optic neuropathy after the surgery.

Garrity et al. described an average proptosis reduction of 4.7 mm with only a transantral (antral-ethmoidal) approach (13). A transfrontal approach for orbital decompression after the failure of a transantral decompression has also been described to improve visual outcomes (14).

Contraindications/Alternative Approaches

While indeed a powerful procedure for achieving broad access to the orbit, a combined orbitofrontal with direct orbitotomy may not be the optimal approach for all orbital pathology. Many orbital lesions, particularly those extending superiorly, laterally, and inferiorly, may be anterior enough to be approached solely by an oculoplastic surgery approach (i.e., a lateral orbitotomy) with far less morbidity. In addition, a medial orbitotomy through an eyelid or caruncle incision, possibly combined with nasal endoscopy, is sufficient for lesions in the medial orbit (15,16).

Preoperative Planning

The optimal surgical approach is one that targets the lesion using the most direct route while minimizing morbidity. This evaluation, as for any condition, begins with a thorough history and physical examination. The nature of the lesion and goals of the surgery should then be further elucidated. For example, does the surgical plan call for total resection, biopsy, or debulking?

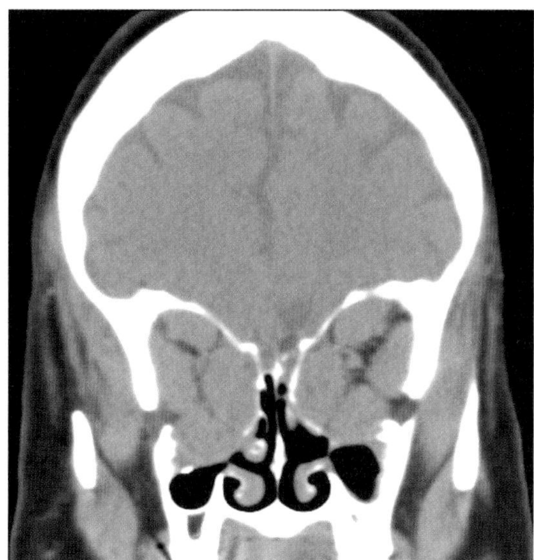

Figure 9.3 Coronal CT of a patient with severe Graves' orbitopathy. Note the extremely large rectus muscles compressing the optic nerves. This patient underwent bilateral transantral decompression but had persistent optic neuropathy. In such cases, an orbito-frontal craniotomy to decompress the roof and lateral wall of the orbit is indicated as salvage therapy.

What are the goals of the patient? Determining the answer to these is critical to choosing the appropriate technique.

Imaging plays a crucial role in the preoperative evaluation of a patient undergoing surgical intervention. Computerized tomography (CT) and magnetic resonance imaging (MRI) are essential for determining important characteristics of the lesion as well as determining the precise size, location, and intraorbital/intracranial relationships (Figure 9.4). CT studies for stereotactic navigation may be beneficial for complex lesions. MRI studies may be particularly helpful in evaluating lesions in the orbital apex, optic canal, anterior cranial fossa, or at the orbito-cranial junction.

Surgical Anatomy

• Orbitofrontal Craniotomy

From a hemicoronal incision or from various periorbital incisions (Figure 9.5), a craniotomy can be performed for access to the anterior cranial

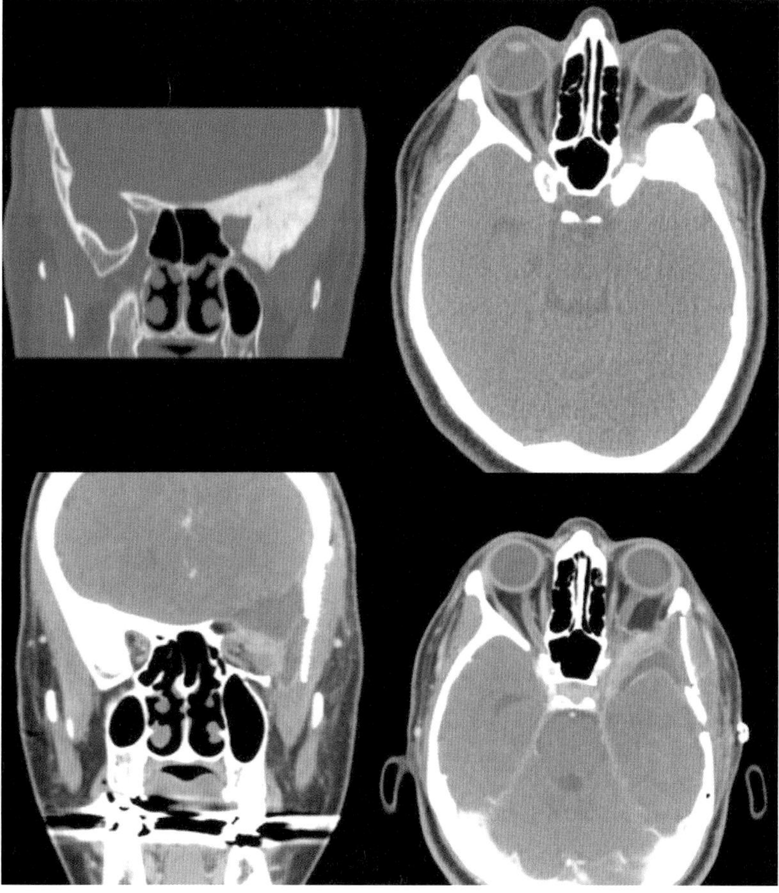

Figure 9.4 CT scan of a 41-year-old female with a history of progressive left optic neuropathy. She was found to have left optic nerve edema on ophthalmic exam. This scan shows the wide extent of her sphenoid wing meningioma in the top two pre-operative images. The intracranial-intraorbital relationship of the tumor is evident. The patient has notable optic nerve compression at the orbital apex. Postoperative CT scan (bottom 2 images) demonstrates resection of the tumor with decompression of the nerve at the orbital apex.

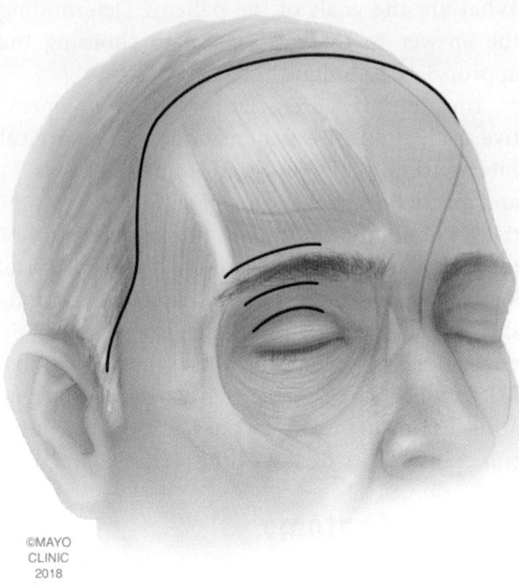

Figure 9.5 Schematic illustration showing the most frequently used skin incisions for the combined orbito-frontal approach. Depending on characteristics such as the size and location of the lesion, there are a variety of options for the incision used. Options include hemicoronal or bicoronal (the uppermost incision), supra-brow, sub-brow, eyelid crease, and periorbital. The periorbital incisions can be extended along relaxed skin tension lines to the lateral canthus and toward the helix of the ear for greater access to the lateral orbital wall and zygoma. An alternate incision includes a frontal crease incision, which is more commonly used in elderly patients (not shown here).

fossa or orbital apex or for greater access to the orbital roof. The periosteum is elevated and the scalp flap is reflected to give sufficient exposure. A burr hole is made a few millimeters above the frontosphenoidal suture, and a craniotome is used to create the bone flap, which may be extended to remove the superior orbital rim up to the frontozygomatic suture. The bone flap can be removed en bloc with the orbital roof. If necessary, the dura is opened in a semilunar fashion and reflected inferiorly along the orbital base (Figure 9.6) (3,8). From here, the dissection can be performed under microscopic or endoscopic visualization to the point of interest. For lesions in which a corticectomy is needed along the basal frontal surface, basal cisterns such as the carotid-ophthalmic, lamina terminalis, or Sylvian cisterns may be opened to drain cerebrospinal fluid for brain relaxation (17). Alternatively, a lumbar drain with or without early administration of mannitol may also be beneficial (18). It is also important to note that the gyrus rectus, olfactory sulcus, and orbital gyri are respectively located on the medial to lateral inferior surface of the frontal lobe.

Superior Orbitotomy

In addition to the incision described previously, the orbit may be accessed through a variety of direct incisions. A suprabrow, subbrow, or eyelid crease incision extending from the supraorbital notch as the medial border to the lateral canthus or beyond may be the preferred approach when combined with an orbitofrontal craniotomy (Figure 9.5). For both incisions, it is important to carry the incision through the skin and orbicularis oculi muscle (pars orbitalis, if creating an eyebrow incision, and pars palpebralis, if creating an eyelid crease incision) without violation of the orbital septum to prevent fat herniation. The dissection from here can be carried to the superior orbital rim, where the arcus marginalis is identified. The arcus marginalis is the periosteal attachment of the orbital septum along the orbital rim. The arcus marginalis is incised, and the periorbita is carefully reflected away from the roof of the orbit. The periosteum can also be elevated superiorly toward the frontalis to widely expose the frontal bone. Care must be taken near the orbital apex to protect the frontal nerve, which divides into the supraorbital and supratrochlear nerves. The supraorbital nerve then exits the orbit from the supraorbital foramen or notch, lies in close proximity to the periosteum, and runs deep to the orbicularis, corrugator, and frontalis muscles. As the supraorbital nerve travels superiorly along the forehead, its branches become more superficial and penetrate the muscle to the subcutaneous plane (19). Once the periorbita is sufficiently reflected away from the orbital roof, it can be incised appropriately to expose the orbital lesion, or for fat mobilization or removal in cases of Graves' orbitopathy.

For a medial intraconal lesion, the orbital fat can be gently retracted. The trochlear nerve to the superior oblique muscle exits the superior orbital fissure, travels outside the annulus of Zinn, and can be identified passing medially and above the levator and superior rectus muscles. It penetrates the superior oblique along the posterior third of

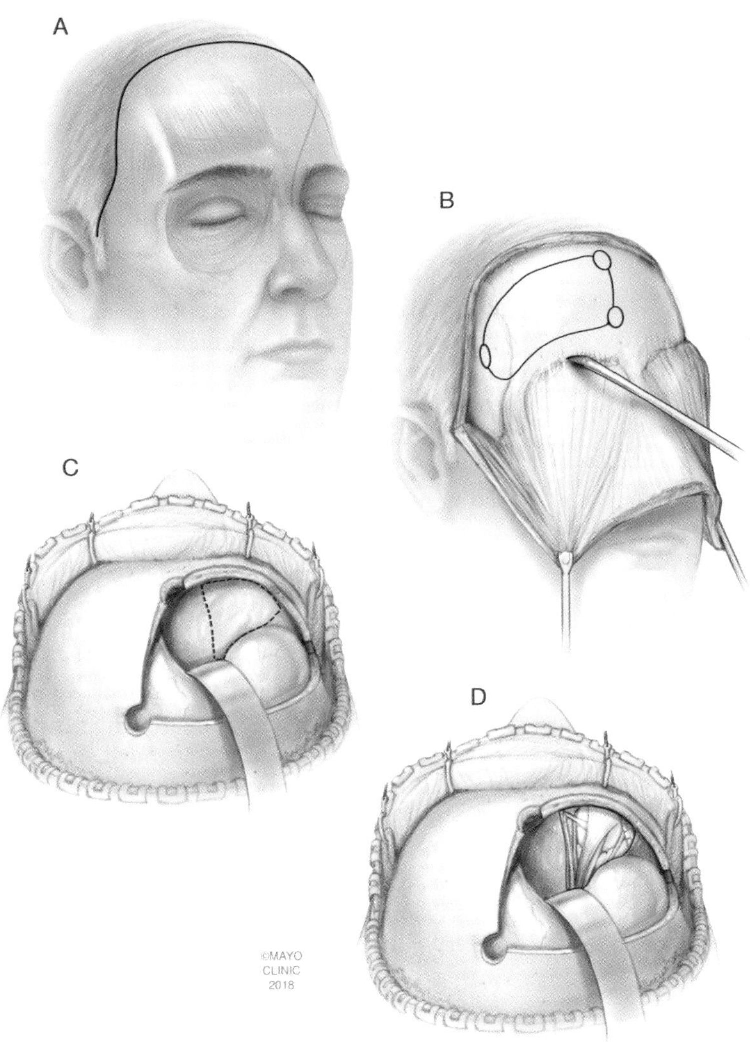

Figure 9.6 Schematic illustration showing the main steps of the orbitofrontal craniotomy via a hemi/bicoronal incision. (A) The incision is usually made behind the hairline for cosmesis and follows the shape of the widow's peak. (B) Bone is exposed after meticulous subcutaneous dissection. The number and location of burr holes may vary depending on the patient characteristics such as age, frontal sinus anatomy, and previous surgeries. (C) After the craniotomy is performed, retraction of the frontal lobe exposes the orbital roof, which may be drilled to approach the periorbita. Such retraction can be done in an extradural or intradural fashion. (D) Illustration showing the view of the orbital compartment obtained after exposure and drilling of the orbital roof.

the muscle. The superomedial intraconal space can be accessed by gently retracting the superior rectus and superior oblique muscles.

The superolateral intraconal space can be accessed by retracting the superior rectus medially and the lateral rectus inferiorly. Careful retraction of the fat can again help in identifying a deep lesion; however, there are critical structures that should be identified as early as possible in the dissection so care can be taken when navigating around these structures. The superior ophthalmic vein travels just medially and then inferiorly to the superior rectus muscle in the anterior orbit to the mid-orbit and then courses along the lateral border as it enters the superior orbital fissure and continues into the cavernous sinus. One must also be cognizant of the ciliary ganglion that resides along the lateral aspect of the optic nerve, which can be found approximately 1 cm anterior to the optic canal. Parasympathetic fibers synapsing at the ciliary ganglion can be damaged, thus causing mydriasis.

Also important to note is the course of the ophthalmic artery, which carries the major blood supply to the globe and orbit. The ophthalmic artery originates from the internal carotid artery just beneath the intracranial portion of the optic nerve and travels within the subdural space. The artery enters the optic canal inferior to the optic nerve then enters the orbit inferolateral to the optic nerve. From here, the branching of the ophthalmic artery can vary. It generally crosses over, but may cross under, the optic nerve to course medially, where it gives off the central retinal artery, usually as the first branch. Other major lateral or medial branches of the posterior ciliary arteries may also be identified (8,19).

Additional exposure to the lateral orbit can be gained by extending the subbrow or eyelid crease incision laterally over the lateral canthus along relaxed skin tension lines. The lateral orbital rim and the superior rim may be removed for greater access.

Surgical Technique

Neurosurgical Procedure (Figure 9.6)

- The patient is placed under general anesthesia and intubated with an endotracheal tube.
- The head is positioned 15–30 degrees to the contralateral side of the craniotomy site.
- The frontal craniotomy is performed.
- The dura is elevated from the orbital roof.
- The orbital roof is opened and removed, extending medially to the ethmoid sinus, anteriorly to the frontal sinus, and posteriorly to the optic foramen.
- The lateral wall (frontal bone, greater wing of sphenoid, and zygoma) are drilled down.
- After completion of the procedure, the dura of the frontal lobe is returned to its native position over the orbital contents.
- The bone flap is replaced.

• Oculoplastics/Orbital Surgical Procedure

- The periorbita is inspected using two cotton-tipped dissectors.
- The frontal nerve, which can often be seen through the periorbita, is identified.
- Longitudinal incisions are made both medial and lateral to the frontal nerve with the anterior extent near the posterior aspect of the globe.
- When the orbit is under pressure, as is the case in severe Graves' orbitopathy, fat will typically readily prolapse once the periorbita has been opened. In such cases, perform the following:
- Mobilize the fat such that it adequately protrudes through the incisions to decrease pressure on the optic nerve.
- If needed, the fat can also carefully be excised while ensuring hemostasis to reduce the risk of postoperative retrobulbar hemorrhage.
- Intraconal tumors can also be exposed for removal from this incision with basic microsurgical techniques under direct visualization.

Complications

Orbital Complications

Complications can vary, depending on the disease process being treated and the technical demands of the case. In cases of severe Graves' orbitopathy, for which a combined orbitofrontal craniotomy with direct orbitotomy may be indicated, there may be an incomplete treatment of the proptosis. To prevent this, it is important to review preoperative imaging and to correlate these images with the intraoperative anatomy to ensure sufficient bony removal. Residual proptosis may also be a result of inadequate fenestration of the periorbita, particularly in patients with expanded fat compartments, compared with patients with primarily enlarged muscle compartments. In some cases, it may be required to augment the procedure with orbital fat removal to improve the proptosis.

When working within the orbit there is also the risk of diplopia due to iatrogenic extraocular muscle injury. Another potential complication is nerve injury. Various nerves travel around and within the orbit. Cautious dissection should be performed near the supraorbital neurovascular bundle and supratrochlear nerve superiorly. Laterally, when working on the external surface of the orbit, caution should be taken near the temporal branch of the facial nerve. When working within the lateral orbit, there is a possibility of injury to the zygomaticofacial and zygomaticotemporal neurovascular bundles, which can result in temporary numbness. In the dissections outlined in this chapter, it would be unusual to encounter the external aspects of the zygomaticofacial and zygomaticotemporal neurovascular bundles.

Finally, there is a risk of retrobulbar hemorrhage. Perioperative anticoagulant and antiplatelet agents should be held for as long as safely possible. Wound healing generally begins immediately with clot formation and hemostasis. The initial clots continue to evolve and slowly resorb until approximately five days postoperatively, when fibroblasts are recruited to the site and maximum collagen production begins (20). If possible, consider delaying the resumption of anticoagulant or antiplatelets until after this time to reduce the risk of delayed hemorrhages.

Neurosurgical Complications

In a large study by Rolston et al. of more than 10,000 patients undergoing intracranial operations, two of the most frequently described complications were blood loss requiring transfusion (5.4%) and reoperation within 30 days (7.3%). Another potential complication of cranial surgery is the inability to wean the patient from mechanical ventilation for more than 48 hours after the surgery, which was noted in 7.6% of patients in the described study. It was also noted that African Americans were significantly more likely to experience any complication compared with Caucasians, with a relative risk of 1.24 (21). Racial and socioeconomic disparities in surgical complications have been described across various surgical specialties ranging from ophthalmology to otolaryngology (22,23). The sources of these disparities are not entirely clear, though it is important to note the potential for higher complication rates in minorities. The study by Rolston et al. evaluated all intracranial surgeries from the American College of Surgeons National Surgical Quality Improvement Program database. Limitations such as the lack of specificity do exist when utilizing a national database, although this data still offers helpful insight into potential complications.

Another potential complication associated with orbitofrontal craniotomy includes cerebrospinal fluid (CSF) leak. Large sinuses may also be a potential concern; in cases where the sinuses have been entered, CSF leak may occur due to inadequate dural closure. This can be prevented with adequate reconstruction. Dural closure in a watertight fashion is of paramount importance. Direct closure with non-resorbable suture is the preferable option. Should the dural edges not be directly suturable, autologous pericranial or myofascial grafts may be utilized. Heterologous dural grafts (suturable and non-suturable) and biologic glues are alternatives, although economic implications and the risk of developing a foreign body reaction should be taken into account. Cranialization and/or sealing of opened sinuses (especially the frontal sinus) are also crucial to conduct when indicated in order to minimize the risk of postoperative misadventures other than CSF leak, such as epidural/subdural empyema, brain abscess, osteomyelitis, or chronic infections.

Postoperative Considerations

In addition to typical postoperative wound care, frequent neurological and vision checks are important to detect any potential complications early. Postoperative nausea and vomiting (PONV) is also a common concern. Latz et al. described a series of 229 patients in which the overall incidence of PONV was 47% after craniotomy, while other studies report rates ranging from 10% to 74%. Inadequate nausea control may be harmful because of the risk of intracranial bleeding. Perioperative nausea control should begin with prophylaxis such as preoperative dexamethasone and continued with postoperative anti-emetics (24,25).

Other general postoperative considerations include elevating the patient's head to help improve swelling, avoiding strenuous activity, avoiding alcohol, and encouraging early ambulation as tolerated. Patients should also be advised of the signs and symptoms of potential complications such as fevers, intolerable nausea or vomiting, severe pain, significant changes in vision, loss of bladder or bowel function, or sudden changes in mentation. Very rarely, patients may also describe postoperative globe pulsations that are typically not problematic and resolve spontaneously over time.

Key Points and Clinical Pearls

The surgical management of complex intraorbital and intracranial lesions or Graves' orbitopathy requires precise planning and often collaboration with other subspecialties to ensure optimal outcomes. The key points to a successful outcome are highlighted:

- Begin with a comprehensive history and physical exam.
- Perform preoperative imaging with CT and/or MRI.
- Identify the nature and precise location of the lesion as well as the goals of surgery (biopsy versus resection versus debulking/ decompression).
- Discuss potential complications with the patient.

- Arrange preoperative medical evaluation for risk stratification and management of any anticoagulant or antiplatelet medications.
- Ensure proper patient positioning in the operating room.
- Discuss nausea/vomiting prophylaxis with the anesthesia team.
- Ensure that all instrumentation is available and set up appropriately.
- Be flexible intraoperatively, and change your preoperative surgical plan as needed.
- Ensure adequate decompression in cases of Graves' orbitopathy; at times, orbital fat excision may be necessary.
- Postoperatively, closely monitor vision and neurological status.
- Discuss signs and symptoms of complications with the patient and his or her family.

References

1. Jane JA, Park TS, Pobereskin LH, Winn HR, Butler AB. The supraorbital approach: technical note. *Neurosurgery*. 1982;**11**(4):537–42.
2. Delashaw JB, Jane JA, Kassell NF, Luce C. Supraorbital craniotomy by fracture of the anterior orbital roof. *J Neurosurg*. 1993;**79**(4):615–18.
3. Shanno G, Maus M, Bilyk J, et al. Image-guided transorbital roof craniotomy via a suprabrow approach: a surgical series of 72 patients. *Neurosurgery*. 2001;**48**(3):559–68.
4. Paluzzi A, Gardner PA, Fernandez-Miranda JC, et al. Round-the-clock surgical access to the orbit. *J Neurol Surgery, Part B: Skull Base*. 2015;**76**(1):12–24.
5. Wang Y, Tooley AA, Mehta VJ, Garrity JA, Harrison AR, Mettu P. Thyroid Orbitopathy. *Int Ophthalmol Clin*. 2018;**58**(2):137–79.
6. Srinivasan A, Bilyk JR. Transcranial approaches to the orbit. *Int Ophthalmol Clin*. 2018;**58**(2):101–10.
7. Bejjani GK, Cockerham KP, Kennerdel JS, Maroon JC. A reappraisal of surgery for orbital tumors. Part I: extraorbital approaches. *Neurosurg Focus*. 2001;**10**(5):1–6.
8. Abuzayed B, Kucukyuruk B, Tanriover N, et al. Transcranial superior orbitotomy for the treatment of intraorbital intraconal tumors: surgical technique and long-term results in single institute. *Neurosurg Rev*. 2012;**35**(4):573–82.
9. Bradley EA, Bartley GB, Garrity JA. Surgical management of Graves' ophthalmopathy. In Bahn RS, ed. *Thyroid Eye Disease*. Boston: Springer; 2001: 219–33.
10. Naffziger HC. The surgical treatment of progressive exophthalmos following thyroidectomy. *J Am Med Assoc*. 1932;**99**(8):638.
11. Stranc M, West M. A four-wall orbital decompression for dysthyroid orbitopathy. *J Neurosurg*. 1988;**68**(5):671–7.
12. Linnet J, Hegedus L, Bjerre P. Results of a neurosurgical two-wall orbital decompression in the treatment of severe thyroid associated ophthalmopathy. *Acta Ophthalmol Scand*. 2001;**79**(1):49–52.
13. Garrity JA, Fatourechi V, Bergstralh EJ, et al. Results of transantral orbital decompression in 428 patients with severe Graves' ophthalmopathy. *Am J Ophthalmol*. 1993;**116**(5):533–47.
14. Fatourechi V, Bartley GB, Garrity JA, Bergstralh EJ, Ebersold MJ, Gorman CA. Transfrontal orbital decompression after failure of transantral decompression in optic neuropathy of Graves' disease. *Mayo Clin Proc*. 1993;**68**(6):552–5.
15. Maroon JC, Kennerdell JS. Surgical approaches to the orbit: indications and techniques. *J Neurosurg*. 1984;**60**(6):1226–35.
16. Cockerham KP, Bejjani GK, Kennerdell JS, Maroon JC. Surgery for orbital tumors. Part II: transorbital approaches. *Neurosurg Focus*. 2001;**10**(5):E3.
17. Ditzel Filho LFS, McLaughlin N, Bresson D, Solari D, Kassam AB, Kelly DF. Supraorbital eyebrow craniotomy for removal of intraaxial frontal brain tumors: a technical note. *World Neurosurg*. 2014;**81**(2):348–56.
18. Owusu Boahene KD, Lim M, Chu E, Quinones-Hinojosa A. Transpalpebral orbitofrontal craniotomy: a minimally invasive approach to anterior cranial vault lesions. *Skull Base*. 2010;**20**(4):237–44.
19. Jordan DR, Mawn LA, Anderson RL. *Surgical Anatomy of the Ocular Adnexa*, 2nd ed. Oxford: Oxford University Press; 2012.
20. Greenfield L, Mulholland M, Doherty G, eds. *Greenfield's Surgery: Scientific Principles and Practice*. 4th ed. New York: Lippincott Williams & Wilkins; 2005.
21. Rolston JD, Han SJ, Lau CY, Berger MS, Parsa AT. Frequency and predictors of complications in neurological surgery: national trends from 2006 to 2011. *J Neurosurg*. 2014;**120**(3):736–45.
22. Ling JD, Mehta V, Fathy C, et al. Racial disparities in corneal transplantation rates, complications, and outcomes. *Semin Ophthalmol*. 2016;**31**(4):337–44.

23. Sosa JA, Mehta PJ, Wang TS, Yeo HL, Roman SA. Racial disparities in clinical and economic outcomes from thyroidectomy. *Ann Surg.* 2007;**246**(6):1083–91.

24. Latz B, Mordhorst C, Kerz T, et al. Post-operative nausea and vomiting in patients after craniotomy: incidence and risk factors. *J Neurosurg.* 2011;**114**(2):491–6.

25. Gan TJ, Meyer T, Apfel CC, et al. Consensus guidelines for managing post-operative nausea and vomiting. *Anesth Analg.* 2003;**97**(1):62–71.

Chapter 10

Transbasal and Transfacial Approach for Paranasal and Anterior Cranial Fossa Tumors

Michael J. Link and Eric Moore

Introduction

The transbasal approach (TBA) was first defined during the early 1970s, and multiple possible extensions were also later described (1). This versatile approach provides access to the anterior fossa, orbit, nasal cavity, paranasal sinuses, pterygopalatine fossa, and pituitary fossa. The concept of a combined craniofacial and transbasal approach was first introduced by Cushing in 1939. Almost two decades later, Smith et al. provided the first description of utilization of the combined approach against paranasal tumors with intracranial invasion that had responded poorly to radiotherapy. The addition of a transfacial route to the TBA allows excellent direct visualization and, therefore, access to deeper structures with minimal brain retraction and risk to important neural and vascular structures.

Given the complexity of the approach, oftentimes necessitating multiple surgical specialties collaborating, most craniofacial surgeries (CFS) take place in academic medical centers. Early on, many patients with pathologies amenable to CFS were previously treated with radiotherapy and/or chemotherapy without satisfactory treatment outcomes. However, a multidisciplinary approach and sophisticated modern surgical techniques give skull base surgeons the ability to achieve negative margin resections with significantly lower morbidity and mortality rates.

The indication for this combined approach, and intended extent of resection, depends on a case-by-case analysis and a multidisciplinary discussion. Thus the approach mentioned here may not be straightforwardly applied to each case. However, for the purpose of this chapter, indications, anatomical, and surgical details are directed toward the CFS approach to treat benign and malignant neoplasms involving the anterior skull base, paranasal sinuses, and potentially the orbits.

Indications

The surgical strategy and the specific transfacial route (e.g., Le Fort, lateral rhinotomy) vary, depending on the location and origin of the lesion. The most common indication for CFS with a combined TBA is a malignant neoplasm invading both the extracranial and intracranial compartments of the anterior skull base. However, the tumor may have its origins in adjacent structures such as the maxillary sinus, sphenoid sinus and/or the nasal cavity. Achieving negative margins in all surrounding biopsies is crucial. Primary examples of such tumors in these locations include esthesioneuroblastoma, chordoma or chondrosarcoma, atypical or frankly malignant meningioma, sarcoma, sinonasal carcinoma, mucosal melanoma, and other metastatic carcinomas.

A combined TBA + CFA approach can also be appropriate for extremely large and highly vascular tumors that are not suitable for endoscopic removal or when broad exposure of the orbit, paranasal sinuses, and/or sphenoid region is needed. An example of an ideal clinical scenario would be a tumor invading the orbit or paranasal sinuses, potentially causing visual symptoms and proptosis, without clear evidence of metastasis, in a patient without significant comorbidities that would preclude them from surgery.

As an illustrative example, here we present the surgical description of a case of an esthesioneuroblastoma extending through the cribriform plate to the frontal lobes and the paranasal sinuses.

Contraindications

The main contraindication to this approach is the presence of medical comorbidities that would make a long surgery too dangerous to conduct. Giving neoadjuvant therapy, such as undergoing chemotherapy or radiation therapy preceding surgery should be considered carefully to avoid surgical complications such as cerebrospinal fluid (CSF) leak, wound dehiscence, and wound infection. Diffusely metastatic disease and life expectancy less than 6 months would also make a combined TBA and CFA approach contraindicated.

Preoperative Planning

CT and MRI with and without contrast of the head, face, and neck are mandatory to accurately identify the extent of the tumor, and to guide decision-making regarding whether a margin negative resection can be achieved. Most patients also undergo a PET-CT to investigate for metastatic disease that might make an extensive craniofacial resection contraindicated. Rarely, preoperative cerebral angiography followed by possible embolization is used in the case of highly vascular tumors.

Anatomy

Anterior Cranial Fossa

- The bones that form the anterior cranial base are the ethmoid, sphenoid, and frontal bones. The floor of the anterior fossa is composed bilaterally and anteriorly by the frontal bone and posteriorly by the sphenoid bone.
- The middle portion of the floor of the anterior cranial fossa is formed by the superior surface of the ethmoid bone and the cribriform plate. In the midline, the articulation of the crista galli with the frontal crest marks the foramen cecum. This forms the entrance of an emissary vein from the nose to the superior sagittal sinus.
- The olfactory bulbs (CN I) are located immediately above the cribriform plate, and the nerve terminal fibers pass through the cribriform plate to form the olfactory epithelium at the roof of the nasal cavity.

Sinonasal Cavity

The nasal cavity is roofed by the frontal bone anteriorly, the ethmoid bone medially, and the body of the sphenoid posteriorly. In the midline, the perpendicular plate of the ethmoid bone articulates inferiorly with the vomer bone and, together with a cartilaginous structure, forms the nasal septum. The lateral walls are composed of the superior, middle, and inferior turbinates. While the inferior is a separate bone, the superior and middle turbinates are appendages of the ethmoid bone. The nasal cavity connections are as follows:

- The sphenoid sinuses drain posterior to the superior turbinate through the sphenoid-ethmoidal recess
- The posterior ethmoidal air cells of the ethmoidal labyrinth drain into the superior turbinate through the superior meatus
- The anterior ethmoidal cells and frontal sinus drain between superior and middle turbinates through the middle meatus
- Below the inferior turbinate, the inferior meatus receives the nasolacrimal duct

Posteriorly the nasal cavity opens through the choana to the nasopharynx. The choana is surrounded by the vomer medially, inferiorly by the palatine bones, laterally by the pterygoid plate of the sphenoid bone, and superiorly by the body of the sphenoid bone. The anterior opening of the nasal cavity is known as the pyriform aperture, limited by two superior nasal bones and the maxilla.

Surgical Technique

Positioning

Under general anesthesia, the patient is positioned supine, with the head slightly extended and fixed in a three-point pinion head holder. It is important to make sure the pins are placed in a retroauricular fashion, so as not to obstruct the surgical incision. The bifrontal area and entire face down to the upper lip, and either side of the lateral thigh (to allow for a fascia lata graft), are shaved, prepped, and draped.

Transbasal Tumor Resection Craniotomy

- A modified Souttar incision is made behind the hairline, and the scalp and pericranium are turned forward to the orbital rims, taking great care not to injure the pericranium.
- A burr hole is placed on each side of the superior sagittal sinus (SSS) approximately 7 cm superior to the nasion. It is important to place these burr holes at least one centimeter lateral to the edge of the SSS to avoid injury to any arachnoid granulation, which then makes stripping the dura away from the bone very

difficult. Additional burr holes are placed laterally over each orbital roof just medial to the anterior-most attachment of the temporalis muscle. The frontal dura is carefully dissected free from the inner calvarium of the skull, and a bifrontal craniotomy is turned. It is important to note that the anterior cranial fossa extends very low medially to the level of the cribriform plate. The inferior bone cut should be made as close to parallel to this as possible – staying just above the orbital roofs laterally and then curving inferiorly medially. Additionally, if the frontal sinuses are very large, as the posterior sinus wall separates from the anterior wall, the spiral bit and footplate attachment on the craniotome may not be long enough to complete this cut. In such cases, only the anterior wall of the frontal sinus can be cut. The posterior wall will often simply crack when the rest of the craniotomy is complete, or an osteotome may be needed to fracture the posterior wall to allow safe removal of the bone flap. Of note, the craniotomy does not need to extend more than 6 or 7 cm superior to the nasion (Figure 10.1).

- After the dura is tacked to the bone margin posteriorly, the subfrontal dura is elevated off of the orbital rims bilaterally from laterally to medially toward the cribriform plate. A tumor is usually encountered coming through the cribriform plate and invading the dura. The olfactory dura is incised circumferentially to free up the dura posteriorly to the planum sphenoidale. Then the tumor-infiltrated dura, including the cribriform plate and part of the planum sphenoidale, is extensively removed. If the approach is used in the case of suspected cancer, the bilateral olfactory tracts will need to be divided and margins sent for frozen pathologic analysis to check for tumor involvement.
- Oftentimes, the tumor has a preserved arachnoid plane with the frontal lobes; and at times, the tumor is found to directly invade the brain.
- Multiple biopsies of the dural margins, olfactory tracts, and frontal lobes are obtained in cancer cases to ensure gross total resection intracranially.

Dural Reconstruction

The authors prefer to repair the skull base defect with a fascia lata graft. This is trimmed to an appropriate size and shape, and sewn to the dura in a watertight fashion using a running, double-armed 5–0 or 6–0 Prolene suture to replace the large area of excised dura. The fascia lata graft is used as an inlay graft such that it is at least 1 cm larger than the dural defect circumferentially.

Transfacial Tumor Resection (Collaboration with Ophthalmology and ENT)

- A lateral rhinotomy incision is made and the soft tissues are elevated off of the lamina papyracea. The tumor is detached from the periorbita. The anterior ethmoidal artery is ligated.
- The soft tissues are then elevated off the face of the maxilla. The maxillary sinus is entered and the maxillary mucosa is sent to for neuropathological analysis.
- An incision is then made along the pyriform aperture, dividing the upper lateral cartilages to the septum to open up the nasal cavity. The frontal process of the maxilla is then removed with a rongeur. The bone in the region of the lacrimal sac is then removed, and the lacrimal duct is divided. The bone inferiorly between the nose and the maxillary sinus is usually removed back to the posterior wall of the antrum.
- Bone cuts are then made from above using typically a 3 mm diamond burr or osteotome with the frontal cut just behind the frontal sinus and anterior to the cribriform, laterally over the roof of each orbit, and posteriorly through the planum sphenoidale to enter the sphenoid sinus. Cuts are then made in the nasal septum beneath the tumor back to the rostrum of the sphenoid. The craniofacial specimen is removed in an en bloc fashion.
- Once completely negative margins are obtained based on frozen section neuropathologic analysis, often the remaining fascia lata is laid in as an onlay graft to cover the native dura and the inlay fascia lata graft that had previously been sewn in. The pericranium, which is left vascularized

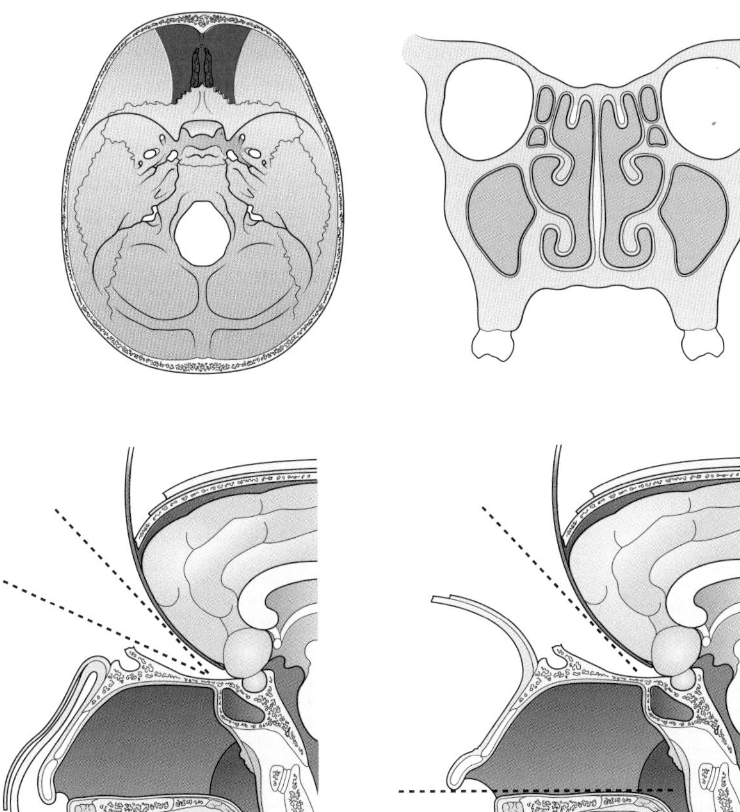

Figure 10.1 Drawings providing an overview of the anterior cranial fossa anatomy and the surgical approaches

anteriorly, is then freed from the scalp flap and swung in and tacked to the planum sphenoidale with two interrupted 5–0 Prolene sutures to act as a vascularized barrier between the nasal cavity and the intracranial cavity. Thus, from the nasal side, the barriers to a CSF leak are the vascularized pericranium, an onlay fascia lata graft, and a sewn-in inlay fascia lata graft.

- The rhinotomy incision is closed in layers after first approximating the medial canthal tendon to the periosteum. The proximal portion of the lacrimal duct is opened, and left open, to drain into the wound. Soft tissues are closed with interrupted sutures, and the skin incision is closed with a running 5–0 fast-absorbing chromic stitch.

Complication Avoidance

1. CSF leak: Careful attention to watertight dural closure with an autologous fascia lata graft and multilayer reinforcement including the use of a vascularized pericranial graft is essential to avoid this frustrating and dangerous complication.
2. Meningitis: To avoid ascending infection following TBA, we typically give triple antibiotics with vancomycin, cefepime, and metronidazole perioperatively while the drains are in place, until at least postoperative day 3.
3. Perioperative seizure management: All patients receive a loading dose of levetiracetam at the time of induction of anesthesia and are typically kept on a low-maintenance dose of 500 mg orally twice a day for 2 weeks postoperatively.

Postoperative Considerations

The majority of patients who undergo TBA present with malignant neoplasm, and the associated complexity of these surgeries requires multidisciplinary involvement of neurosurgery, ENT, radiation oncology, and medical oncology. Serial follow-up imaging is typically obtained following the completion of radiation therapy, and then every 3–6 months for the first 5 years after resection.

Clinical Pearls

- Extension of craniotomy, as well as the removal of orbital frontal rims, depends on the extension of the tumor.
- Multiple negative margin checks are necessary for optimal surgical outcome in cases of cancer.
- A vascularized pedicle flap with pericranium is useful to separate the nasal cavity from the cranium.
- Watertight dural closure with fascia lata graft is important for avoiding CSF leaks.
- Optimal perioperative use of multiple antibiotics is likely beneficial for avoiding procedure-related infections.

Addendum

Multiple variations are described for the TBA approach. Feiz-Erfan and Spetzler (2) defined four main categories:

- **Level 0:** Consists of classic bifrontal craniotomy above orbital rim, avoiding any osteotomy of the nasion. There are three other extended variations of the TBA.
- **Level I:** Includes detachment of olfactory bulb from cribriform plate and release of the supraorbital and supratrochlear neurovascular complexes. The supraorbital bar is released as a second bone flap, including detachment of the superior periorbital wall. The orbital roof can be detached as close to the orbital apex, anteriorly or posteriorly, to the cribriform plate as much as needed. This provides a more basal trajectory that minimizes brain retraction and improves access to the central skull base (Figure 10.2).
- **Level II:** The nasal cut is extended inferiorly to the superior piriform aperture. The nasolacrimal duct must be identified and preserved. This more caudal bony extension requires detachment of the medial canthal ligament, which attaches to the nasion below the frontonasal suture. The main advantage of this variation is avoiding TFA for tumors with minimal sinonasal extension. Cribriform plate osteotomy (CPO; Figure 10.5 can optimally be applied with this extension. The application of this technique is optional and especially suitable for those patients who prioritize olfaction preservation,

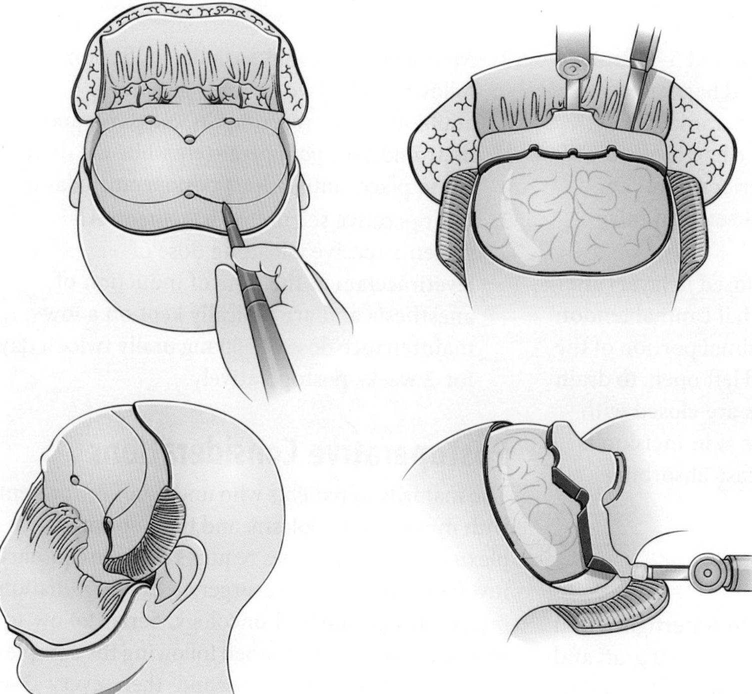

Figure 10.2 Left: Bifrontal craniotomy, Right: Removal of the supraorbital bar. n = nerve.

although the authors remain skeptical this goal can actually be reliably achieved.

- **Level III:** Consists of the same medial cut as Level II, with extended lateral bony resection including complete lateral orbital wall and zygomatic arch (Figure 10.4). This extension is indicated for tumors located mainly in the maxillary sinus, and when combined with a TFA, a sublabial Le Fort I approach, for better cosmetic results (Figure 10.3).

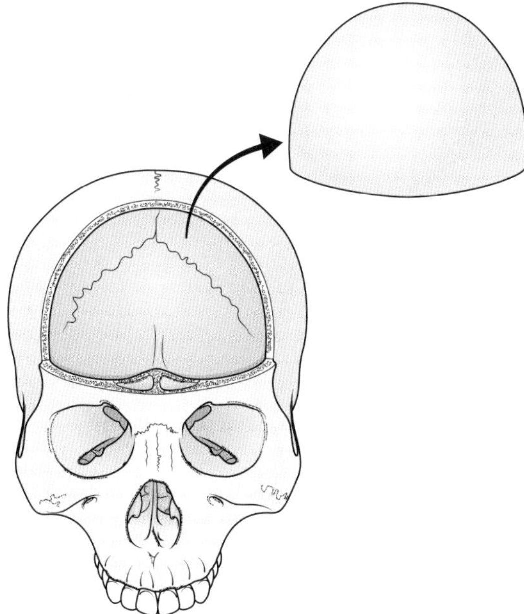

Figure 10.3 Level 0 TBA

In our experience, more frequently a Level 0 or a Level I craniotomy, in combination with a selected transfacial or endoscopic transnasal route, is used when broader paranasal access is needed. This nearly always provides a sufficient surgical corridor.

Through the TBA the upper nasal cavity can be exposed by widely removing the ethmoid and sphenoid sinus roofs. The posterior nasal septum can be removed as well if needed. By drilling the posterior portion of the superior-medial orbital wall, access to the orbital apex and optic nerve is achieved. Through this medial corridor, the pituitary gland and sella can be accessed.

The addition of a transfacial craniotomy supplements the TBA by providing access to more lateral or posteriorly located lesions. In the context of lesions with intracranial invasion, various transfacial routes can be utilized as follows:

- Caldwell Luc sinus osteotomy: Useful if additional access only to maxillary sinus is needed
- Transfacial swing osteotomy, Weber Ferguson incision: Indicated for large tumors with total invasion of the paranasal sinuses, such as in esthesioneuroblastoma
- Lateral rhinotomy
- Le Fort I craniotomy: Provides access to the maxillary sinus. In addition, it can be used as a transmaxillary route through the sphenoid sinus toward the sella turcica, where the cavernous sinus can be accessed inferiorly

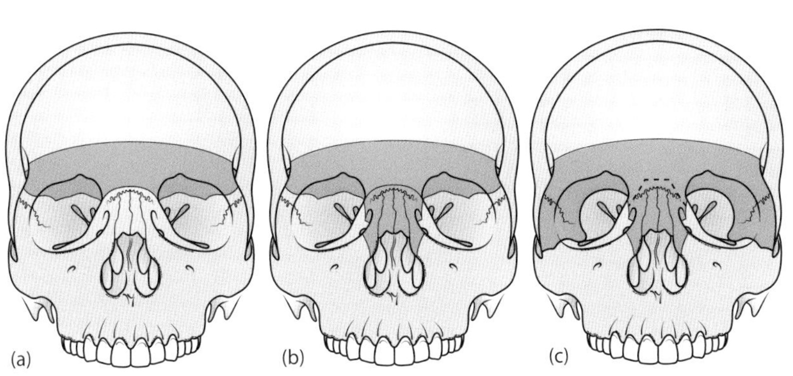

Figure 10.4 Extended Level I (A); Level II (B); Level III (C)

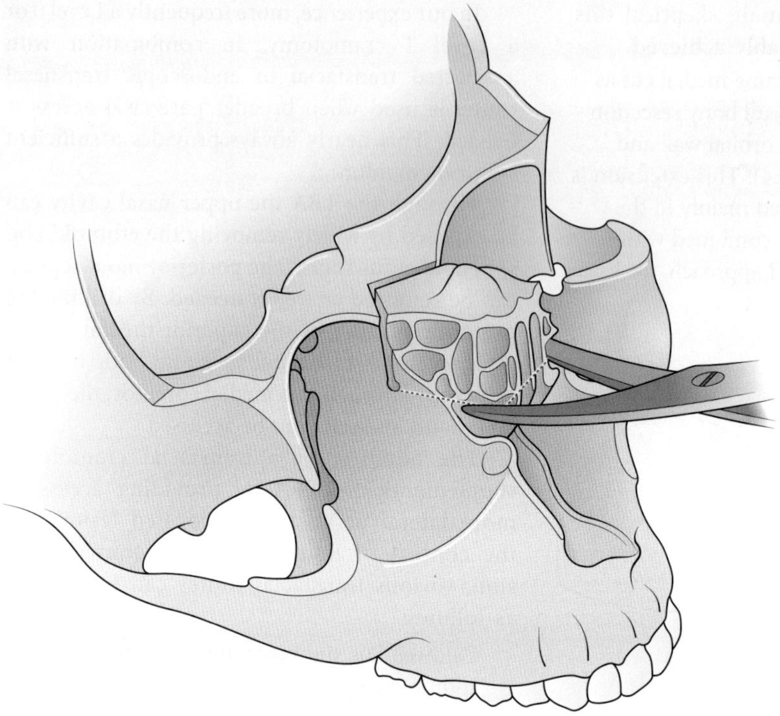

Figure 10.5 CPO technique

References

1. Patel SG, Singh B, Polluri A, et al. Craniofacial surgery for malignant skull base tumors. *Cancer*. 2003;**98**(6):1179–87.
2. Feiz-Erfan I, Spetzler RF, Horn EM, et al. Proposed classification for the transbasal approach and its modifications. *Skull Base*. 2008;**18**(1):29–47.
3. Jittapiromsak P, Wu A, Deshmukh P, et al. Comparative analysis of extensions of transbasal approaches: effect on access to midline and paramedian structures. *Skull Base*. 2009;**19**(6):387–99.
4. Kim SR, Lee JW, Han YS, Kim HK. Transfacial surgical approaches to secure wide exposure of the skull base, transfacial surgical approaches to secure wide exposure of the skull base. *Arch Craniofac Surg*. 2015;**16**(1):17–23.
5. Spetzler RF, Herman JM, Beals S, Joganic E, Milligan J. Preservation of olfaction in anterior craniofacial approaches. *Journal of Neurosurgery*. 1993;**79**(1):48–52.

Chapter 11

Combined Middle Fossa Craniotomy and Mastoidectomy for Cerebrospinal Fluid Leak Repair and Encephalocele Resection

Kevin Li and Howard Moskowitz

Introduction

Lateral skull base meningoencephalic herniations (MEH) are rare instances where dura mater (meningocele) or cerebral tissue (encephalocele) protrudes through the skull base dehiscences, commonly in the tegmen tympani or mastoideum. The etiology of tegmen defects is variable and divided into congenital and acquired, with acquired further subdivided into non-traumatic, traumatic, or spontaneous. Potential etiologies for non-traumatic tegmen defects include chronic otitis media with or without cholesteatoma and neoplasia, while traumatic etiologies include head trauma with temporal bone fracture and history of otologic surgery (1-3). A MEH may also have a concomitant cerebrospinal fluid (CSF) leak characterized by the egress of CSF from the intracranial cavity through an osteodural defect, in which case the defect is categorized as a true encephalocele (1,3-5). In the literature, there is confounding nomenclature due to the variability in the contents of the herniations. The terms "meningocele," "meningoencephalocele," "encephalocele," and "arachnoid diverticulum," among others, are commonly interchanged. However, since herniation contents can often only be visually verified through microscopic examination, variability in the terminology remains (6).

Before the modern era of antibiotics, MEHs were commonly thought to be a result of prior surgical treatment for sigmoid sinus thrombophlebitis or temporal bone cholesteatoma, with the highest incidence resulting from mastoidectomies (5,7). Other authors theorized that encephaloceles may be the result of a failed union of the temporal and sphenoid bone ossification centers, erosion due to pressure, or arachnoid granulations protruding through the tegmen (8,9). This last theory is supported by a Sanna et al. series showing patients presenting with spontaneous herniation at a mean age of 57 years, suggesting that natural defects in the tegmen erode the dura over time and lead to herniation (1). The recent increase in rates of spontaneous CSF leaks and encephaloceles may be related to increased rates of obesity and intracranial hypertension. Stucken et al. found a statistically significant difference in BMI among patients who presented with spontaneous versus non-spontaneous CSF leaks, indicating that obesity may play a role (10). Sugarman et al. took it one step further by hypothesizing that the increased abdominal pressure from obesity directly leads to increased intrapleural pressure, which decreases cardiac filling. The decreased cardiac filling results in increased CSF pressure due to decreased venous return from the brain (11). Obstructive sleep apnea is also a known risk factor for developing spontaneous CSF leaks, and a systematic review by Bakhsheshian et al. showed 4.7 times greater odds of developing a CSF fistula with obstructive sleep apnea (12). It is currently believed that encephaloceles are due to a multifactorial process that results from increased intracranial pressure in an anatomically predisposed patient, eventually leading to herniation of brain tissue into the middle ear or mastoid cavity with possible CSF otorrhea (13). Encephaloceles and CSF leaks carry great risk, as they provide a potential pathway from the middle ear to the subarachnoid space and can lead to harmful sequelae such as otogenic cerebral abscesses, meningitis, and encephalitis (1,5). Moreover, for encephaloceles, herniated cerebral tissue has been shown to predispose patients to epilepsy (1,14). Thus early detection and surgical repair of encephaloceles or CSF leaks are imperative.

Pertinent Microanatomy

The tympanic cavity is an air-filled space in the middle ear of the temporal bone that contains the malleus, incus, and stapes with their attached muscles. The roof of the tympanic cavity is formed by the tegmen tympani and is the boundary between the tympanic cavity and the MCF contents. The tegmen tympani itself is formed by both the petrous and the squamous portions of the temporal bone, with the petrosquamous suture line remaining unossified in young individuals. This suture line does not completely ossify until adulthood, and is a potential cause of encephaloceles and CSF leaks. Moreover, this suture also transmits veins from the middle ear to the superior petrosal sinus. The tegmen tympani extends anteriorly to cover the semicircular canals and posteriorly to the roof of the tympanic antrum (14,15). The lateral edge of the tegmen tympani is the remnant of the petrosquamous suture and develops from membranous ossification. The medial part develops from the otic capsule during chondral ossification (16). The MCF is formed from the greater wing of the sphenoid bone and the squamous and petrous portions of the temporal bone. It houses the temporal lobe and also transmits many important neurovascular structures such as the second and third divisions of the trigeminal nerve through the foramen rotundum and foramen ovale, respectively, both of which are contained within the greater wing of the sphenoid bone. The middle meningeal artery also runs through the foramen spinosum near the junction of the greater wing of the sphenoid and the petrous temporal bone.

Surgical Approaches

When an encephalocele or CSF leak is diagnosed, surgical repair is the definitive treatment option. There are a variety of surgical approaches that can be used to correct tegmen defects, but there are no accepted guidelines for the management of temporal defects. Typical surgical approaches for lateral skull base encephaloceles are based on surgeon experience and include the transmastoid (TM), middle cranial fossa (MCF), and combined transmastoid and middle cranial fossa approach, which incorporates steps from both procedures. The surgical approach for repair of a tegmen defect depends on the size and location of the bony defect, the status of the ossicular chain and hearing, and the preference of the surgeon.

The TM approach repairs the defect from below and is typically indicated for smaller defects or spontaneous etiologies. Many authors prefer the transmastoid approach, as it is easier to perform, gives access to the entire tegmen and the posterior fossa plate, and allows for repair of dehiscence without manipulation or elevation of the middle cranial fossa dura (17-21). If herniation is through a posterior fossa plate defect, the TM approach is necessary to access the lesion (1). This approach is advantageous because it avoids the need for craniotomy, compared with the MCF and combined approach. Gioacchini et al. showed in a subgroup meta-analysis of 76 procedures that the TM approach had a success rate of 97.1% for CSF leaks (22). However, if there is a wide dural defect, the TM approach has a higher failure rate because it may not provide adequate space to achieve successful repair, and a more invasive surgical procedure such as the middle cranial fossa or the combined approach may be preferred (4,22). Defects in the tegmen tympani may not be readily accessible and may require removal of the incus and possibly the head of the malleus (23). Mayeno et al. recommend the TM approach for any defect smaller than 1 cm and limited to the tegmen mastoideum. For larger defects or lesions anterior to the tegmen tympani, they recommend the MCF approach or the combined approach (21). Moreover, if there are contracted mastoids, tympanomastoid infection, history of failed repairs, or risk factors for poor healing such as prior radiation, the MCF or combined approach is preferred (19,24).

The MCF approach repairs the defect from above and gives a more direct route and improved exposure to the entire tegmen, avoids potential manipulation of the ossicular chain, and allows for easier multilayered repairs. Thus it is indicated for patients who present with normal hearing without middle-ear or mastoid infections. Many authors consider the MCF a good initial approach for all defects (4,19,22,25). Gioacchini et al. found in a subgroup of 146 patients that the MCF had a success rate of 94.1%. The success rate is slightly lower than the TM approach and is most likely due to the larger size of the defects repaired in the MCF approach, however, the authors note that this difference is not statistically significant.

The combined approach incorporates both the TM and MCF approaches. This approach permits management of the repair from above the tegmen defect and gives access both intracranially and extradurally. Once the dura is elevated, a wide bed is created for graft placement. Gioacchini et al. also found that, in a subgroup of 97 procedures, the combined approach had a success rate of 97.9%, greater than both the TM and MCF approaches (22). The authors also found that the middle cranial fossa approach had a higher rate of post-surgical complication (meningitis, prolonged postoperative headache, epidural or subdural hematoma, temporal lobe edema, and speech difficulty), in general, with 9.1% compared with the combined approach with 1.9% and the TM approach with 1.3%. It should be noted that these complication rates are calculated from five studies, and neither the success rate nor the complication rate of the MCF approach were found to be statistically significant in comparison to the TM and combined approaches (22). Hoang et al. believe that cases with significant middle-ear pathology such as a cholesteatoma require the combined approach, as the addition of a mastoidectomy allows for better visualization of the ossicles and safer removal of pathology (26). Careful selection of repair techniques may not only reduce surgical time, but also reduce hospital stay and recovery time, ultimately minimizing morbidity, complications, and costs (21).

In general, the TM approach is used for small defects of the mastoid tegmen smaller than 1 cm and is generally favored because it is minimally invasive and does not require manipulation of the dura. For larger defects, the MCF or combined approach is the procedure of choice. The MCF requires a craniotomy and temporal lobe retraction, so there is a higher risk of complications during the postoperative period. The combined approach allows for the safe repair of large tegmen defects and exposes the dehiscence adequately with either a limited or standard craniotomy, and minimal temporal lobe retraction (24). Marchioni et al. believe that the TM is the preferred approach for small defects and can be converted to the combined approach if necessary. If the defect is large, the combined approach is the preferred procedure, especially in patients with normal hearing (4). Carlson et al. believe that a middle fossa craniotomy with a multilayer bone and fascia overlay provides the best long-term repair and minimal morbidity (24). In our institution, the patient characteristics are carefully weighed in a multidisciplinary fashion before a particular approach is selected (Figure 11.1).

Alternative Approaches

Besides the TM, MCF, and combined approaches, middle-ear obliteration (MEO) can also be performed to repair encephaloceles and CSF leaks. Middle-ear obliteration typically consists of a TM or MCF approach with a blind-sac closure of the external auditory canal; complete removal of the external auditory canal skin, tympanic membrane, mastoid and tympanic cavity mucosa, and malleus and incus; and the creation of an open cavity. Any herniated tissue is reduced using bipolar coagulation and cut with microscissors. The opening is then obliterated with abdominal fat, and the eustachian tube is then packed with muscle or cartilage (1,22,27). This approach is most suited for patients with poor hearing in the affected ear and is typically reserved for recurrent cases of CSF leak or encephalocele with no alternative solution (1). If there is a concomitant cholesteatoma, however, clinical monitoring is not possible, and radiological surveillance is necessary with high-resolution CT or MRI. When there is no possibility of hearing preservation or rehabilitation, Sanna et al. believe an MEO is the safest surgical approach over the TM and MCF approach for the repair of CSF leaks or encephaloceles, as an MEO has very low recurrence rates and provides definitive treatment (Figure 11.1) (1).

Preoperative Planning

Encephaloceles and CSF leaks are difficult to diagnose, because patients often present with non-specific clinical symptoms such as aural fullness, tinnitus, headaches, and imbalance. The most common complaints are conductive or mixed hearing loss with serous otitis media or a draining ear (5,28). Clinical examination may reveal middle-ear effusions, pulsatile movement of the tympanic membrane, rhinorrhea, or otorrhea (28). Audiometric tests may demonstrate conductive hearing loss due to CSF or herniated brain tissue in the middle ear, but these findings are non-specific (1). However, if a CSF leak or encephalocele is masked by symptoms related to the primary pathology, such as chronic otitis media, the diagnosis may be an unintended intraoperative finding (29). Therefore, a high

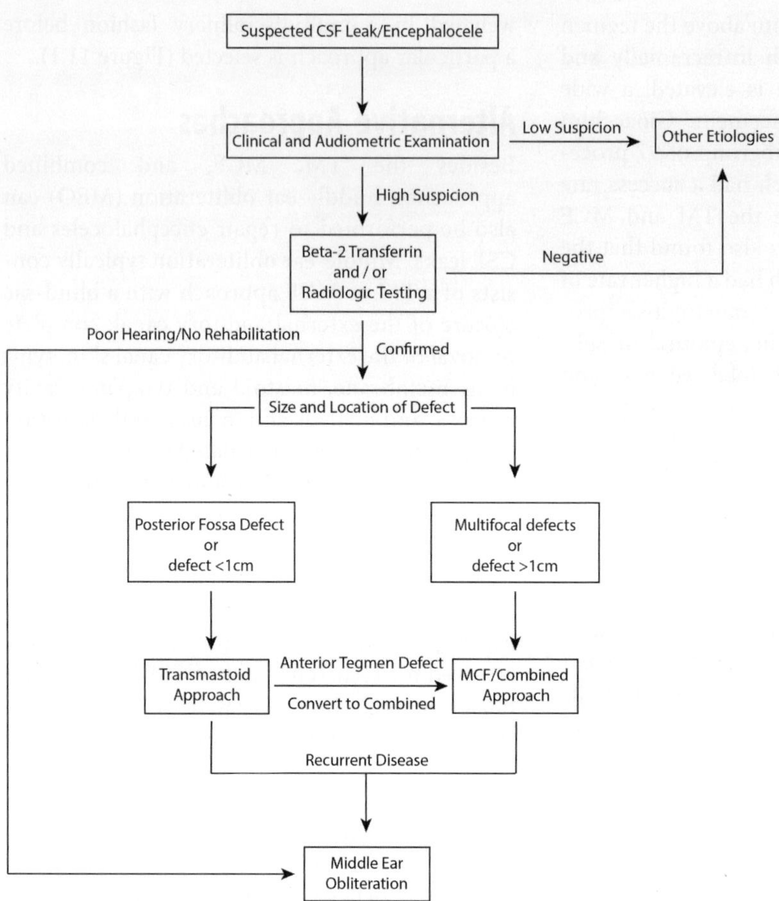

Figure 11.1 Algorithm for combined surgical management of cerebrospinal fluid leaks and encephaloceles.

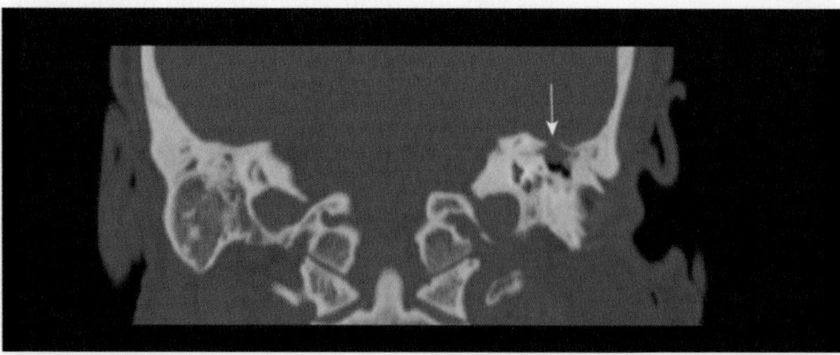

Figure 11.2 A preoperative coronal CT scan revealing a posterior tegmen defect suitable for a transmastoid approach.

degree of clinical suspicion is needed to properly diagnose patients with encephaloceles and CSF leaks. Suspected encephaloceles or CSF leaks can first be assessed by obtaining a sample of otological secretion when possible and performing a β2-transferrin and β-trace protein analysis (23).

A thorough radiological assessment is also performed to confirm the diagnosis, evaluate for the underlying cause, and identify the location of the osteodural defect (30). High-resolution computed tomography (CT) in axial and coronal planes provides imaging of soft tissue herniation through the tegmen (Figures 11.2–11.3). The axial view is useful for the rare cases of posterior cranial fossa herniation, but the coronal view is preferred for middle cranial fossa herniation. Not only does

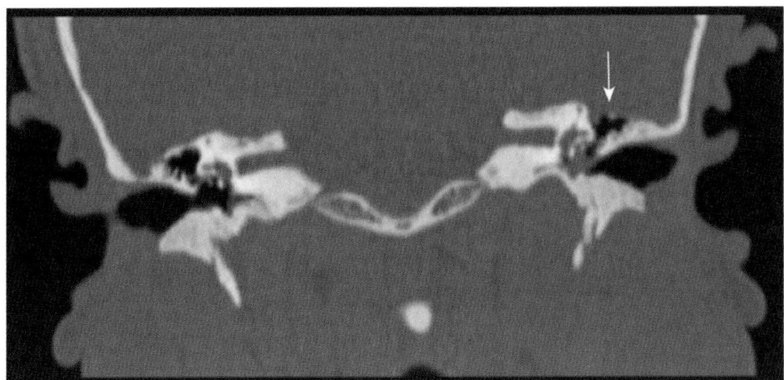

Figure.11.3 A preoperative coronal CT revealing an anterior tegmen defect suitable for a middle cranial fossa approach.

high-resolution CT provide evidence of an encephalocele or CSF leak, but also it can also provide information on the location, number, and size of the bony defects (1). If the exact site of CSF leak cannot be identified, a radionuclide cisternography with intrathecal fluorescein injection can be used. This will confirm the presence of a CSF leak, and a CT cisternography can localize the defect (31). High-resolution CT is limited in that it only demonstrates non-enhancing soft tissue and cannot differentiate between a cholesteatoma, cholesterol granuloma, granulation tissue, or other soft-tissue masses of the middle ear. Therefore, magnetic resonance imaging (MRI) can be used to help differentiate the etiologies of the defect (Figure 11.1) (7). MEH appears as a non-enhancing contiguous mass isotense to the brain. In contrast, a cholesteatoma will appear hyperintense on T2-weighted images, and a cholesterol granuloma will appear hyperintense in both T1- and T2-weighted images. Typically, T2-weighted coronal sections are the most useful for identifying MCF herniations (32,33). Preoperative high-resolution CT with 0.5-mm contiguous coronal reconstructions and MRI with and without contrast enhancement are recommended for all patients (5). Moreover, imaging should be carefully evaluated for possible geniculate ganglion, petrous carotid, or superior semicircular canal dehiscence (24).

Detailed Surgical Technique

General Surgical Techniques

Patients are placed in a supine position, and depending on surgeon preference, a shoulder roll placed underneath their ipsilateral shoulder, with their heads turned 60 degrees to the contralateral side. Obese patients can be placed in a lateral position, and a Mayfield three-pin head holder can be used for patients with poor cervical rotation. Patients are then induced with general anesthesia and may undergo a lumbar drain at the surgeon's discretion (5). However, note that an intraoperative lumbar drain could register an opening pressure value that appears normal, even in the presence of increased intracranial pressure due to the presence of a CSF leak. Some authors avoid lumbar CSF drainage because it allows for a temporal lobe subarachnoid space cushion and provides protection during the procedure (14). Brain relaxation can alternatively be achieved using mannitol. Prophylactic antibiotics and anti-epileptic medications are also routinely administered, and antibiotics should be appropriately re-dosed. Bipolar facial electromyography electrodes can be placed in the orbicularis oculi and oris muscles for continuous intraoperative monitoring of facial nerve integrity and detection of the greater superficial petrosal nerve on the floor of the middle fossa (24,34). Additionally, Carlson et al. recommend that intraoperative auditory brainstem response monitoring be considered if superior semicircular canal dehiscence is suspected (24).

Transmastoid Approach

The TM approach begins with a postauricular incision with a canal-wall-up mastoidectomy and transmastoid atticotomy. If a previous canal-wall-down mastoidectomy has been performed, a revision is often necessary, and in cases of chronic otitis media, disease needs to be eradicated. The tegmen defect is located and isolated,

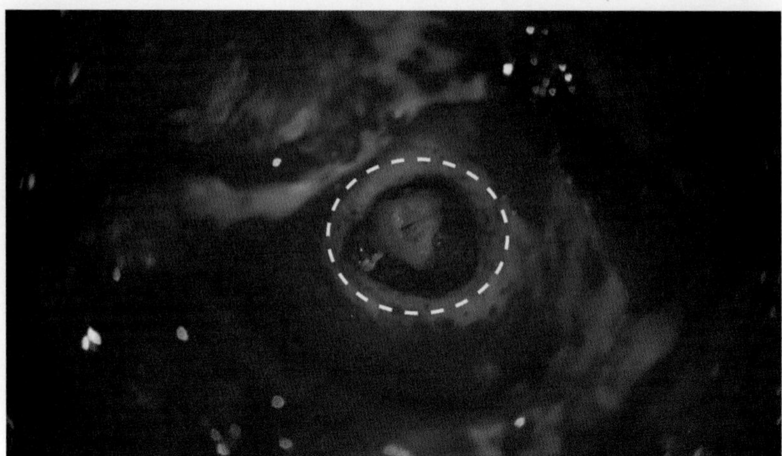

Figure 11.4 Encephalocele visualized during transmastoid approach.

and the operative field can be irrigated with antibiotic solution (35). Using gentle, blunt dissection, dural margins are exposed by elevating the dura in the epidural plane. If an encephalocele is found, it is fulgurated at its stalk and excised (Figure 11.4). Many authors prefer to excise the encephalocele to prevent potential intracranial dissemination of infection (36). In the "overlay" technique, a cartilage-perichondrium graft is glued to the surface of the defect. While this leaves the intracranial compartment untouched, it is also prone to dislodging into the mastoidectomy under the pressure of CSF if it is not properly supported by other filling materials. The "inlay" technique is a variation where the middle cranial fossa dura is detached with blunt dissection approximately 3–4 mm from the bony border of the defect. This uses a slightly larger implant, as it allows for overlapping of the implant between the dura and the petrous bone. The graft is held in place by gravity and physiological intracranial pressure (35). Finally, the surgeon may use a "sandwich" technique for watertight sealing by placing a cartilage-perichondrium graft directly against the dural defect and applying a temporalis fascia overlay held in place with fibrin glue (Figure 11.5). Fascia is also draped over the aditus to prevent fat herniation into the middle-ear cavity. The mastoid cavity may be obliterated with an abdominal fat graft, and fibrin glue is placed between the layers. Finally, a watertight periosteal closure is performed, and a mastoid dressing is applied and kept in place for 48 hours with strict CSF leak precautions (20,35).

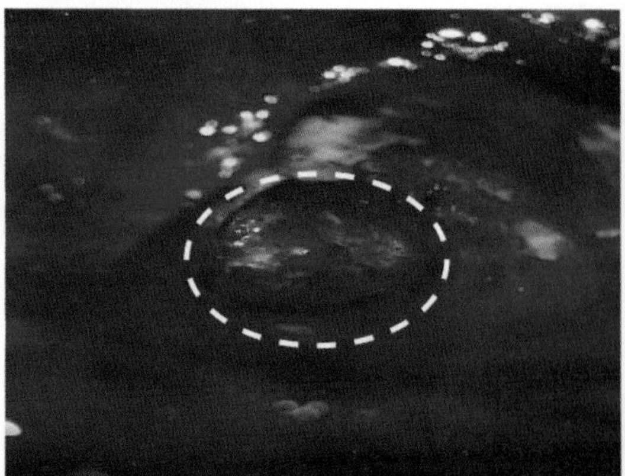

Figure 11.5 Tegmen defect repaired with a combined cartilage and perichondrial graft.

Middle Cranial Fossa Approach

The MCF approach begins with a pre-auricular lazy-S incision, depending on if a combined approach will be utilized. This allows for wide exposure of the bone for a temporal craniotomy. Then, a temporalis fascia graft is harvested for later use in closing the inner ear canal. It is at this point that 0.5–1.0 g/kg of mannitol can be delivered intravenously to reduce intracranial pressure. The temporalis muscle is then divided, with care taken to leave a small cuff of muscle along the superior temporal line for easier wound approximation. From here, the squamous temporal bone is exposed in a sub-periosteal fashion and the tegmen can be exposed, with care taken to avoid creating new areas of dural dehiscence. Depending on the size and location of singular or multiple defects, either a limited craniotomy (3 × 3 cm) for a single large defect or a standard craniotomy for multifocal defects (a 5 × 5 cm craniotomy, superior to the zygomatic root and positioned approximately one-third posteriorly and two-thirds anteriorly to the external ear canal) is performed. A single burr hole is placed in the inferior temporal region and is usually sufficient, but a second burr hole is often used to prevent dural violation if the dura cannot be easily dissected away from the bone (34). Care must be taken to avoid causing an incidental durotomy by drilling the bone flush to the floor of the middle fossa. This improves visualization and minimizes the amount of temporal lobe retraction. Using a microscope, the dura is elevated in a posterolateral-to-anteromedial direction from the middle cranial fossa floor until the defect is visualized. Key anatomical landmarks to identify are the middle meningeal artery anteriorly, the greater superficial petrosal nerve medially, and the arcuate eminence posteriorly. Rarely, the middle meningeal artery needs to be coagulated and divided, as defects are typically located lateral and posterior to the foramen spinosum. Any encephaloceles identified are dissected and then coagulated and sharply cut at the stalk. Intracranial hemostasis is maintained, and dural defects are repaired using an interrupted or running 6-0 monofilament suture. If dural defects are numerous or the dura is of poor quality, a layer of fascia followed by cartilage or bone is draped over the defect. Carlson et al. have found that creating a "sandwich" of fascia, cartilage, and bone and placing the entire "sandwich" as a single unit for repair is useful (24). The muscle and fascia are then closed and the bone plate is secured, and the wound is closed in anatomical layers (24,37).

Combined Middle Cranial Fossa and Transmastoid Approach

The combined approach is a combination of the TM and MCF approach, often utilizing a keyhole craniotomy. As described by Marchioni et al., the combined approach begins with a traditional retroauricular incision extending superiorly to below the superior temporal line. This allows for a wide exposure of the mastoid bone and exposure of the mastoid tegmen superiorly and sigmoid sinus posteroinferiorly. Additionally, the sinodural angle can be fully exposed, and any site of CSF leakage or encephalocele can be identified. The bony defect is located, and an anterior epitympanotomy is performed to preserve the ossicular chain, if possible. This also exposes the lateral epitympanum and the whole tegmen tympani. The authors note that some cases require an endoscopic procedure to expose the dural defect. Mastoidectomy also allows for confirmation of the pathology, facilitation of the dissection of the encephalocele from the ossicles or the tympanic segment of the facial nerve, and optimization of craniotomy placement. From here, if an encephalocele or MEH is found, bipolar cautery is used to gently reduce the dehiscence until the entrance of the dural defect is located. This allows for visualization of the base of the cerebral material and subsequent cutting with microscissors. If there is only CSF leakage without concomitant MEH, the bony wall is removed as described above. Next, a craniotomy is performed along the temporal squama, and the MCF dura mater is exposed. If a single large defect exists, a limited craniotomy centered over the dehiscence can be performed (Figure 11.6). However, if there are multiple dehiscence points or the location is medial, a more "standard" craniotomy can be performed. The dura is gently elevated off the floor of the MCF. Having both extradural and intracranial elevation of the dura allows for exposure of the floor of the mastoid and tegmen intracranially (4,24).

Depending on the size of the defect, the repair is performed using different materials. DuraGen grafts or temporal fascia grafts can be used in a single layer in most cases, but for large defects, multilayer repair is preferred. Some authors believe that autogenous graft material is superior, and the temporal fascia is used most often (7,38). Marchioni et al. suggest using a DuraGen graft or temporal fascia graft as the initial layer and subsequently placing a cortical mastoid graft as the second layer to reconstruct the whole tegmental defect. The graft is then shaped and inserted through the craniotomy between the MCF floor and the temporal lobe dura to cover the tegmen defect in the epidural space. A split thickness bone graft from the craniotomy bone flap can be placed over the repair site to cover the tegmental defect and fixed in place with fibrin glue for stabilization. The mastoid is then filled with Gelfoam and the closure is completed in a multilayered fashion (4). Alternatively, some authors seal the tegmen plate,

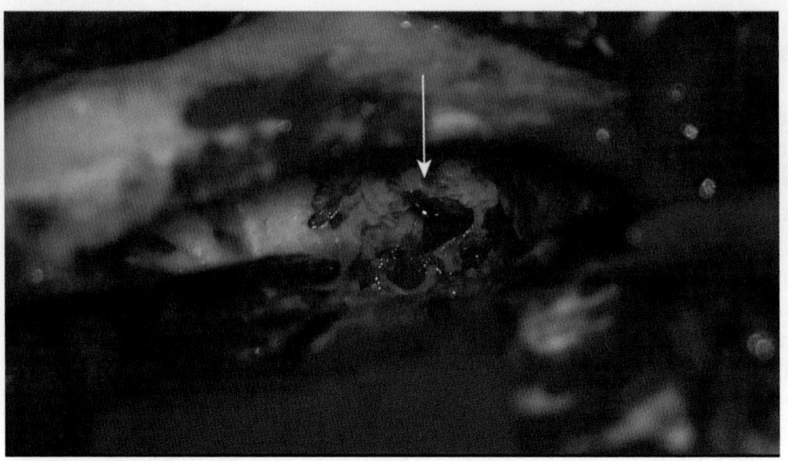

Figure 11.6 Middle cranial fossa approach reveals dehiscence overlying the middle ear.

posterior fossa plate, and otic capsule defects with hydroxyapatite cement (23), titanium mesh (36), and/or MEDPOR (26).

Complication Avoidance

If the TM approach fails, it can be converted intraoperatively into the combined approach for better access. Some authors report that a recurrent CSF leak following the TM approach may be attributed to having a more anteriorly located defect that was not noticed on the initial repair (29). CSF leak or encephalocele recurrence can also be repaired at a later time with either the MCF or combined approach. Paradoxically, the most common complication for the MCF approach is CSF leak (reported up to 13%), but facial nerve palsy, meningitis, hydrocephalus, and ataxia are also seen. CSF leak typically presents within the first few postoperative days as leakage into the wound or posterior rhinorrhea (39,40). Gonen et al. found in a review of 19 publications from 1986 to 2013 that the rate of recurrent CSF leaks postoperatively ranged from 0% to 28.5%. Many studies in this group had no recurrence rates, but two studies showed higher recurrence rates of 27% and 28.5% with noticeably smaller sample size (34). As mentioned, it typically presents as leakage into the wound or as posterior rhinorrhea and is thought to be due to the opening of well-pneumatized temporal bone cells above the superior semicircular canal and the internal auditory canal (37). Scheich and Hagen described resolution of CSF leak in up to 70% of cases through stepwise conservative treatment, including bed rest, pressure dressings, and IV antibiotics. If conservative treatment measures fail, a spinal lumbar drain can be placed, and surgical re-exploration is indicated. Teachey et al. found in a systematic review that there was a statistical difference in successful closure of anterior skull base CSF leaks in patients with active management of increased intracranial pressure compared with no management. Active management was defined as any intervention that measured intracranial pressure, such as lumbar puncture, drain, or ventriculostomy, and long-term management with acetazolamide or CSF diversion with a ventriculoperitoneal or lumbo-peritoneal shunt (41). There is currently no comparison study for lateral skull base CSF leaks or encephaloceles, but managing intracranial hypertension may also be an effective method of reducing recurrence rates. Other complications are very rare but include meningitis, hemorrhage, and pulmonary embolism (37). Kutz et al. also noted that 12.5% of their patients had concomitant superior semicircular canal dehiscence, which is associated with a thin tegmen. They recommend that an intraoperatively identified superior canal dehiscence be plugged with bone wax and then covered with bone cement. They note that no patient in their series showed any negative long-term sequelae (23).

Postoperative Considerations

Gonen et al. found in a review of 284 cases that the MCF approach had an overall complication rate of 5% that included facial palsy, seizures, expressive aphasia, and subdural hematoma. Complications were commonly due to inadvertent dural tears during the craniotomy, and no permanent neurological sequelae resulted (34). Due to the potential complications, the MCF approach has a need for close observation postoperatively, often involving the use of an intensive care unit stay (23). Some authors recommend the use of antiepileptics perioperatively, which can be discontinued at a follow-up appointment approximately two weeks after the procedure (26). If idiopathic intracranial hypertension is believed to be the cause of CSF leaks or encephaloceles, repair of the skull base defect may lead to progression of symptoms, as the intracranial pressure may have been previously normalized by the egress of CSF. Therefore, Kutz et al. recommend that patients obtain a lumbar puncture six weeks postoperatively to assess for idiopathic intracranial hypertension, which is diagnosed with an opening pressure greater than 25 cm/H_2O (23). One drawback of the MCF approach is the need for temporal lobe retraction and the associated potential complications. Venous infarction from prolonged temporal lobe retraction has been reported, but short operative times and intermittent relaxation of retractors has been shown to reduce the risk of this complication. Although lumbar drains are used variably between institutions, CSF drainage can facilitate temporal lobe relaxation and minimize the amount of retraction needed (34). If a lumbar drain is used during the perioperative period there are additional complications to watch for, including tension pneumocephalus, subdural or subarachnoid hemorrhages, retained catheter, meningitis, headaches, radiculopathy, and local wound infection (42). Wound infections are treated with a wound washout with the removal of the craniotomy bone flap, in order to address potential osteomyelitis, often followed by IV antibiotics. Facial nerve or greater superficial petrosal nerve injury is also uncommon with manifestations of facial nerve weakness or eye dryness. Haong et al. noted that most facial nerve symptoms improved by three months, and complete resolution was noted by one year (26). The potential complications of the combined approach include the same risks as the MCF approach (4). Marichioni et al. recommend that a postoperative CT scan be performed one day after combined TM and MCF surgery and for patients to maintain a head elevated position for at least two days with antibiotic and corticosteroid therapy. Kutz et al. recommend a follow-up diffusion-weighted MRI between 18 and 24 months after surgery, due to the risk of cholesteatoma formation if external canal skin is left behind (23). Notably, the transmastoid approach and both the MCF and combined approaches have also been shown to improve hearing in patients postoperatively. This was shown as both subjective improvements and objective improvements in audiogram evaluations and preserved integrity of the ossicular chain postoperatively (4,14,43).

Clinical Pearls

- Encephaloceles and CSF leaks carry great risk because they provide a potential pathway from the middle ear to the subarachnoid space. Potential sequelae include cerebral abscesses, meningitis, encephalitis, and epilepsy.
- A high degree of clinical suspicion is needed to properly diagnose patients with encephaloceles and CSF leaks. The most common complaints are conductive or mixed hearing loss with serous otitis media or a draining ear.
- Suspected encephaloceles or CSF leaks should be assessed by with a β2-transferrin and β-trace protein analysis and a thorough radiological assessment with both high-resolution (CT) and (MRI).
- The TM approach can be used for defects smaller than 1 cm and is minimally invasive without dural manipulation. The TM approach can be converted to the combined approach, if necessary.
- Larger defects require the MCF or combined approach. Both require a craniotomy and temporal lobe retraction. The combined approach allows for the safe repair of large tegmen defects and exposes the dehiscence adequately with either a limited or standard craniotomy, or minimal temporal lobe retraction.
- When there is no possibility of hearing preservation or rehabilitation, an MEO can be considered due to low recurrence rates and definitive treatment.

Key Points

- CSF leaks and encephaloceles are rare herniations of dura mater or brain tissue through skull base defects, commonly in the tegmen tympani or mastoideum.
- Encephaloceles and CSF leaks are difficult to diagnose, because patients often present with

non-specific clinical symptoms. A high degree of clinical suspicion is needed, and a thorough radiologic assessment is performed to confirm the diagnosis and location of bony defects.

- The surgical approach for repair of a tegmen defect depends on the size and location of the bony defect, the status of the ossicular chain and hearing, and the preference of the surgeon.
- Typical surgical approaches include the transmastoid, middle cranial fossa, and combined approaches. Middle-ear obliteration is an alternative approach for refractory cases or definitive treatment.
- Our institution prefers the combined transmastoid and keyhole middle cranial fossa approach.

References

1. Sanna M, Fois P, Russo A, Falcioni M. Management of meningoencephalic herniation of the temporal bone: personal experience and literature review. *Laryngoscope* 2009;**119**:1579–85.
2. Egilmez OK, Hanege FM, Kalcioglu MT, Kaner T, Kokten N. Tegmen tympani defect and brain herniation secondary to mastoid surgery: case presentation. *Case Rep Otolaryngol* 2014;**2014**:756280.
3. Alonso RC, de la Pena MJ, Caicoya AG, Rodriguez MR, Moreno EA, de Vega Fernandez VM: Spontaneous skull base meningoencephaloceles and cerebrospinal fluid fistulas. *Radiographics* 2013;**33**:553–70.
4. Marchioni D, Bonali M, Alicandri-Ciufelli M, Rubini A, Pavesi G, Presutti L. Combined approach for tegmen defects repair in patients with cerebrospinal fluid otorrhea or herniations: our experience. *J Neurol Surg B Skull Base* 2014;**75**:279–87.
5. Jeevan DS, Ormond DR, Kim AH, et al. Cerebrospinal fluid leaks and encephaloceles of temporal bone origin: nuances to diagnosis and management. *World Neurosurg* 2015;**83**:560–6.
6. Schuknecht B, Simmen D, Briner HR, Holzmann D. Nontraumatic skull base defects with spontaneous CSF rhinorrhea and arachnoid herniation: imaging findings and correlation with endoscopic sinus surgery in 27 patients. *AJNR Am J Neuroradiol* 2008;**29**:542–9.
7. Souliere CR, Jr., Langman AW. Combined mastoid/middle cranial fossa repair of temporal bone encephalocele. *Skull Base Surg* 1998;**8**:185–9.
8. Byrne RW, Smith AP, Roh D, Kanner A. Occult middle fossa encephaloceles in patients with temporal lobe epilepsy. *World Neurosurg* 2010;**73**:541–6.
9. Gacek RR, Gacek MR, Tart R. Adult spontaneous cerebrospinal fluid otorrhea: diagnosis and management. *Am J Otol* 1999;**20**:770–6.
10. Stucken EZ, Selesnick SH, Brown KD. The role of obesity in spontaneous temporal bone encephaloceles and CSF leak. *Otol Neurotol* 2012;**33**:1412–17.
11. Sugerman HJ, DeMaria EJ, Felton WL, 3rd, Nakatsuka M, Sismanis A. Increased intra-abdominal pressure and cardiac filling pressures in obesity-associated pseudotumor cerebri. *Neurology* 1997;**49**:507–11.
12. Bakhsheshian J, Hwang MS, Friedman M. Association between obstructive sleep apnea and spontaneous cerebrospinal fluid leaks: a systematic review and meta-analysis. *JAMA Otolaryngol Head Neck Surg* 2015;**141**:733–8.
13. Woodworth BA, Prince A, Chiu AG, et al. Spontaneous CSF leaks: a paradigm for definitive repair and management of intracranial hypertension. *Otolaryngol Head Neck Surg* 2008;**138**:715–20.
14. Braca JA, 3rd, Marzo S, Prabhu VC. Cerebrospinal fluid leakage from tegmen tympani defects repaired via the middle cranial fossa approach. *J Neurol Surg B Skull Base* 2013;**74**:103–7.
15. Parisier SC. The middle cranial fossa approach to the internal auditory canal – an anatomical study stressing critical distances between surgical landmarks. *Laryngoscope* 1977;**87**:1–20.
16. Toth M, Helling K, Baksa G, Mann W. Localization of congenital tegmen tympani defects. *Otol Neurotol* 2007;**28**:1120–3.
17. Semaan MT, Gilpin DA, Hsu DP, Wasman JK, Megerian CA. Transmastoid extradural-intracranial approach for repair of transtemporal meningoencephalocele: a review of 31 consecutive cases. *Laryngoscope* 2011;**121**:1765–72.
18. Rao AK, Merenda DM, Wetmore SJ. Diagnosis and management of spontaneous cerebrospinal fluid otorrhea. *Otol Neurotol* 2005;**26**:1171–5.
19. Dutt SN, Mirza S, Irving RM. Middle cranial fossa approach for the repair of spontaneous cerebrospinal fluid otorrhoea using autologous bone pate. *Clin Otolaryngol Allied Sci* 2001;**26**:117–23.
20. Perez E, Carlton D, Alfarano M, Smouha E. Transmastoid repair of spontaneous cerebrospinal

fluid leaks. *J Neurol Surg B Skull Base* 2018;**79**:451–7.

21. Mayeno JK, Korol HW, Nutik SL. Spontaneous meningoencephalic herniation of the temporal bone: case series with recommended treatment. *Otolaryngol Head Neck Surg* 2004;**130**:486–9.
22. Gioacchini FM, Cassandro E, Alicandri-Ciufelli M, et al. Surgical outcomes in the treatment of temporal bone cerebrospinal fluid leak: A systematic review. *Auris Nasus Larynx* 2018;**45**:903–10.
23. Kutz JW, Jr., Husain IA, Isaacson B, Roland PS. Management of spontaneous cerebrospinal fluid otorrhea. *Laryngoscope* 2008;**118**:2195–9.
24. Carlson ML, Copeland WR III, Driscoll CL, et al. Temporal bone encephalocele and cerebrospinal fluid fistula repair utilizing the middle cranial fossa or combined mastoid-middle cranial fossa approach. *J Neurosurg* 2013;**119**:1314–22.
25. Brown NE, Grundfast KM, Jabre A, Megerian CA, O'Malley BW Jr., Rosenberg SI. Diagnosis and management of spontaneous cerebrospinal fluid-middle ear effusion and otorrhea. *Laryngoscope* 2004;**114**:800–805.
26. Hoang S, Ortiz Torres MJ, Rivera AL, Litofsky NS. Middle cranial fossa approach to repair tegmen defects with autologous or alloplastic graft. *World Neurosurg* 2018;**118**:e10–e17.
27. Sanna M, Dispenza F, Flanagan S, De Stefano A, Falcioni M. Management of chronic otitis by middle ear obliteration with blind sac closure of the external auditory canal. *Otol Neurotol* 2008;**29**:19–22.
28. Leonetti JP, Marzo S, Anderson D, Origitano T, Vukas DD. Spontaneous transtemporal CSF leakage: a study of 51 cases. *Ear Nose Throat J* 2005;**84**:700,2–4, 6.
29. Wootten CT, Kaylie DM, Warren FM, Jackson CG. Management of brain herniation and cerebrospinal fluid leak in revision chronic ear surgery. *Laryngoscope* 2005;**115**:1256–61.
30. Lloyd KM, DelGaudio JM, Hudgins PA. Imaging of skull base cerebrospinal fluid leaks in adults. *Radiology* 2008;**248**:725–36.
31. Gubbels SP, Selden NR, Delashaw JB Jr., McMenomey SO. Spontaneous middle fossa encephalocele and cerebrospinal fluid leakage: diagnosis and management. *Otol Neurotol* 2007;**28**:1131–9.
32. Bovo R, Ceruti S, Padovani R, Martini A. Temporal bone brain herniation. *Otol Neurotol* 2006;**27**:576–7.
33. De Foer B, Vercruysse JP, Bernaerts A, et al. Detection of postoperative residual cholesteatoma with non-echo-planar diffusion-weighted magnetic resonance imaging. *Otol Neurotol* 2008;**29**:513–7.
34. Gonen L, Handzel O, Shimony N, Fliss DM, Margalit N. Surgical management of spontaneous cerebrospinal fluid leakage through temporal bone defects–case series and review of the literature. *Neurosurg Rev* 2016;**39**:141–50; discussion 50.
35. Zanetti DG, Werner G, Gaini L. Transmastoid repair of temporal meningoencephaloceles and cerebrospinal fluid otorrhea. *Otorhinolaryngology Clinics: An International Journal* 2011;**3**:31–41.
36. Jackson CG, Pappas DG Jr., Manolidis S, et al. Brain herniation into the middle ear and mastoid: concepts in diagnosis and surgical management. *Am J Otol* 1997;**18**:198–205; discussion 206.
37. Zanoletti E, Mazzoni A, Martini A, et al. Surgery of the lateral skull base: a 50-year endeavour. *Acta Otorhinolaryngol Ital* 2019;**39**:S1–S146.
38. Sergi B, Passali GC, Picciotti PM, De Corso E, Paludetti G. Transmastoid approach to repair meningoencephalic herniation in the middle ear. *Acta Otorhinolaryngol Ital* 2013;**33**:97–101.
39. Scheich M, Ginzkey C, Ehrmann Muller D, Shehata Dieler W, Hagen R. Complications of the Middle Cranial Fossa Approach for Acoustic Neuroma Removal. *J Int Adv Otol* 2017;**13**:186–90.
40. Scheich M, Ginzkey C, Ehrmann-Muller D, Shehata-Dieler W, Hagen R. Management of CSF leakage after microsurgery for vestibular schwannoma via the middle cranial fossa approach. *Eur Arch Otorhinolaryngol* 2016;**273**:2975–81.
41. Teachey W, Grayson J, Cho DY, Riley KO, Woodworth BA. Intervention for elevated intracranial pressure improves success rate after repair of spontaneous cerebrospinal fluid leaks. *Laryngoscope* 2017;**127**:2011–16.
42. Governale LS, Fein N, Logsdon J, Black PM. Techniques and complications of external lumbar drainage for normal pressure hydrocephalus. *Neurosurgery* 2008;**63**:379–84; discussion 384.
43. Kim L, Wisely CE, Dodson EE. Transmastoid approach to spontaneous temporal bone cerebrospinal fluid leaks: hearing improvement and success of repair. *Otolaryngol Head Neck Surg* 2014;**150**:472–8.

Transcochlear and Extended/Combined Transcochlear Approaches for Complex Tumors of the Skull Base and Posterior Cranial Fossa

Emily Guazzo, Arturo Solares, and Ben Panizza

Introduction

The number of skull base approaches described in the literature highlights that no single approach is superior for all pathologies and locations. A skull base surgeon must tailor their surgery to both the tumor and the patient to optimize conditions for tumor removal while minimizing morbidity. Surgical approaches traversing the temporal bone, also known as lateral skull base approaches, are an attractive option to access the skull base given the direct surgical access to the lower cranial nerves, the intra- and extratemporal internal carotid artery (ICA), and the venous sinuses (1). Lateral skull base approaches can be broadly classified as otic capsule-sparing and otic capsule-sacrificing. Otic capsule-sacrificing approaches, including the translabyrinthine, transotic, and transcochlear approaches, often provide superior access to the internal auditory canal (IAC) and petrous apex. However, this is often at the expense of both auditory and vestibular function and poses varying degrees of risk to the facial nerve. Otic capsule-preserving approaches include those extending superiorly, inferiorly, anteriorly, or posteriorly to the cochlear and labyrinth and ideally preserve both hearing and balance. Surgical access when preserving the otic capsule may be suboptimal, and/or the patient may be exposed to differing surgical morbidities such as those encompassed by a craniotomy (2). Complex tumors may not be adequately addressed with a single surgical approach and require a combination or modification of the aforementioned techniques. In this chapter, we will describe transcochlear approaches and how they can be modified to provide extended skull base access (Table 12.1).

Patient Selection

- Selecting the appropriate surgical approach for an individual patient is perhaps the most challenging aspect of skull base surgery. The surgeon needs to consider and balance the access required to achieve tumor removal against the morbidity of the surgical approach.
- Ideal patients for transcochlear/extended transcochlear approaches are patients with no functional hearing and who have a competent vestibular system on the contralateral side.

Contraindications

- Transcochlear/extended transcochlear approaches are contraindicated for patients with serviceable hearing in whom another skull base approach will provide similar access; for example, patients with a meningioma or lower cranial nerve schwannoma may be amenable to a petro-occipital transsigmoid approach with preservation of middle-ear function and without the morbidity of transposing the facial nerve.
- These approaches are also contraindicated for patients in whom similar degrees of tumor control can be obtained with less potential morbidity to the patient; for example, radiotherapy may be indicated for some tumors, and some tumors can be debulked and do not require en-bloc resection, such as epidermoids.

Preoperative Planning

- Obtain comprehensive preoperative patient history and perform preoperative examination

Table 12.1 Skull Base Approaches

Otic Capsule-Sacrificing Approaches	Description
Translabyrinthine approach	A wide mastoidectomy is performed followed by a labyrinthectomy, and the internal acoustic meatus and cerebellopontine angle are accessed. The facial nerve is left in situ.
Transotic approach	This is an anterior extension of the translabyrinthine approach. It is identical to the transcochlear approach except the facial nerve is left in situ. The cochlea is removed and bone is drilled between the internal carotid artery (ICA) and the geniculate ganglion of the facial nerve via the petrous apex to reach the posterior fossa dura.
Transcochlear approach	Similar to the transotic approach except the facial nerve is transposed posteriorly, allowing wider access to the posterior fossa. The surgeon is not restricted by the facial nerve posteriorly and superiorly and thus can achieve much wider access to the posterior cranial fossa and prepontine region.
Otic Capsule-Preserving (Extralabyrinthine and Extracochlear) Approaches	**Description**
Above the otic capsule	Middle cranial fossa, extended middle cranial fossa, and middle fossa transpetrous approaches.
Passing behind the otic capsule	Retrosigmoid, retrolabyrinthine, and retrolabyrinthine transtentorial approaches.
Passing inferiorly to the otic capsule	Infratemporal fossa type A and extreme lateral approaches.
Passing posteriorly-inferiorly to the otic capsule	Petro-occipital transsigmoid (POTS) approach.
Passing anteriorly to the otic capsule	Infratemporal fossa type B and C and subtemporal preauricular infratemporal approaches.

including clinical examination of hearing, vestibular function, and cranial nerve function.

- Perform audiological evaluation including pure tone audiometry, speech discrimination, and tympanometry.
- Perform vestibular testing, including calorics and electronystagmography (ENG).
- Obtain preoperative imaging, including:
  - CT of petrous temporal bones to assess tumor and radiological features, which determine the degree of surgical access. These include the pneumatization of the mastoid, dehiscence or prominences of the sigmoid or the tegmen, facial nerve position, and any aberrant anatomy.
  - Contrasted MRI to provide superior soft tissue definition; to define the presence and extent of any intracranial extension or cranial nerve involvement; and to assess the proximity and/or infiltration of major vascular structures, including the internal carotid artery, basilar artery, and brainstem perforators.
  - Contrasted imaging to ensure patency of the torcula and to determine the side of dominant intracranial venous drainage. Collateral drainage within the skull base is not as robust as that encountered within the head and neck. Venous infarction or secondary hydrocephalus can occur with ligation or occlusion of the dominant drainage system, resulting in devastating neurological sequelae. Occlusion of the dominant intracranial venous drainage may also result in raised intracranial pressure and increased risk of CSF leak (3).
- Discuss treatment strategies at a multidisciplinary skull base meeting (MDT), including radiation oncologists, medical oncologists, neurosurgeons, otorhinolaryngologists, and head and neck surgeons, to provide the patient with a consensus regarding the best clinical treatment paradigm.
- Obtain thorough informed consent about potential complications and expected postoperative course of treatment.

Transcochlear Approach

Originally described by Drs. House and Hitselberger in 1976, the transcochlear approach is an extension of the translabyrinthine approach to the cerebellopontine angle (CPA) (4). The approach is similar to the transotic approach, with the addition of posterior facial nerve transposition. Facial nerve transposition provides wider surgical exposure of the posterior cranial fossa, anterior aspect of the CPA, petrous apex, petrous ICA, and lower cranial nerves, without the need for brain retraction (1,2,5).

Indications

- Extensive petrous apex lesions with facial nerve compromise, including cholesteatomas, large facial nerve hemangiomas/schwannomas, and cholesterol granulomas
- CPA lesions anterior to the IAC extending into prepontine cistern or clivus, including meningiomas, jugulotympanic paragangliomas, chordomas/chondrosarcomas, and (rarely) acoustic neuromas
- Extensive lesions of the clivus or petroclival region (1,2,5,6)

Advantages

- Improved anterior access compared with the translabyrinthine approach through wide exposure of the posterior cranial fossa, and anterior aspect of the CPA, petrous apex, and clivus
- Greater field of access compared with the transotic approach in that the surgeon is not limited by an acutely angulated surgical field between the ICA and the facial nerve; posterior facial transposition means that the surgical field is extended superiorly and posteriorly
- No/limited brain parenchyma retraction and thus lower risk of temporal lobe ischemia/necrosis, intradural bleeding, seizures, and chronic headaches (5)
- Increased vascular control for the surgeon through improved visualization and access for dissection of tumor off of major vascular structures

Disadvantages

- Destruction of the cochlea/vestibule and subsequent loss of auditory and vestibular function (5)
- Postoperative facial nerve dysfunction, with immediate complete facial nerve dysfunction to be expected; long-term facial nerve recovery, even with an experienced surgeon, rarely surpasses a House-Brackmann score of 3 (7)

Surgical Steps

Preoperative Preparation/Patient Positioning

- The patient is placed in a supine position in a Mayfield head clamp with the head turned to the contralateral side.
- The procedure is performed under general anesthesia with short-acting or no paralysis to facilitate facial nerve and other lower cranial nerve electromyography (EMG) monitoring as appropriate.
- Intravenous antibiotics are administered preoperatively and every six hours intraoperatively.
- Anti-embolism stockings are placed to minimize perioperative thromboembolic complications.
- Pressure areas are minimized, given the anticipated length of surgery.

Soft Tissue Dissection/Access

- See Figures 12.1–12.3. A postauricular incision is made 3–4 cm posterior to the sulcus, extending superiorly to the level of the helical root and inferiorly to the mastoid tip.
- Soft-tissue dissection is extended anteriorly until the external auditory canal (EAC) is palpable. A posteriorly based U-shaped mastoid periosteal flap is raised, and the EAC is identified using a Cryer elevator.
- The EAC is transected at the bony-cartilaginous junction and dissection proceeds anteriorly over the parotid fascia to provide circumferential exposure of the EAC.
- Skin of the cartilaginous EAC is carefully dissected off using iris scissors or sharp dissection. The skin is then everted, and a layered closure is performed with 3.0 Vicryl using mattress sutures to create a blind sac closure. It is important to avoid buttonholes of the EAC skin to avoid blind sac necrosis and subsequent risk of CSF leak.
- The epithelium of the bony EAC and the entire tympanic membrane are removed. It is

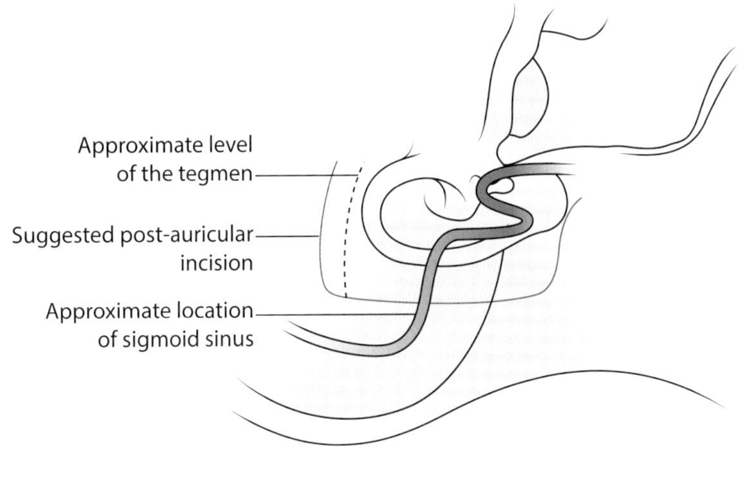

Figure 12.1 Post-auricular incision for transchlear approach

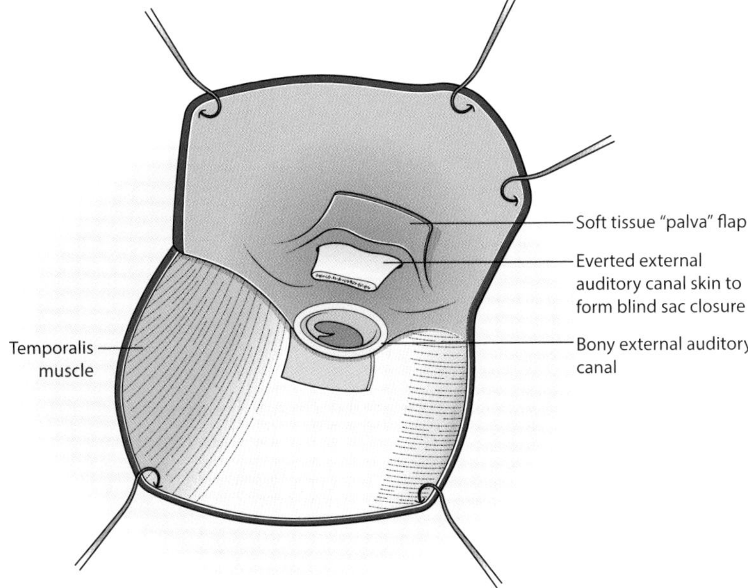

Figure 12.2 The soft tissue layers for the transcochlear approach

important to ensure complete removal of the squamous lining of the EAC and tympanic membrane to prevent long-term iatrogenic implantation cholesteatoma.

- The incudostapedial joint is disarticulated, and the incus and the malleus are removed.

Mastoidectomy

- See Figure 12.4. Complete mastoidectomy is performed with a large cutting burr, ensuring that all mastoid air cells are exenterated. The middle fossa dura, posterior fossa dura, and sigmoid are all exposed and skeletonized.
- The facial nerve is identified using standard mastoidectomy landmarks and traced from the geniculate ganglion to the stylomastoid foramen using a diamond burr with copious irrigation.
- The canals of the labyrinth are identified, and all infralabyrinthine and retrofacial air cells are completely removed.
- The sigmoid sinus is followed retrofacially to allow identification of the jugular bulb.
- The posterior aspect of the EAC wall is drilled flush to the level of the facial nerve, similarly to a canal wall down mastoidectomy. The anterior wall of the external canal wall is

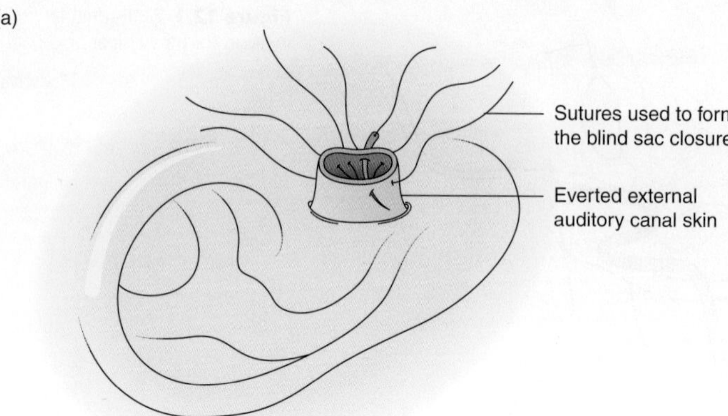

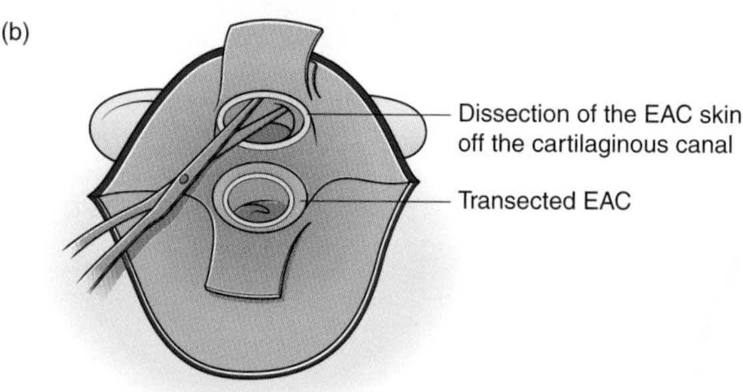

Figure 12.3 The formation of the blind sac closure showing (a) location of the sutures and (b) transected external auditory canal

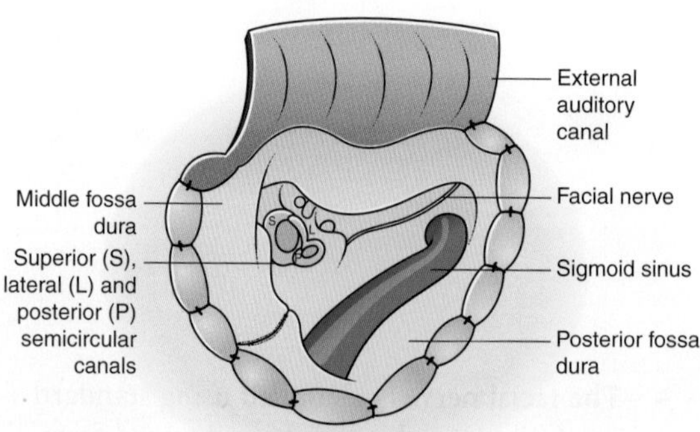

Figure 12.4 Extended mastoidectomy with the identification of facial nerve and semicircular canals

skeletonized, with care taken not to violate the temporomandibular joint (TMJ) capsule.

Labyrinthectomy and Identification of the Internal Acoustic Meatus (IAM)

- See Figures 12.5–12.7. Labyrinthectomy involves complete removal of all the semicircular canals. Using a 4 mm cutting burr, commence the labyrinthectomy at the posterior semicircular canal (PSCC); then continue to the lateral semicircular canal (LSCC) and the superior semicircular canal (SSCC) with identification of the subarcuate artery. During the labyrinthectomy, the anterior wall of the LSCC and the ampulla of the SSCC are initially preserved; these provide protection to the tympanic and labyrinthine portions of the facial nerve and serve as a landmark for the superior vestibular nerve, respectively. Open the vestibule by drilling through the ampulla of the horizontal semicircular canal (HSCC).
- Next, the IAC is identified. This starts with delineation of the superior and inferior boundaries of the canal at the porus acusticus by following the posterior fossa dura forward to the fundus. The SSCC ampulla is a useful landmark for identifying the superior vestibular nerve and superior border of the IAC at the fundus.

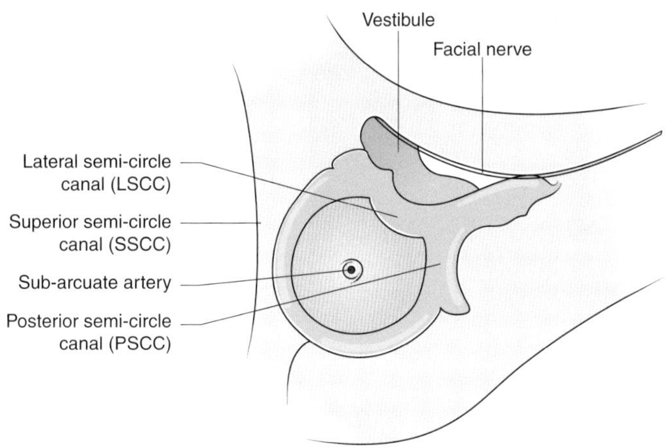

Figure 12.5 Identification and opening of the superior semicircular canal and subarcuate artery

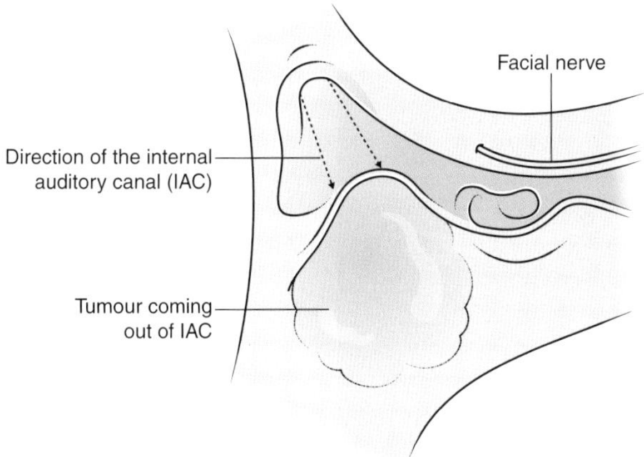

Figure 12.6 Identification of the internal auditory canal

- At the end of the labyrinthectomy, the superior and inferior extent of the IAC are clearly identified, and 270 degrees of the dura is visible. The IAC is opened, and its contents are determined by their relationship to the transverse crest and Bill's bar.
- Identify the facial nerve in the IAC by first identifying the superior vestibular nerve. The superior vestibular nerve is transected and mobilized posteriorly, allowing the facial nerve to be visualized in the anterior-superior location. This is subsequently confirmed on EMG with facial nerve stimulation, if needed (2,4-8).

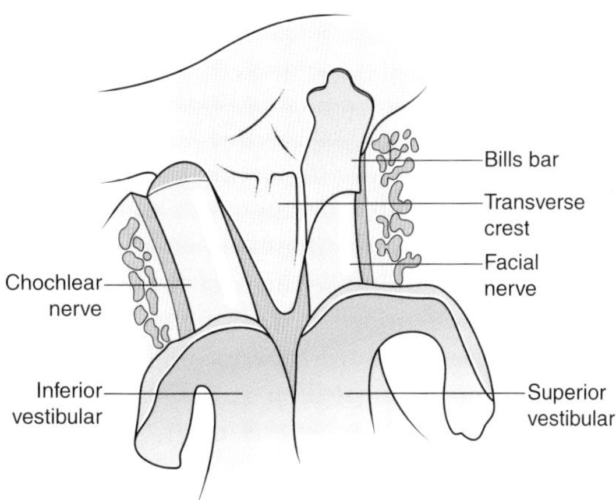

Figure 12.7 Exposure after opening of the internal auditory canal and identification of the facial nerve

Facial Nerve Mobilization

- See Figures 12.8–12.11. Complete decompression of the facial nerve from the IAC to the stylomastoid foramen is important to allow posterior facial nerve transposition. Facial nerve decompression is usually

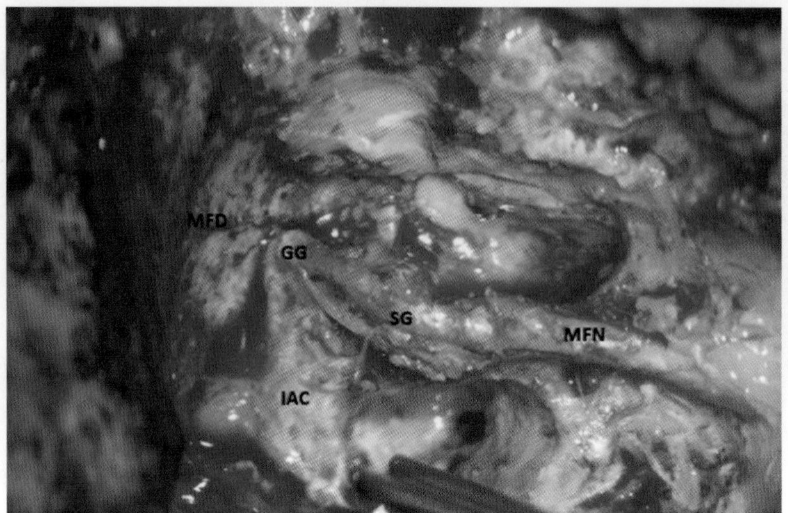

Figure 12.8 Intraoperative photograph of the exposure and decompression of the full length of the facial nerve. MFD = middle fossa dura, GG = geniculate ganglion, SG = second genu, MFN = meatal segment of facial nerve, IAC = internal auditory canal.

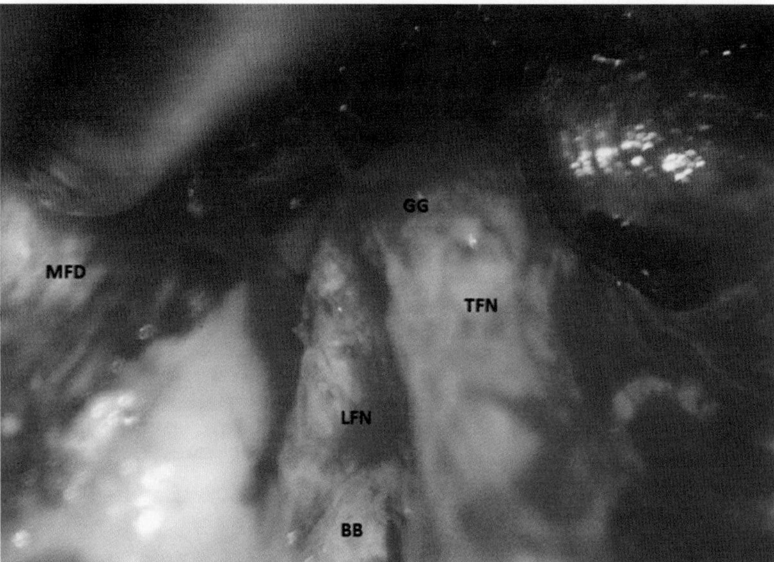

Figure 12.9 Intraoperative increased magnification view of the geniculate ganglion (GG). MFD = middle fossa dura, BB = Bill's bar, LFN = labyrinthine segment of facial nerve, TFN = tympanic segment of facial nerve.

performed with a diamond burr and copious irrigation to avoid thermal injury.

- The labyrinthine segment of the facial nerve is identified at the fundus of the IAC and traced upward superiorly to identify the geniculate ganglion at the superior aspect of the tympanic segment. Anterior to the geniculate ganglion, the greater superficial petrosal nerve (GSPN) and the petrosal branch of the middle meningeal artery are identified prior to their entry into the middle cranial fossa via the facial hiatus. To improve visualization of these structures, the middle cranial fossa dura can be elevated. The GSPN and its accompanying artery are then cut with bipolar cautery to allow mobilization of the geniculate ganglion. The acute angulation of the nerve, as well as the reduced blood supply, make the geniculate and labyrinthine segments particularly vulnerable to injury.
- The complete length of the facial nerve, from the IAC to the stylomastoid foramen, is mobilized from the underlying bone using a right-angled hook or a small sickle knife. Protect the mobilized segment of facial nerve by placing it on the posterior fossa dura

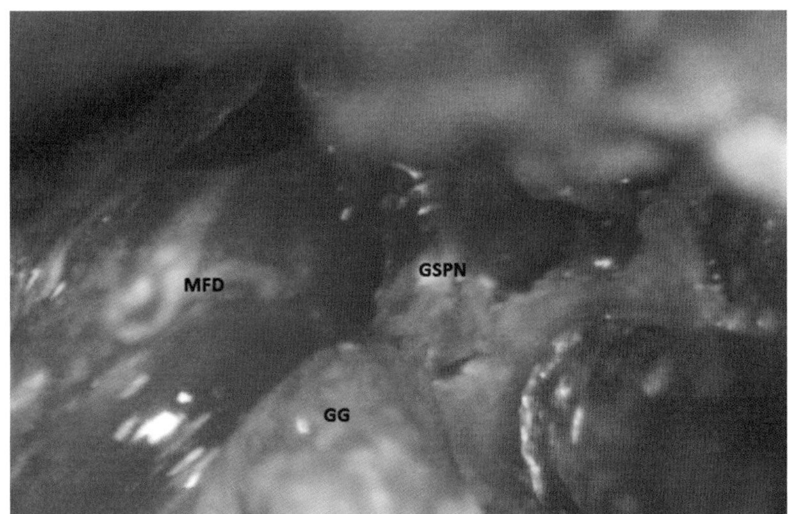

Figure 12.10 Intraoperative increased magnification view again displaying the geniculate ganglion (GG) and the greater superficial petrosal nerve (GSPN). MFD = middle fossa dura.

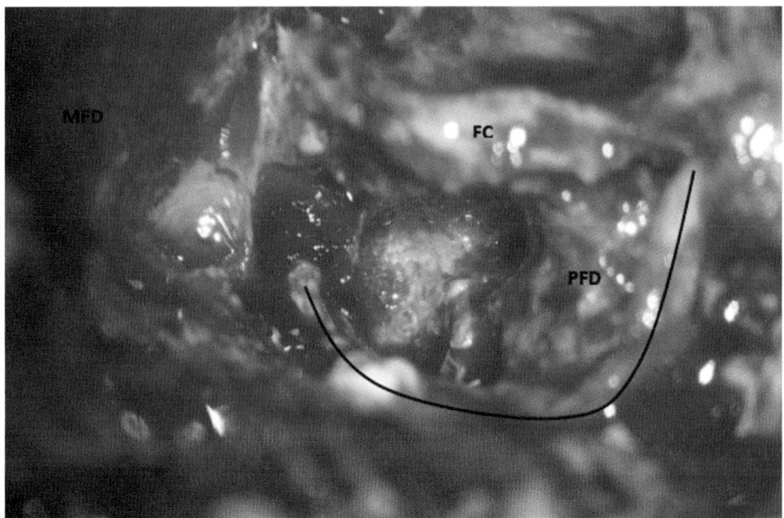

Figure 12.11 Intraoperative view showing posterior translocation of the facial nerve (solid black line). MFD = middle fossa dura, FC = fallopian canal, PFD = posterior fossa dura.

anterior to the sigmoid and posterior to the jugular bulb and securing it with fibrin glue and/or covering it with silastic sheeting.

Transcochlear Surgical Steps

- See Figures 12.12–12.13. The posterior translocation of the facial nerve ensures much wider surgical access than in the transotic approach. All bone is removed between the ICA anteriorly, the jugular bulb inferiorly, the tegmen superiorly, and the translocated facial nerve posteriorly. This involves the complete destruction of the cochlea.
- It is important to identify the ICA in the middle ear to avoid causing injury to it. The ICA is immediately medial to the floor of the eustachian tube (ET), and they are separated by a thin bony lamina. Careful dissection is important in this region, as in 2% of patients the ICA is dehiscent. The carotid lies anterior and medial to the cochlea; however, this relationship is quite variable, ranging from 1 mm to 5 mm between structures.
- The cochlea is drilled and the tensor tympani muscle is sacrificed to ensure complete cochlear exenteration. Drilling continues through the petrous apex and clivus until the posterior fossa dura is exposed. The inferior petrosal sinus marks the junction between the petrous apex and the clivus and often must be packed with Surgicel for hemostatic control. It is important to ensure that the sinus is packed as loosely as possible while still providing

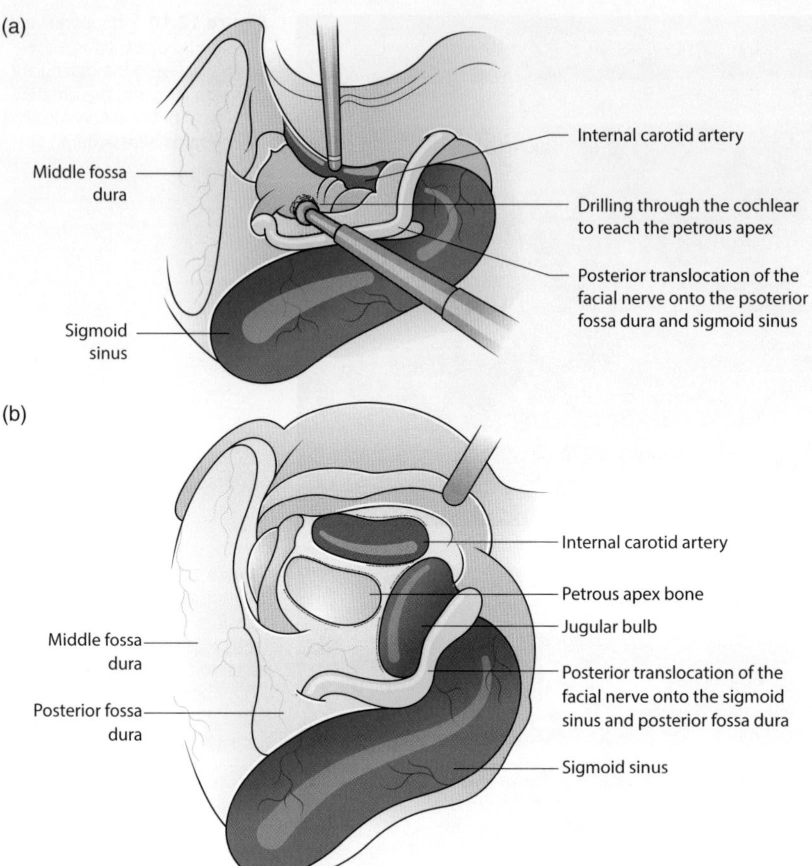

Figure 12.12 Drilling through the cochlear to reach the petrous apex (a) with magnified view (b)

adequate hemostasis, as "overpacking" can result in glossopharyngeal nerve injury.

- Intradural tumor can be removed via an incision in the dura anterior to the IAC to avoid iatrogenic injury to the facial nerve. Once the dura is incised, one obtains excellent access to the basilar artery and the prepontine cistern. Inferiorly, both vertebral arteries can be seen, and superiorly, with retraction, the middle cranial fossa, the superior cerebellar artery, and the trigeminal nerve can be visualized.

Defect Reconstruction and Closure

- It is important to close as much dura as possible to create the smallest possible dural defect to minimize the risk of CSF leak. A generous amount of fat is harvested from the abdomen to obliterate the operative cavity. The eustachian tube is tightly occluded with muscle and fascia usually harvested from the temporalis region. The soft tissues are closed in a layered fashion, and a head wrap with a mastoid pressure dressing is applied and left in situ for three to five days.

Clinical Pearls

- To create additional space for improved surgical access, the sigmoid sinus and middle fossa dura can be decompressed.
- The geniculate ganglion is especially vulnerable to injury, so care must be taken to avoid causing damage during the transposition of the facial nerve.
- Difficulty in facial nerve mobilization is usually secondary to inadequate facial nerve decompression and subsequently compromises surgical access.
- Removal of the bone separating the IAC segment of the facial nerve from the superior vestibular nerve, known as Bill's bar, is often the key to commencing facial nerve mobilization.

(a)

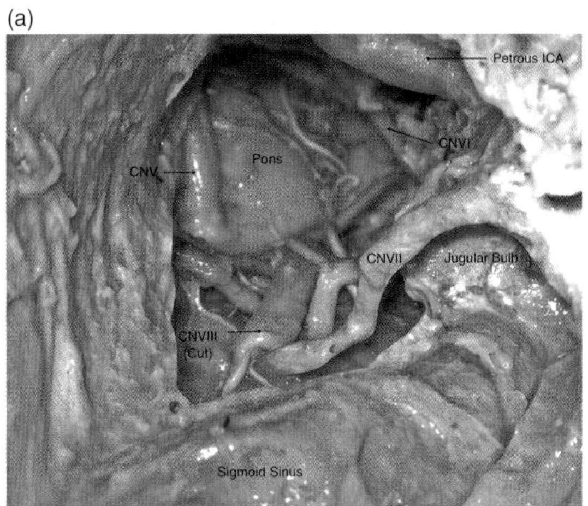

(b)

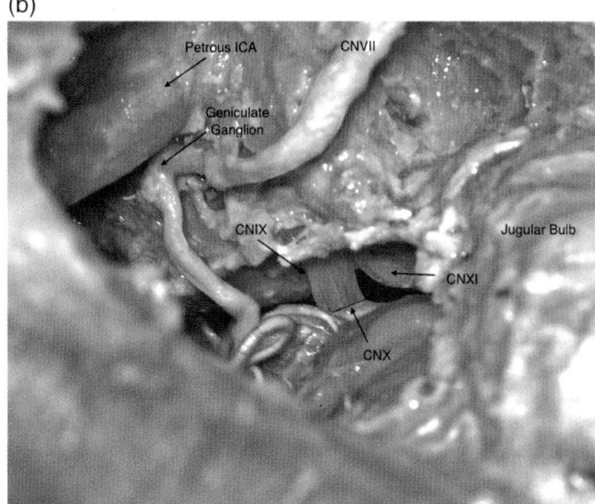

Figure 12.13 Cadaver view of incisions made in the posterior fossa dura (a) with magnified view (b)

- Given the fibrous attachments to the fallopian canal, it may be necessary to sharply dissect the mastoid segment of the facial nerve using a right-angled hook, sickle knife, or microscissors.
- Decompression is continued to the stylomastoid foramen, and all tissue around the foramen is freed to allow tension-free posterior translocation of the facial nerve and access to the inferior border of the tumor.
- Decompressing and depressing the jugular bulb can assist in visualization of the lower cranial nerves and the vertebrobasilar junction.
- The ICA always needs to be identified but is only mobilized to the extent necessary for tumor removal. Often, the majority of the dissection is deep to the ICA. However, if further anterior exposure is required, the artery can be skeletonized and mobilized in its vertical and horizontal segmentals, respectively, and transposed anteriorly. The surgeon must be mindful that with increased carotid mobilization the potential for intracranial ischemic complications increases accordingly.
- When drilling is extended to the anteromedial aspect of the clivus, the abducens nerve is at risk in Dorello's canal. Using Dorello's canal and the inferior petrosal sinus as the anterior limit of the posterior cranial fossa, exposure should protect the abducens nerve from iatrogenic injury. However, often these landmarks are obliterated by the tumor. In this situation, abducens monitoring and/or careful examination of the abducens position on preoperative imaging is essential.
- For benign tumors or unresectable tumors with intact facial nerve function, consider leaving the tumor on the facial nerve and observing for ongoing tumor growth or treating with radiotherapy.

Further Anterior Access Required: Combined Transcochlear and Infratemporal Fossa Fisch Type B or C Approach

Indications

- Tumors involving both the temporal bone and the infratemporal fossa/parapharyngeal space
- Benign or malignant lesions with circumferential involvement of the ICA
- Petroclival lesions that extend in a limited fashion to the contralateral side
- Intracranial lesions extending down into the parapharyngeal space or infratemporal fossa

Advantages

- Access anteriorly to the infratemporal fossa, parapharyngeal space, clivus, and nasopharynx

- Inferior control of major vascular structures: exposure and control of the ICA extra- and intratemporally, and exposure of the entire course of the sigmoid sinus, jugular bulb, and internal jugular vein (IJV).
- Access to the lower cranial nerves from the skull base to the periphery.
- In the Type B approach, wide access to the clivus via inferior reflection of the zygomatic arch and temporalis muscle, removal of the middle fossa skull base, and anterior mobilization of the ICA.
- In the Type C approach, access to the nasopharynx via resection of the pterygoid plates; however, staged surgery – usually more appropriate given a resection from the prepontine cistern directly into the nasopharynx – is undesirable.

Disadvantages

- Morbid surgery; staged surgery with access to the anterior aspect of the tumor should be considered
- Entry into the nasopharynx or sphenoid sinus, which results in high rates of CSF leak into the sinonasal cavity unless the surgery is staged

Surgical Steps

Surgery proceeds per the transcochlear approach with the modifications described below. Extend or modify your postauricular incision as needed to provide adequate access.

Combined with Type B Infratemporal Approach: Wide Access to the Clivus

- The facial nerve is located preauricularly at the stylomastoid foramen using the standard landmarks. The upper branch of the facial nerve is traced in a similar manner to a parotidectomy to the level of the frontalis branch. While protecting the frontal branch of the facial nerve, perform osteotomies of the zygomatic arch anteriorly and posteriorly. The removed segment of the zygoma is kept and often replaced at the end of the operation to assist in facial contouring.
- The anterior wall of the bony EAC is drilled, and the capsule of the TMJ is identified and separated. The mandibular condyle is exposed by removing the TMJ articular disk. A Fisch infratemporal fossa retractor is used to retract the ascending ramus of the mandible, which is displaced antero-inferiorly.
- The middle fossa dura in the subtemporal region is skeletonized until the foramen ovale is reached. The middle meningeal artery and mandibular division of the trigeminal nerve are coagulated/divided at the foramen spinosum and foramen ovale, respectively, to permit greater surgical exposure.
- The ICA is exposed in the middle ear at its genu and followed along the medial aspect of the ET. The entire vertical and horizontal segments of the ICA are skeletonized. The horizontal ICA is followed anteromedially to the level of the pterygoid process. This allows the ICA to be transposed anteriorly, allowing for improved access to both the petrous apex and clivus.

Combined with Type C Infratemporal Approach: Access to the Nasopharynx

- Initial surgical steps are the same as the Type B infratemporal fossa approach.
- The ICA is exposed over both its vertical and horizontal segments, and the bony eustachian tube is removed until the osseocartilaginous junction is exposed.
- Subperiosteal dissection of the lateral pterygoid allows for elevation and lateralization of all lateral pterygoid attachments.
- The pterygoid process and body are removed until the sphenoid sinus mucosa is visible and the middle fossa dura is identified.
- For tumors involving the nasopharynx, access can be obtained by removing the medial pterygoid plate. Usually, this would require a staged approach and would be considered for benign or low-grade malignancies (2,9,10).

Superior Extension: Subtemporal Exposure

Indications

- Posterior fossa tumors that extend into the middle fossa via direct tentorial invasion through Meckel's cave or the tentorial notch

Advantages

- Access to tumors extending into the middle cranial fossa anterior to the pons and midbrain
- Minimal temporal lobe retraction in combination with a craniotomy

Disadvantages

- Increased middle cranial fossa exposure with increased risks of intracranial injury, bleed, and CSF leak

Surgical Steps

Surgery proceeds per the transcochlear approach with the modifications described as follows.

Subtemporal Extension

- See Figures 12.14–12.16. During the mastoidectomy, perform a wide exposure of the middle cranial fossa dura to obtain extended superior access. Usually, 3–5 cm of the middle cranial fossa is exposed; however, this is dependent on the extent of the tumor present above the tentorial notch.
- The middle fossa dural incision is placed superior and parallel to the superior petrosal sinus, and the sinus is subsequently incised and obliterated with Surgicel or a surgical clip.
- The tentorium is incised anterior to the junction of the sigmoid and the superior petrosal sinus. The surgeon then continues in an anterior-medial direction until the tentorial notch is reached. It is important to avoid injury to the trochlear nerve and oculomotor nerve by excising posterior to where the nerves enter the tentorium. If the tentorium is involved with tumor, then it is excised (2,10).

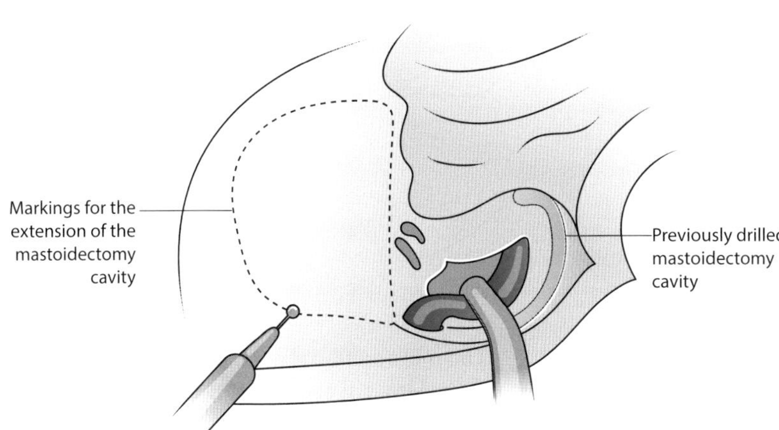

Figure 12.14 Superior extension of the mastoidectomy (shaded in blue)

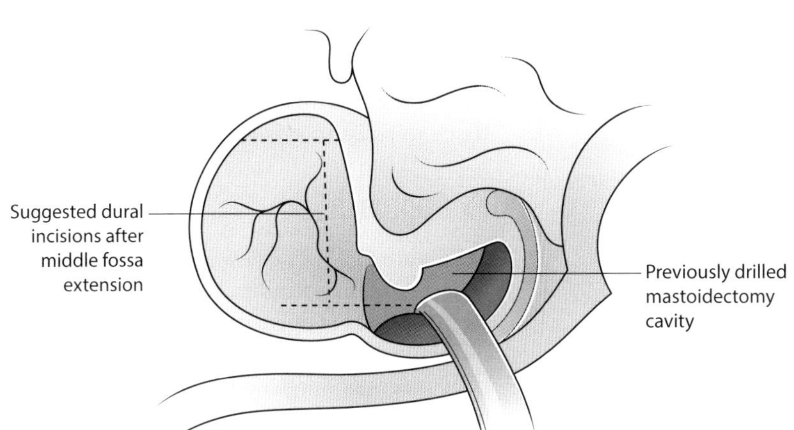

Figure 12.15 Middle fossa dura incision

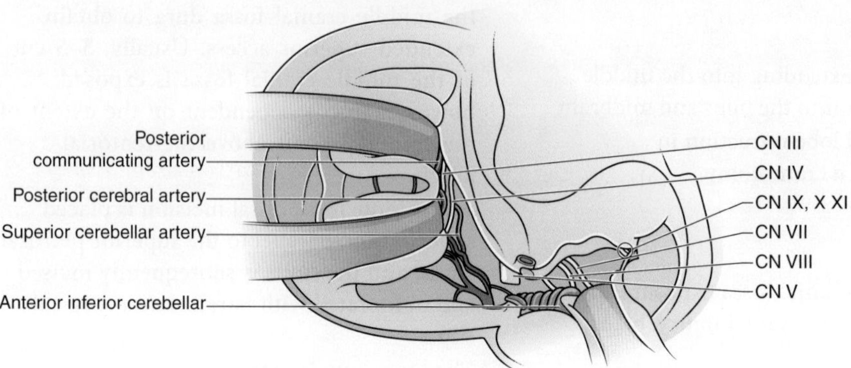

Figure 12.16 Final exposure after the tentorium is incised

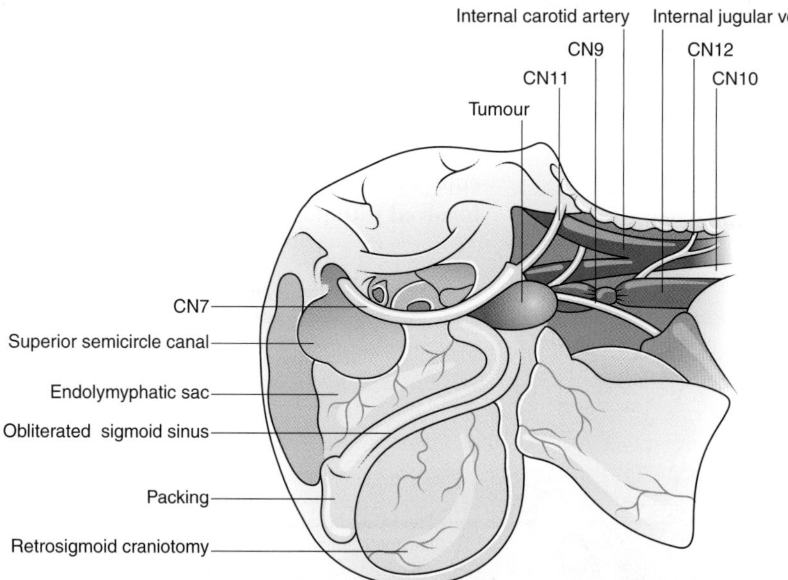

Figure 12.17 Final exposure achieved by the petro-occipital trans-sigmoid approach

Inferior Extension: Petro-occipital Transsigmoid Approach (POTS)

Indications

- Lesions of the middle and lower clivus
- Lesions extending into the jugular foramen and upper neck

Advantages

- Improved access to the jugular bulb, jugular foramen, and foramen magnum
- Access to the clivus more inferiorly than possible with a transcochlear approach

Surgical Steps

Surgery proceeds per the transcochlear approach with the modifications described as follows.

- The incision is extended inferiorly 2 cm below the mastoid. Take care not to extend this incision too far into the neck, as this increases the chance of postoperative CSF leak. If CSF leak into the neck does occur, the CSF usually resolves spontaneously, given its limited space to drain.
- The fascia and muscle are incised in a U-shape, based inferiorly to allow preservation of soft tissue to assist in closure.

POTS Approach

- See Figure 12.17. The flow in the sigmoid sinus is decreased by extradural compression. The sigmoid sinus is opened and packed intraluminally proximally and distally with large pieces of Surgicel. Proximal packing is done initially to eliminate blood flow. Distal

packing commences at the sigmoid but is progressively advanced to the jugular bulb.
- Bleeding can be encountered from the inferior petrosal sinus, which is identified within the lumen of the jugular bulb. However, in cases requiring a POTS, the inferior petrosal sinus is often already occluded by the tumor. Care must be taken, as overzealous packing may result in glossopharyngeal nerve injury.
- The sigmoid incision can be continued down the lateral wall of the internal jugular vein (IJV) for extended access. It is important not to disrupt the medial wall of the IJV to protect the integrity of the glossopharyngeal and vagus nerves.
- The sternocleidomastoid muscle (SCM) is dissected out of the investing fascia and retracted laterally and posteriorly. The carotid sheath is identified superiorly in the neck, and the IJV, ICA, and hypoglossal and accessory nerves are identified in the neck.
- Once vascular control has been achieved, the dura can be opened. A retrosigmoid craniotomy can be performed for improved posterior access; however, when this approach is combined with a transcochlear approach, a small retrosigmoid craniotomy will already have been performed with 2–3 cm of bone already removed posterior to the sigmoid. The dura is opened at the posterior aspect of the sigmoid. With this exposure, the lower cranial nerves, vertebral artery, and basilar artery are exposed.
- After resection of the tumor is complete, the dura is closed as much as possible, and the residual defect is obliterated with abdominal fat and fascia until a watertight seal is achieved (2,11-14).

Further Inferior Extension: Extreme Lateral Approach

Indications

- Lesions involving the whole clivus with inferior extension into the foramen magnum or hypoglossal canal or further inferiorly toward the craniocervical junction.

Advantages

- Vertebral artery can be seen throughout its intracranial course and controlled both proximally and distally.
- Good access to the anterolateral aspect of the brainstem.

Disadvantages

- Such wide extension carries a high risk of postoperative CSF leak because of the connection between the soft tissues of the neck and the subarachnoid space. Provided the neck wound is limited, a majority of these leaks settle spontaneously.

Surgical Steps

Surgery proceeds per the transcochlear approach with the modifications described as follows.

- Extend the skin incision inferiorly into the posterior aspect of the neck to provide the additional access needed for the extreme lateral approach.

Extreme Lateral Approach

- See Figure 12.18. The mastoid process is identified, and its muscular attachments – the SCM, splenius capitis, longissimus capitis, and semispinalis capitis – are detached to expose the suboccipital triangle (2,15).
- The transcochlear approach is performed as described earlier in this chapter.
- The occipital artery (located in the roof of the suboccipital triangle) is ligated.
- The vertebral artery extends from the foramen transversarium of the C1 vertebrae and runs along the floor of the suboccipital triangle prior to piercing the atlanto-occipital membrane. Identify it by detaching the superior and inferior oblique muscles off the transverse process of the C1 vertebrae and reflecting them posteriorly.
- The transverse process of the C1 vertebrae is identified, and the foramen transversarium is exposed. Within the foramen, the vertebral artery is surrounded by a rich venous plexus. To avoid troublesome bleeding, perform dissection in a subperiosteal plane until the vertebral artery is mobilized.
- The spinal accessory nerve, extradural posterior spinal artery, and posterior inferior cerebellar artery are closely related to the vertebral artery as it enters the dura. Care

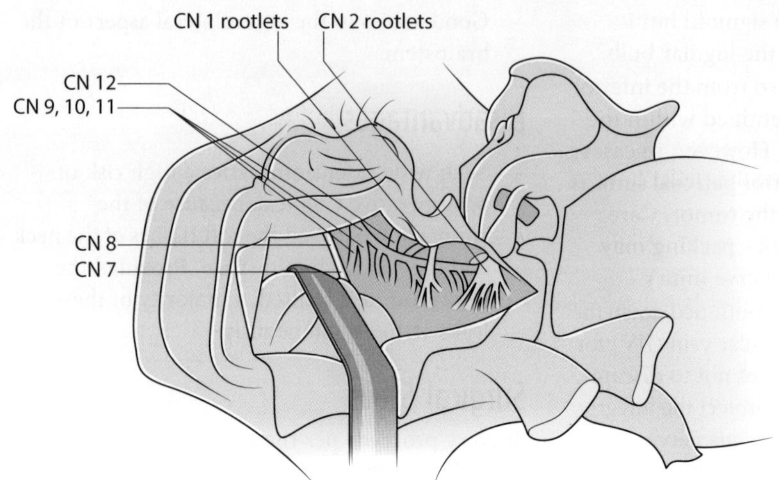

Figure 12.18 Final exposure achieved by the extended lateral approach

must be taken to avoid iatrogenic injury to these structures.

- Drilling is continued downward to provide access to the lateral rim of the foramen magnum.
- The lateral aspect of the occipital condyle is removed with a high-speed drill and a cutting burr. When drilling the occipital condyle, little bleeding is encountered from the cortical layer; however, once the cancellous layer is reached, Surgicel and bone wax may be required to achieve hemostasis.
- If more than one-third of the condyle is removed, craniocervical junction instability may occur and operative fixation should be considered. Total condylectomy does not significantly increase petroclival exposure and results in significant craniocerebral junction instability and is therefore not advised.
- A malleable retractor is used to protect the cervical spinal cord dura, and the bone of the C1 and C2 vertebrae are removed. Care is taken not to injure the cervical spinal nerves or the vertebral artery.
- The posterior fossa dura is opened longitudinally posterior to the sigmoid sinus. It may be necessary to cauterize the marginal sinus prior to opening the dura. As the vertebral artery enters the intracranial cavity, the dura is often very adherent; a cuff may be left behind to preserve vascular integrity.

Dressings and Postoperative Care

- The wound is closed in a watertight fashion and dressed with a tight head bundle. The head bundle should remain in situ for at least 72 hours to minimize wound disturbance and subsequent CSF leak.
- The patient is transferred to an ICU or high-acuity facility.
- If the patient is extubated postoperatively, they must be closely monitored with routine neurological checks and vital signs.
- Subcutaneous heparin is commenced on the first-day post-operation, and TEDS and intermittent pneumatic compression devices are instituted both intra- and postoperatively.
- IV prophylactic antibiotics are routinely administered for 48 hours after the surgery.
- Physiotherapy is instituted on day one, and all barriers to mobilization – such as an indwelling catheter – are removed if the patient's mental status permits.
- A CT head scan without contrast is performed 24 hours postoperatively, or at any time there is neurological dysfunction during the postoperative course.

Complications

CSF Leak

CSF leak rates following lateral skull base surgery vary in the literature from 2% to 30% (16-19). This complication can be minimized by ensuring watertight dural closure/repair, adequate eustachian tube blockage, and careful blind sac closure. Certain patients are at increased risk, including patients with large/complex tumors with both intra- and extradural components, patients who have had revision surgery or irradiated surgical fields, or patients in whom the venous drainage has been obstructed by the tumor. Staged procedures should be considered for tumors with intra- and extradural components (20). Free flap reconstruction should be considered in high-risk cases to reinforce dural closure. Following lateral skull base surgery, CSF leaks usually manifest as either (1) discharge from the postauricular wound leaking from a dehiscent blind sac closure or (2) rhinorrhea. The timely identification and management of a CSF leak are important, as leaks represent a potential portal for infection, which may result in meningitis and neurological sequelae.

Management

Conservative Management

The rate of spontaneous resolution of CSF leak, with conservative management, is high (19,21,22). Conservative measures usually include bed rest, head elevation, administration of stool softeners and acetazolamide, and placement of compressive dressings over the surgical site. Acetazolamide (Diamox), a diuretic that reduces CSF production and thus intracranial pressure, is used in many institutions as part of a conservative paradigm. While it is logical to suspect that reducing intracranial pressure encourages arachnoid repair and resolution of CSF leaks, the evidence supporting the use of acetazolamide in lateral skull base surgery is limited (23-25). Pressure dressings are thought to work by pushing the fat obliterating the mastoid/middle-ear space back into the dural defect (26). If a subcutaneous CSF collection is present, sterile aspiration may be considered prior to the application of a pressure dressing. All other conservative measures are aimed at reducing intracranial pressure to encourage closure of the arachnoid.

Lumbar Drain

A lumbar drain may be used in conjunction with, or after failure of, conservative measures. It is effective in resolving CSF fistulas following lateral skull base surgery in 31–83% of cases; however, it is not without complications (22,26-28). Minor complications, including headaches, nausea, and vomiting, have been reported in up to 59% of patients. More severe complications such as tentorial herniation, tension pneumocephalus, and severe neurological deterioration are less common (27,28).

Surgical Revision

When conservative measures fail over a period of 48–72 hours, surgical revision and reclosure are indicated. The fat obliterating the dural defect is removed and repacked. A collagen matrix such as DuraGen can be considered to encourage dural closure. The surgeon must ensure that all air cell tracts are completely exenterated and that the eustachian tube has been successfully obliterated. The soft tissues and skin edges must be meticulously closed in an airtight fashion (21,26).

Wound Infection

Wound infections following transcochlear/transotic approaches include simple skin infections or necrosis of the abdominal fat graft used to obliterate the mastoid/middle ear potential space. It is important to identify wound infections early and to instigate appropriate treatment to prevent fat graft infarction and subsequent CSF leak due to inadequate dural repair support. At our institution, postoperative intravenous antibiotics are administered prophylactically and then continued or discontinued at the clinician's discretion.

Facial Nerve Dysfunction

- Posterior rerouting of the facial nerve almost invariably results in complete ipsilateral weakness in the immediate postoperative period (19,29,30). This is likely due to a combination of microsurgical manipulation and ischemic injury following the division of the blood vessels traveling with the GSPN (31). Gradual partial recovery is usually expected, with House-Brackmann grade 3 nerve function seen in 70% of patients undergoing transcochlear approaches in a series by Russo et al. (32).

– Immediately postoperatively, facial nerve dysfunction is managed conservatively with lubricating eye drops and eye closure at nighttime to prevent corneal injury secondary to exposure. Long-term dysfunction can be managed with static or dynamic surgical facial nerve reanimation or rehabilitation as appropriate.

Cranial Nerve Dysfunction

Extended approaches to the lateral skull base may result in lower cranial nerve dysfunction. This may present as postoperative dysphagia and dysphonia, and potentially result in aspiration or respiratory impairment (19,29). Intraoperative identification, careful surgical technique, and EMG monitoring of cranial nerves can potentially minimize postoperative dysfunction. Early involvement of allied health professionals, including speech pathologists, is vital. A proportion of patients may suffer from severe swallowing dysfunction, requiring short- or long-term enteral feeding. Rarely, a tracheostomy may be required for airway protection. The morbidity of iatrogenic cranial nerve palsies is proportional to the age of the patient and the number of cranial nerves with postoperative dysfunction (19,22).

Venous Infarction

Venous infarction is a potentially devastating intracranial postoperative complication of lateral skull base surgery. Preoperative intracranial venography is suggested to assess tumor-related venous obstruction and to assess the development of collateral systems around the skull base. When the torcula is not patent and contralateral flow/development of collateral drainage has not occurred, a venous infarct can arise intraoperatively at the time of vascular control. Chronic venous insufficiency can also occur, and the presentation may be quite subtle. Symptoms can include persistent headaches, disequilibrium, and ataxia.(3)

Temporomandibular Joint Dysfunction

– Anterior extension of the infratemporal approaches requires anterior or inferior displacement of the mandibular condyle after removal of the bone in the region of the glenoid fossa. The mobilization and division of the temporomandibular joint may result in functional limitations that produce impaired occlusions and diminished mandibular excursion. Patients may occasionally present with trismus, masticatory pain, or myofascial pain syndromes, which can be difficult to manage (1,19).

References

1. Oghalai, J.S., and C.L.W. Driscoll, *Atlas of Neurotologic and Lateral Skull Base Surgery*. 1st ed. 2016: Berlin, Heidelberg: Springer.
2. Sanna, M., et al., *Atlas of Microsurgery of the Lateral Skull Base*. 2nd ed. 2007: New York: Thieme.
3. Roberson, J.B., Jr., D.E. Brackmann, and J. N. Fayad, Complications of venous insufficiency after neurotologic-skull base surgery. *Am J Otol*, 2000. **21**(5): pp. 701–5.
4. House, W.F., and W.E. Hitselberger, The transcochlear approach to the skull base. *Arch Otolaryngol*, 1976. **102**(6): pp. 334–42.
5. Goddard, J.C., and T.R. McRackan, Transcochlear approach to cerebellopontine angle lesions, in *Otologic Surgery*, D.E. Brackmann, C. Shelton, and M.A. Arriaga, eds. 2016: Amsterdam: Elsevier; pp. 557–66.
6. Chawla, S, and J.B. Bowman, The transotic and transcochlear approaches. *Operative Techniques in Otolaryngology – Head and Neck Surgery*, 2013. **24** (3): pp. 157–62.
7. Angeli, S.I., A. De la Cruz, and W. Hitselberger, The transcochlear approach revisited. *Otology & Neurotology*, 2001. **22**(5): pp. 690–5.
8. Sanna, M., et al., Surgical management of jugular foramen schwannomas with hearing and facial nerve function preservation: a series of 23 cases and review of the literature. *Laryngoscope*, 2006. **116**(12): pp. 2191–204.
9. Fisch, U., Infratemporal fossa approach to tumors of the temporal bone and base of the skull. *Journal of Laryngology & Otology*, 1978. **92**(11): pp. 949–67.
10. Chan, J., et al., Anterior and subtemporal approaches to the infratemporal fossa, in *Otologic Surgery*, D.E. Brackmann, C. Shelton, and M.A. Arriaga, eds. 2016: Amsterdam: Elsevier; pp. 557–66.
11. Anderson, S.B., and B.M. Panizza, Petro-occipital transsigmoid approach. *Operative Techniques in Otolaryngology – Head and Neck Surgery*, 2013. **24** (3): pp. 163–8.
12. Mazzoni, A., et al., Lower cranial nerve schwannomas involving the jugular foramen. *Annals of Otology, Rhinology & Laryngology*, 1997. **106**(5): pp. 370–9.

13. Mazzoni, A., and M. Sanna, A posterolateral approach to the skull base: the petro-occipital transsigmoid approach. *Skull Base Surg*, 1995. **5** (3): pp. 157–67.
14. Mann, W.J., et al., Transsigmoid approach for tumors of the jugular foramen. *Skull Base Surg*, 1991. **1**(3): pp. 137–41.
15. Tucci, D.L., D.M. Kaylie, and T. Fukushima, Extreme lateral infrajugular transcondylar approach for resection of skull base tumors, in *Otologic Surgery*, D.E. Brackmann, C. Shelton, and M.A. Arriaga, eds. 2016: Amsterdam: Elsevier; pp. 634–45.
16. Lazard, D.S., et al., Early complications and symptoms of cerebellopontine angle tumor surgery: a prospective analysis. *Eur Arch Otorhinolaryngol*, 2011. **268**(11): pp. 1575–82.
17. Darrouzet, V., et al., Vestibular schwannoma surgery outcomes: our multidisciplinary experience in 400 cases over 17 years. *Laryngoscope*, 2004. **114**(4): pp. 681–8.
18. Samii, M., and C. Matthies, Management of 1000 vestibular schwannomas (acoustic neuromas): the facial nerve–preservation and restitution of function. *Neurosurgery*, 1997. **40**(4): pp. 684–94; discussion 694–5.
19. Schick, B., and J. Dlugaiczyk, Surgery of the ear and the lateral skull base: pitfalls and complications. *GMS Current Topics in Otorhinolaryngology, Head and Neck Surgery*, 2013. 12: p. Doc05.
20. Russel, A., et al., Can the risks of cerebrospinal fluid leak after vestibular schwannoma surgery be predicted? *Otol Neurotol*, 2017. **38**(2): pp. 248–52.
21. Fishman, A.J., et al., Prevention and management of cerebrospinal fluid leak following vestibular schwannoma surgery. *The Laryngoscope*, 2009. **114** (3): pp. 501–5.
22. Heman-Ackah, S.E., J.G. Golfinos, and J.T. Roland, Management of surgical complications and failures in acoustic neuroma surgery. *Otolaryngologic Clinics of North America*, 2012. **45** (2): pp. 455–70.
23. Teachey, W., et al., Intervention for elevated intracranial pressure improves success rate after repair of spontaneous cerebrospinal fluid leaks. *The Laryngoscope*, 2017. **127**(9): pp. 2011–16.
24. Chaaban, M.R., et al., Acetazolamide for high intracranial pressure cerebrospinal fluid leaks. *International Forum of Allergy & Rhinology*, 2013. **3**(9): pp. 718–21.
25. Rubin, R.C., et al., The production of cerebrospinal fluid in man and its modification by acetazolamide. *J Neurosurg*, 1966. **25**(4): pp. 430–6.
26. Wilkinson, E.P., D.E. Brackmann, and J.E. Lupo, Management of postoperative cerebrospinal fluid leak, in *Otologic Surgery*, D.E. Brackmann, C. Shelton, and M.A. Arriaga, eds. 2016: Amsterdam: Elsevier; pp. 646–52.
27. Allen, K.P., et al., Lumbar subarachnoid drainage in cerebrospinal fluid leaks after lateral skull base surgery. *Otol Neurotol*, 2011. **32**(9): pp. 1522–4.
28. Crowson, M.G., et al., Preoperative lumbar drain use during acoustic neuroma surgery and effect on CSF leak incidence. *Ann Otol Rhinol Laryngol*, 2016. **125**(1): pp. 63–8.
29. Poe, D.S., et al., Long-term results after lateral cranial base surgery. *Laryngoscope*, 1991. **101**(4 Pt 1): pp. 372–8.
30. Brackman, D., S. Kinney, and K. Fu, Glomus tumor: diagnosis and management. *Head Neck Surg*, 1987. **9**(5): pp. 306–11.
31. Sanna, M., et al., Petrous bone cholesteatoma: classification, management and review of the literature. *Audiol Neurootol*, 2011. **16**(2): pp. 124–36.
32. Russo, A., et al., Anterior and posterior facial nerve rerouting: a comparative study. *Skull Base*, 2003. **13**(3): pp. 123–30.

Chapter

13 Combined Retrosigmoid and Orbitozygomatic Approach

Michael A. Mooney and Robert F. Spetzler

Introduction

With advances in the operative microscope, the integration of neuronavigation, and continued refinement of microsurgical techniques, skull base principles can be maintained with the combination of less extensive, open surgical approaches. Through the combination of the orbitozygomatic (OZ) and retrosigmoid (RS) approaches, the vast majority of anterior, middle, and posterior fossa pathology can be accessed, and lesions spanning these compartments can be successfully resected. Over the past several decades at our institution, the OZ and RS approaches and their modifications have largely replaced the more traditional transpetrosal approaches, with the two-stage OZ-plus-RS approach being utilized when necessary (1).

Approach Selection and Indications for the Combined Oz-Plus-Rs Approach

Proper approach selection can be the defining factor in the successful resection of skull base pathology. An extensive body of literature is devoted to the assessment of surgical exposure, surgical freedom, and surgical angles of attack achieved from a wide spectrum of skull base approaches. Consideration of these factors, as well as the individual surgeon's experience with a given approach, ultimately guide what can be achieved in surgery and can determine the outcome of an operation.

Transpetrosal Approaches versus the Two-Stage Approach

The transpetrosal approaches were developed to address lesions in the petroclival region with additional supratentorial extension, and these have been extensively modified and refined over the past several decades (2-10). These approaches lie on a spectrum of increasing temporal bone resection, ranging from the retrolabyrinthine approach, which preserves hearing, to the transcochlear approach, which affords the greatest degree of surgical exposure. However, the approach-related morbidity of transpetrosal techniques is significant, with reports of increased risk for cerebrospinal fluid (CSF) leak, facial nerve dysfunction, and temporal lobe injury (11-15). Given these limitations, approaching select lesions with the use of a two-stage OZ-plus-RS approach can decrease approach-related morbidity for a subset of lesions and can provide the working corridor, exposure, and surgical angles needed to achieve a complete resection.

Individually, the OZ and RS approaches are highly versatile and are considered "workhorse" approaches for the skull base surgeon. Proficiency in these approaches affords the surgeon the ability to tailor each approach to the given patient and pathology and to perform the approach portion of the operation safely and expediently. Studies performed in the skull base dissection laboratory have demonstrated the complementary nature of the OZ and RS approaches for addressing pathology in the petroclival region (16), and these approaches have been compared with the transpetrosal approaches to the skull base (11, 17).

Notably, the OZ and RS approaches provide little redundancy in exposure (16). The RS approach provides a view of the ipsilateral clivus from its cranial to caudal extent below the tentorium, whereas the OZ approach allows for improved visualization of the parasellar region, the tentorial notch, and the contralateral portion of the upper quarter of the clivus. Notably, in studies examining surgical working areas and angles of attack, the RS approach achieved results similar to those for the combined petrosal approach for addressing the petroclival region (17). Cranial nerves II–XI, as well as the critical portions of the internal carotid and vertebrobasilar circulation, are readily accessible through the combination of the OZ and RS approaches, allowing for the extensive surgical exposure and surgical freedom necessary for resection of tumors involving combinations of these structures.

Indications and Approach Modifications

Indications for the two-stage OZ-plus-RS approach include those lesions that span both the supratentorial and infratentorial compartments, extending from the sellar, parasellar, cavernous sinus, or petroclival regions. Permutations of both the OZ and RS approaches can allow for more or less exposure of the supratentorial and infratentorial compartments as needed for a given case.

For the OZ approach, modifications to the orbital and zygomatic osteotomies can be employed to modify the subfrontal and subtemporal trajectories, respectively (18). For the RS approach, additional skeletonization of the transverse sinus, skeletonization of the sigmoid sinus, or removal of additional suboccipital bone can allow for improved trajectories to the cerebellopontine angle and brainstem. If necessary, it is possible to drill the petrous temporal bone from either approach. This takes the form of an anterior petrosectomy in the OZ approach and a suprameatal approach to the middle fossa in the RS approach. These modifications are outlined in more detail below.

Sequence and Timing of the Two-Stage Approach

Depending on the tumor location, morphology, and specific goals of the operation, either the OZ or RS stage of the operation can be performed first. Most often, we designate the approach that will allow the greatest volume of tumor removal as the stage-one approach (e.g., the OZ approach for a predominantly supratentorial lesion and the RS approach for a predominantly posterior fossa lesion). This allows for extensive tumor debulking and a maximum degree of resection from the first approach. Occasionally, favorable tumor consistency and tissue planes may allow for a single approach to achieve a complete resection, even when a two-stage resection was initially planned.

The two stages of the operation are planned to occur on back-to-back days when possible. Performing the second stage of the resection within a short period after the first stage maximizes the opportunity for preserved tissue planes, and it may shorten the overall hospital stay for the patient by reducing the number of recovery days between stages. If any complications are encountered after the first stage of the operation, additional time may be required to optimize the patient's condition before any further operation.

The Approaches: Microsurgical Anatomy and Surgical Technique

Orbitozygomatic Approach

Positioning

The patient is positioned supine with the head turned away from the side with the lesion. The exact degree of rotation should be determined based on the morphology of the lesion, with the goal being to align the long axis of the tumor perpendicularly to the floor if possible. The head should be elevated above the heart, and care should be taken to avoid jugular vein compression to maximize venous return to the right atrium. The head should be slightly extended to allow for gravity-retraction of the frontal and temporal lobes (Video 13.1).

Step-by-Step Approach Description

The skin incision is planned from the level of the tragus extending superiorly behind the hairline to the mid-sagittal plane (Figure 13.1A, solid line). Care is taken to preserve the main trunk of the superficial temporal artery, and the scalp flap is rotated anteriorly to the level of the superficial fat pad, approximately one to two finger breadths posterior to the orbital rim. A subfascial dissection of the temporalis fascia is performed, and the scalp flap is rotated anteriorly to expose the orbital rim and zygomatic arch (Figure 13.1B). The deep layer of the temporalis fascia envelops the zygomatic arch and must be incised to allow for the osteotomy cuts.

Video 13.1 Summary animation of the orbitozygomatic approach, highlighting the versatility and range of access afforded by the approach. *Used with permission from Barrow Neurological Institute, Phoenix, Arizona.*

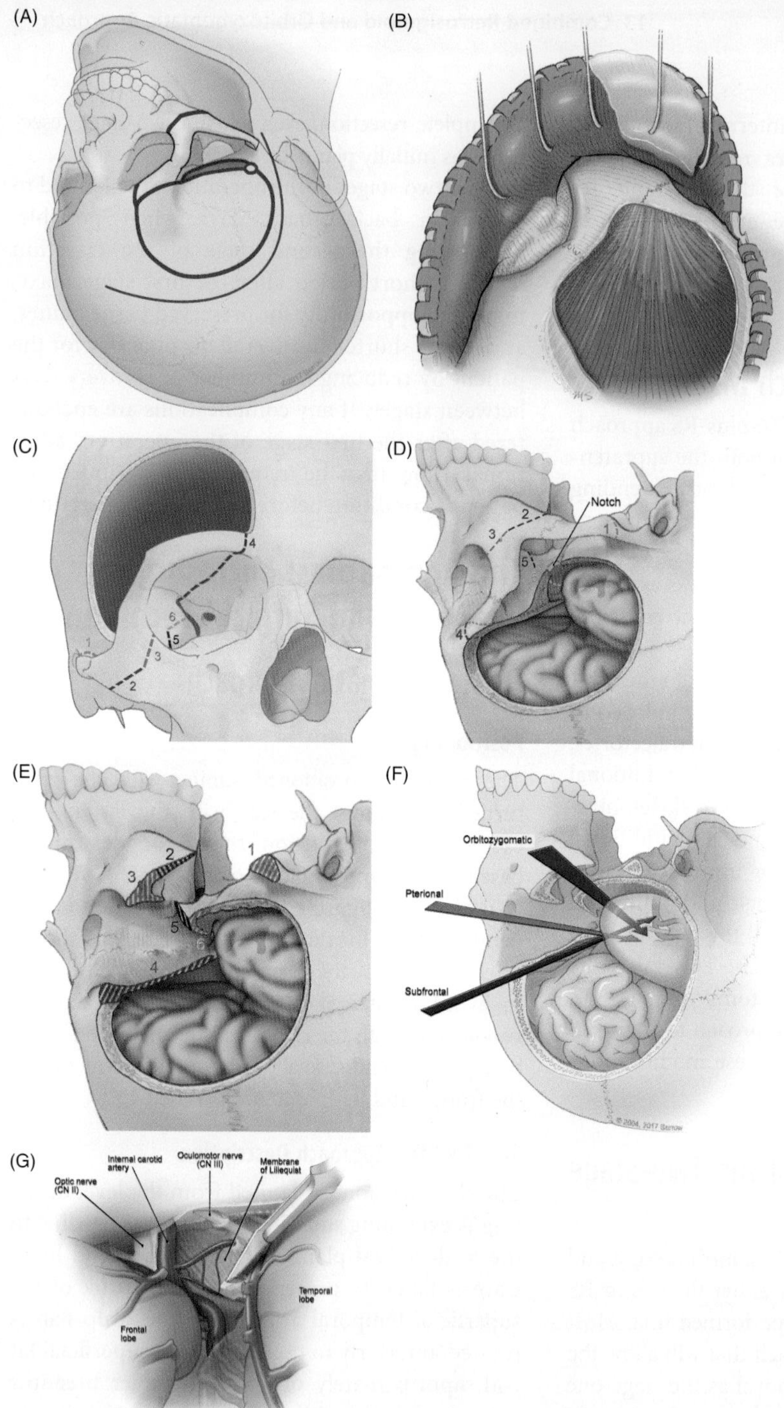

Figure 13.1 Illustration of the key steps of the orbitozygomatic approach. **(A)** Proposed curvilinear skin incision and craniotomy cuts associated with the two-piece orbitozygomatic craniotomy. **(B)** Skin flap reflected anteriorly using a subfascial technique, exposing the lateral orbital rim and zygomatic arch. **(C)** Coronal view, sequential cuts proposed for completing the two-piece orbitozygomatic craniotomy. **(D)** Sagittal view, highlighting the notch at the middle fossa floor that can be used to facilitate the lateral orbital removal. **(E)** Sagittal view, exposure provided by removing the orbitozygomatic unit. **(F)** Surgical trajectories made possible from the orbitozygomatic craniotomy. **(G)** Microsurgical anatomy from the orbitozygomatic craniotomy, highlighting the carotid-oculomotor working corridor. Figure 13.1A,F,G is used with permission from Barrow Neurological Institute, Phoenix, Arizona. Figure 13.1B is modified from Zabramski JM, Kiris T, Sankhla SK, Cabiol J, Spetzler RF: Orbitozygomatic craniotomy. Technical note. J Neurosurg 89:336–341, 1998. Figure 13.1C-E is used with permission from Lekovic GP, Porter RW, Spetzler RF: Supratentorial and infratentorial cavernous malformations. In Winn HR (ed): Youmans Textbook of Neurological Surgery, 6e. Philadelphia: Elsevier, 2011.

The OZ craniotomy can be performed in either one or two pieces. For the two-piece technique, perform a frontotemporal craniotomy. Then perform the OZ osteotomies, which require a total of six distinct cuts to release the OZ unit (Figure 13.1C-E). These cuts can be performed with the sagittal saw, the ultrasonic bone aspirator, or the high-speed drill with a side cutting bit. Cut 1 releases the posterior aspect of the zygomatic arch; care must be taken to avoid entering the temporomandibular joint with this maneuver. Cuts 2 and 3 connect the anterior zygomatic arch with the inferior orbital fissure, with a V-shaped connection approaching the malar eminence. Cut 4 extends through the medial aspect of the orbital rim and posteriorly through the orbital roof. Care should be taken to preserve the supraorbital nerve and vascular bundle, which can be mobilized, if needed, during this step. Cuts 5 and 6 connect the inferior orbital fissure to the middle fossa and the lateral orbital cut to the orbital roof to fully release the OZ unit. Attempts should be made to preserve as much bone as possible from the orbital roof and lateral orbital with the OZ unit to help prevent postoperative enophthalmos. Any remaining bone of the orbital roof or lateral orbit should be removed back to the level of the superior orbital fissure. The sphenoid wing should be drilled to ensure a flat trajectory beneath the frontal lobe and temporal lobes (Figure 13.1F). The dura is then incised and reflected anteriorly, and dural stitches are utilized to reflect the dura over the periorbita and maintain a flat trajectory toward the opticocarotid cistern and cavernous sinus (Figure 13.1G).

Closure

The dura is reapproximated. Dural tack-up sutures should be secured around the periphery of the craniotomy, and central tack-up sutures should be placed as needed for larger exposures. The OZ unit is secured using a cranial plate-fixation system. Care should be taken to eliminate the bone kerf from the craniotomy at the medial-most aspect of the orbital rim as well as medially along the forehead region. Bone cement can be utilized as needed to eliminate additional bony defects. The temporalis muscle should be resuspended to the muscle cuff or secured to the cranium above the superior temporal line. Resuspension of the anterosuperior-most aspect of the temporalis muscle carries the greatest cosmetic importance, and extra attention should be paid to this area during resuspension. A standard galeal closure is then completed, and skin edges are reapproximated with nylon suture or skin staples.

Technical Nuances

Numerous modifications of the OZ approach can be performed, which highlights its utility and versatility (18). The approach can be conceptualized in three distinct pieces: the pterional craniotomy, the orbital osteotomy, and the zygomatic osteotomy. While some lesions require the full OZ approach as described above, some lesions may not require both the orbital and zygomatic osteotomies. Often, the modified OZ approach, or orbitopterional approach, can be sufficient; this approach combines the pterional craniotomy and the orbital osteostomies but leaves the zygoma intact and attached to the temporalis muscle. This modification is suitable for many lesions that will be approached from a subfrontal and transsylvian exposure, and it can spare the time and potential morbidity associated with the zygomatic osteotomy.

Conversely, lesions with supratentorial extension into the middle fossa in the region of the petrous apex may benefit from the zygomatic osteotomy and subtemporal approach but may not require an orbital osteotomy. With experience, surgeons may tailor the OZ approach specifically to the pathology and allow for excellent visualization and surgical freedom while minimizing approach-related morbidity.

Retrosigmoid Approach

Positioning

The patient is positioned in either the lateral decubitus (i.e., "park bench") position or supine with a shoulder roll (Figure 13.2A-D). This decision is made on the basis of the patient's neck flexibility and body habitus. The lateral decubitus position is preferred for some patients for whom neck rotation would significantly compromise venous return. The level of the head should be maintained above the level of the right atrium during the approach to limit posterior fossa swelling (Video 13.2).

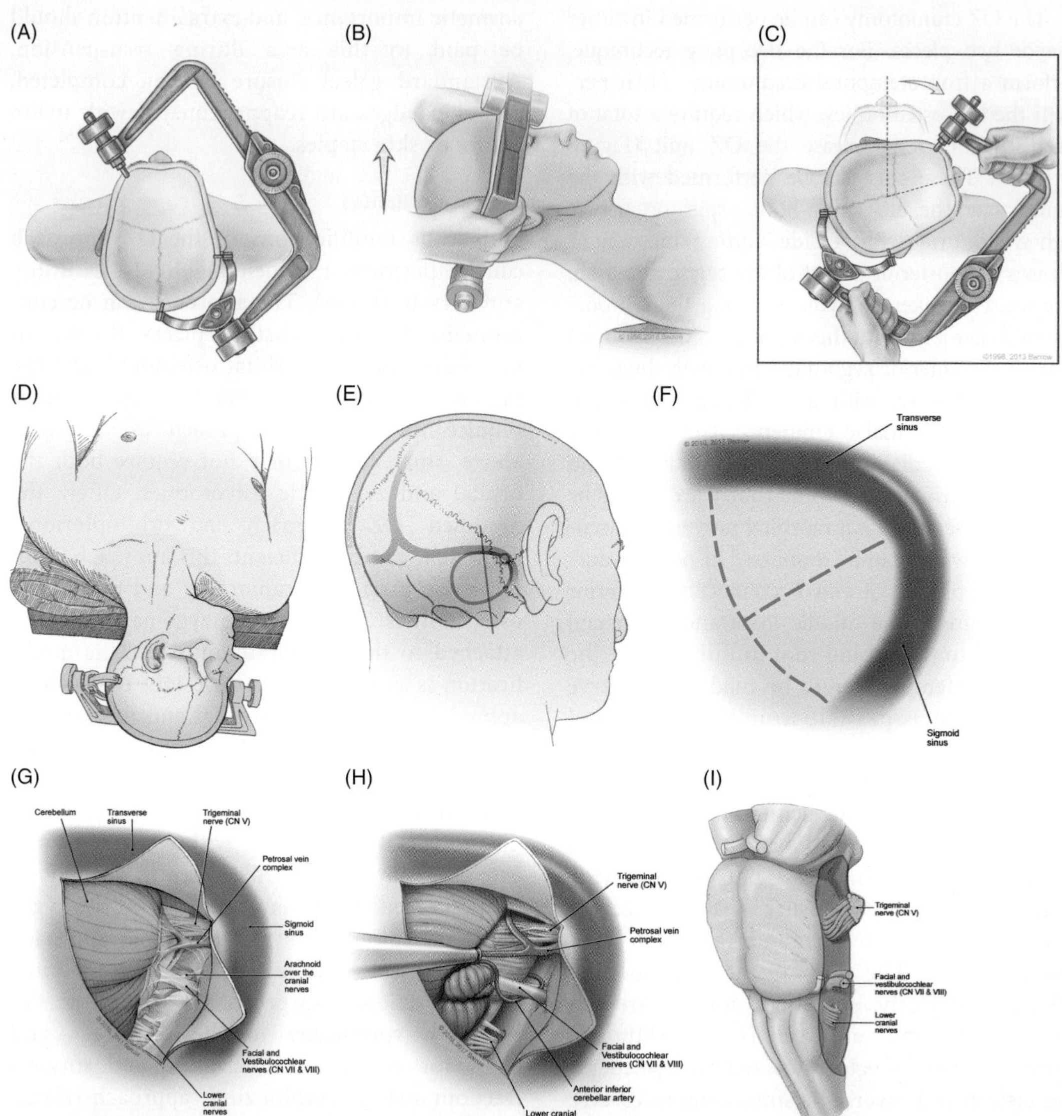

Figure 13.2 Illustration of the key steps of the retrosigmoid approach. **(A)** Mayfield head holder placement for a planned left retrosigmoid approach. **(B)** Elevation of the head above the level of the right atrium to facilitate venous return. **(C)** Head rotation to obtain a working corridor perpendicular to the floor. **(D)** Final position for a left retrosigmoid craniotomy, demonstrating the degree of head rotation and use of an ipsilateral shoulder roll to achieve the working trajectory without over-rotation of the patient's neck. **(E)** Proposed linear skin incision, burr hole, and craniotomy centered at the transverse-sigmoid junction. **(F)** Proposed dural opening, which allows for superior reflection of the transverse sinus and lateral reflection of the sigmoid sinus. **(G and H)** Microsurgical anatomy of the cerebellopontine angle. **(I)** Extent of surgical exposure (blue) along the brainstem afforded by the retrosigmoid approach. Figure 13.2A-C, E-I is used with permission from Barrow Neurological Institute, Phoenix, Arizona. Figure 13.2D is used with permission from Gonzalez LF, Lekovic GP, Kakarla UK, Reis CVC, Weisskopf P, Daspit CP: Surgical approaches to the cerebellopontine angle. Bambakidis NC, Megerian CA, and Spetzler RF (eds). Surgery of the Cerebellopontine Angle. BC Decker and People's Medical Publishing House, Shelton, Connecticut, 2009.

Video 13.2 Summary animation of the retrosigmoid approach, highlighting the relative ease of the approach and the wide surgical corridor. Used with permission from Barrow Neurological Institute, Phoenix, Arizona.

Step-by-Step Approach Description

A linear skin incision is planned from above the level of the transverse sinus and extending inferiorly (Figure 13.2E). A high-speed drill is utilized to create a burr hole at the transverse sigmoid junction, and the RS craniotomy is performed. The dural opening can be tailored to the pathology at hand and centered over the transverse sinus, the sigmoid sinus, or both (Figure 13.2F and 2G).

Release of CSF from the cerebellopontine angle is achieved by dissecting the arachnoid membrane inferiorly, in the direction of the foramen magnum. After sufficient CSF egress, the cerebellum is relaxed, which greatly enhances exposure of the cerebellopontine angle. Care should be taken to avoid any bridging veins and to identify the petrosal vein complex during the initial phase of the approach. Dissection of the arachnoid membranes is then tailored to the pathology to expose the trigeminal nerve, seventh/eighth nerve complex, and lower cranial nerves as needed (Figure 13.2H and 13.2I).

Closure

A watertight closure of the posterior fossa can make the difference between a successful outcome and significant patient morbidity after operation. Every attempt should be made to achieve a primary watertight dural closure. If a defect is present, a muscle plug can be harvested from the suboccipital region. Alternatively, a dural autograft or allograft can be used. Meticulous inspection for entry into the mastoid air cells is required. Bone wax should be generously applied to the anterior aspect of the exposure to seal off any potential sites of communication. If the mastoid is well aerated, a subcutaneous fat graft can be harvested and placed as an additional barrier to CSF leak along the mastoid. The remaining bone flap is plated and secured to the anterior-superior aspect of the defect, and a mesh cranioplasty can be considered for the inferior-posterior aspect of the craniectomy. The suboccipital muscles should be reapproximated and the fascia closed in a watertight fashion. A running nylon suture is used to reapproximate the skin edges.

Technical Nuances

As with the OZ approach, modifications of the standard RS approach can be performed to enhance the surgical exposure and trajectory for certain lesions. For lesions centered at the ambient cistern, tentorial notch, or Meckel's cave, the additional working space of the supracerebellar corridor can be beneficial. In these cases, the craniotomy should be performed more medially along the transverse sinus, and the transverse sinus should be skeletonized. The sinus should be kept moist throughout the operation to prevent sinus thrombosis, particularly if the side of the approach is the dominant drainage site of the posterior fossa.

For lesions extending toward the midline at the brainstem, skeletonization of the sigmoid sinus may be beneficial. Exposure and reflection of the sinus anteriorly can provide a few additional millimeters of exposure to allow identification of the brainstem vascular supply or the arachnoid membrane between the tumor and brainstem, if present.

For lesions extending inferiorly to the level of the medulla and foramen magnum, additional suboccipital bone removal can be performed, which can help with obtaining CSF egress in the initial phase of the operation. For this modification, the linear skin incision can be curved slightly anteriorly toward the inferior aspect of the ear. Care should be taken during dissection of the soft tissue in this region to avoid injury to the vertebral artery.

For tumors extending into the internal auditory canal or middle fossa, additional drilling with the diamond burr can be performed at the internal auditory canal or anterior petrous bone, respectively, to improve access to tumor in these regions.

For large posterior fossa lesions, posterior fossa swelling can accumulate over the course of the resection. The CSF cisterns should be intermittently redrained to obtain cerebellar relaxation and optimize the surgical exposure.

Illustrative Case

A 33-year-old man presented with several months of progressive neurological decline, including weakness and gait instability. An MRI was performed and demonstrated a large, contrast-enhancing supratentorial and infratentorial mass centered at the right parasellar region (Figure 13.3A-D). Notably, the right internal carotid artery terminus was encased in the tumor

Video 13.3 Stage-one orbitozygomatic approach to the supratentorial component of the tumor. Used with permission from Barrow Neurological Institute, Phoenix, Arizona.

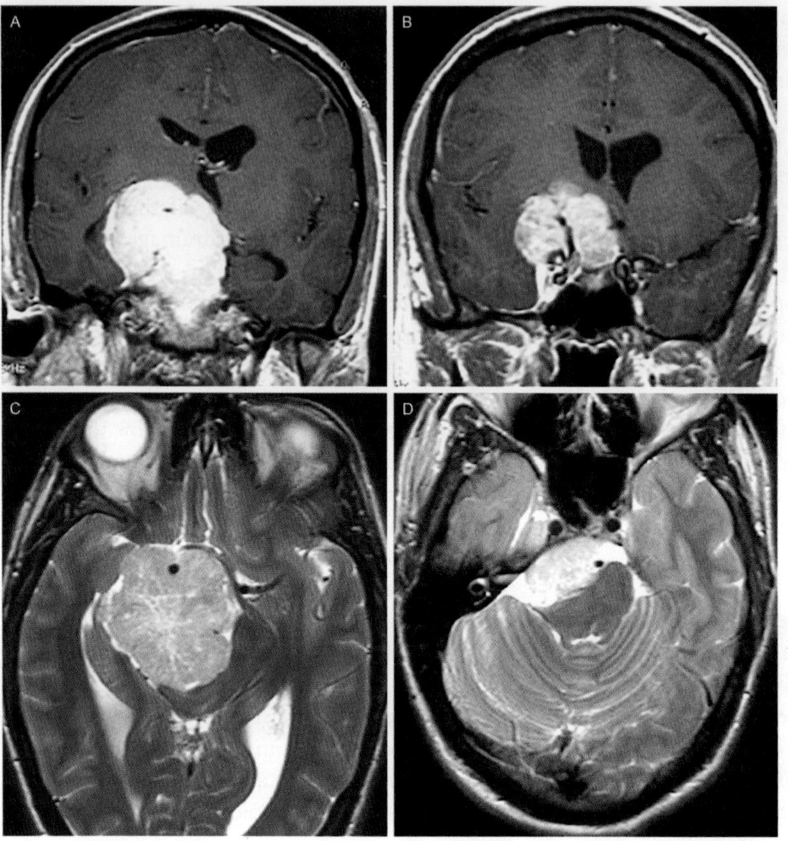

Figure 13.3 Illustrative case preoperative MRI. **(A and B)** T1-weighted contrast-enhanced sequences. **(C and D)** T2-weighted sequences. Used with permission from Barrow Neurological Institute, Phoenix, Arizona.

(Figure 13.3B and 3C), and the basilar artery was displaced contralaterally (Figure 13.3D). A two-stage OZ-plus-RS resection was planned.

Because the majority of the mass was in the supratentorial compartment, the OZ stage of the operation was performed first. The tumor was debulked, and the arachnoid plane was identified and preserved. The tumor consistency was favorable, and it was possible to dissect the tumor from the internal carotid artery terminus and branching vessels (Video 13.3). After stage one, the infratentorial component of the tumor remained; the residual tumor highlights the surgical limits of the OZ approach (Figure 13.4A-D).

A stage-two RS approach was performed on the following day to resect the remainder of the tumor (Video 13.4; Figure 13.5A-C). The patient was neurologically stable following surgery, and his condition progressively improved. Pathological findings indicated that the tumor was a World Health Organization (WHO) Grade I meningioma.

Limitations

Although the OZ and RS approaches are highly versatile and effective, limitations of the two-stage strategy must be acknowledged. Quantitative analyses have demonstrated the inferiority of the RS approach for exposure of the anterior brainstem and access to Meckel's cave in comparison with the combined petrosal approach or Kawase's approach (17, 18). The transotic and transcochlear approaches consistently provide the largest areas of surgical exposure and degrees of surgical freedom at the petroclival region, although at the

Video 13.4 Stage-two retrosigmoid approach to the infratentorial component of the tumor. Used with permission from Barrow Neurological Institute, Phoenix, Arizona.

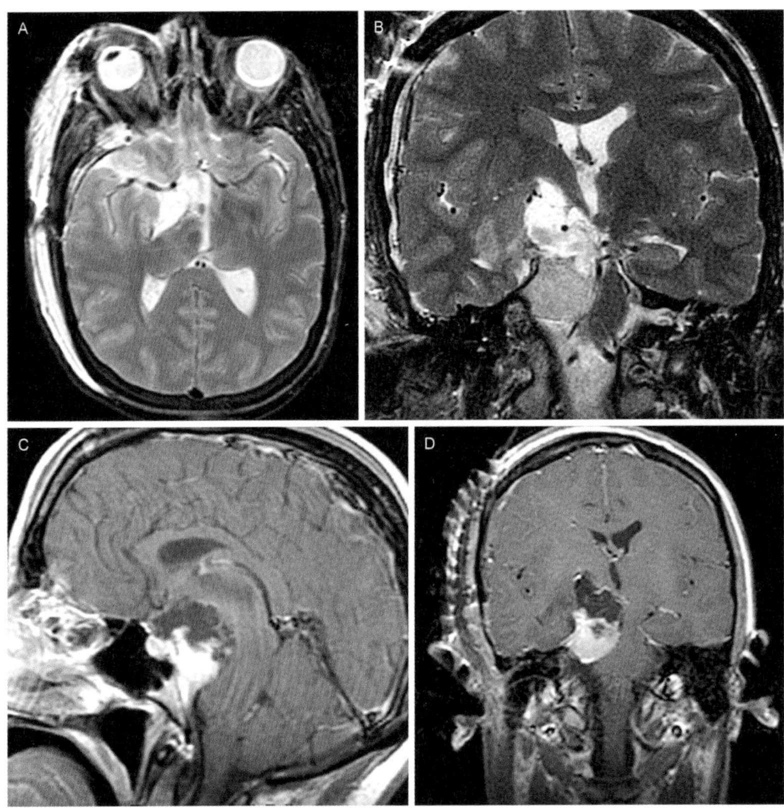

Figure 13.4 Illustrative case postoperative MRI following the stage-one orbitozygomatic approach. T2-weighted axial **(A)** and coronal **(B)** sequences and T1-weighted contrast-enhanced sagittal **(C)** and coronal **(D)** sequences are shown. Used with permission from Barrow Neurological Institute, Phoenix, Arizona.

expense of the patient's hearing, risk to the facial nerve, and increased postoperative CSF-related complications.

In addition, the bony removal accomplished in the transpetrosal approaches may be beneficial in some cases. The transpetrosal approaches can decrease the vascular supply to the lesion early in the operation and may also eliminate disease invading the bone of the skull base during the approach. Additional bony drilling from the OZ or RS approaches would be required to address these aspects of some tumors and must be considered on a case-by-case basis.

Key Points

- The two-stage OZ-plus-RS approach can be used to address some skull base lesions that extend both supratentorially and infratentorially.
- Utilizing the OZ-plus-RS approach rather than the transpetrosal approaches may help limit some of the approach-related morbidity associated with transpetrosal approaches.
- The first stage of the operation is planned to address the larger, more compressive aspect of the lesion; the second stage is planned to occur within one or two days after a successful first operation stage.
- The goals of surgery are complete tumor removal with preservation or improvement of neurological function, and these can be achieved with the two-stage OZ-plus-RS approach in select cases.

Acknowledgments

The authors thank the staff of Neuroscience Publications at Barrow Neurological Institute for assistance with manuscript preparation.

References

1. Bambakidis NC, Kakarla UK, Kim LJ, Nakaji P, Porter RW, Daspit CP, et al. Evolution of surgical approaches in the treatment of petroclival meningiomas: a retrospective review. *Neurosurgery*. 2008;**62**(6 Suppl 3):1182–91.
2. Bernardo A, Evins AI, Visca A, Stieg PE. The intracranial facial nerve as seen through different surgical windows: an extensive anatomosurgical

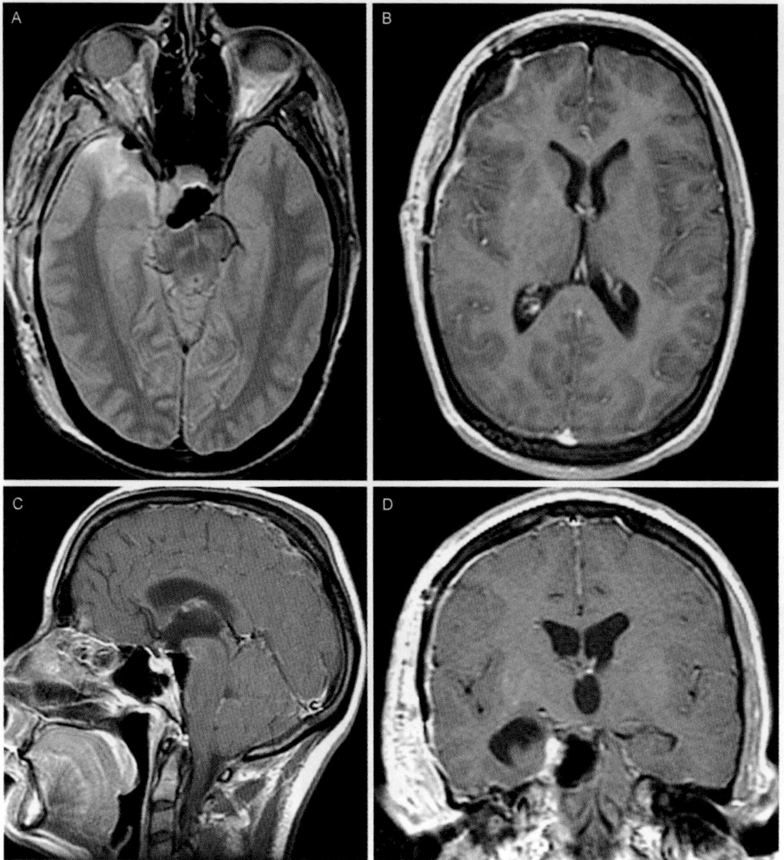

Figure 13.5 Illustrative case postoperative MRI following the stage-two retrosigmoid approach. T2-weighted axial sequences **(A)** and T1-weighted contrast-enhanced axial **(B)**, sagittal **(C)**, and coronal **(D)** sequences are shown. Used with permission from Barrow Neurological Institute, Phoenix, Arizona.

study. *Neurosurgery*. 2013;**72**(2 Suppl Operative): ons194–207.

3. Chanda A, Nanda A. Partial labyrinthectomy petrous apicectomy approach to the petroclival region: an anatomic and technical study. *Neurosurgery*. 2002;**51**(1):147–59; discussion 59–60.
4. Wu CY, Lan Q. Quantification of the presigmoid transpetrosal keyhole approach to petroclival region. *Chin Med J (Engl)*. 2008;**121** (8):740–4.
5. Cho CW, Al-Mefty O. Combined petrosal approach to petroclival meningiomas. *Neurosurgery*. 2002;**51** (3):708–16; discussion 16–18.
6. Horgan MA, Anderson GJ, Kellogg JX, Schwartz MS, Spektor S, McMenomey SO, et al. Classification and quantification of the petrosal approach to the petroclival region. *J Neurosurg*. 2000;**93**(1):108–12.
7. Janjua MB, Caruso JP, Greenfield JP, Souweidane MM, Schwartz TH. The combined transpetrosal approach: anatomic study and literature review. *J Clin Neurosci*. 2017;**41**:36–40.
8. Miller CG, van Loveren HR, Keller JT, Pensak M, el-Kalliny M, Tew JM, Jr. Transpetrosal approach: surgical anatomy and technique. *Neurosurgery*. 1993;**33**(3):461–9; discussion 9.
9. Miller ME, Mastrodimos B, Cueva RA. Facial nerve function after the extended translabyrinthine approach. *J Neurol Surg B Skull Base*. 2015;**76**(1):1–6.
10. Yang J, Zhang F, Xu A, Li H, Ding Z. Comparison of surgical exposure and maneuverability associated with microscopy and endoscopy in the retrolabyrinthine and transcrusal approaches to the retrochiasmatic region: a cadaveric study. *Acta Neurochir (Wien)*. 2016;**158**(4):703–10.
11. Chang SW, Wu A, Gore P, Beres E, Porter RW, Preul MC, et al. Quantitative comparison of Kawase's approach versus the retrosigmoid approach: implications for tumors involving both middle and posterior fossae. *Neurosurgery*. 2009;**64**(3 Suppl):ons44-51.
12. Mason E, Rompaey JV, Solares CA, Figueroa R, Prevedello D. Subtemporal retrolabyrinthine (posterior petrosal) versus endoscopic endonasal

approach to the petroclival region: an anatomical and computed tomography study. *J Neurol Surg B Skull Base*. 2016;**77**(3):231–7.

13. Xu F, Karampelas I, Megerian CA, Selman WR, Bambakidis NC. Petroclival meningiomas: an update on surgical approaches, decision making, and treatment results. *Neurosurg Focus*. 2013;**35**(6):E11.
14. House WF, Hitselberger WE. The transcochlear approach to the skull base. *Arch Otolaryngol*. 1976;**102**(6):334–42.
15. House WF, De la Cruz A, Hitselberger WE. Surgery of the skull base: transcochlear approach to the petrous apex and clivus. *Otolaryngology*. 1978;**86**(5):ORL-770–9.
16. Little AS, Jittapiromsak P, Crawford NR, Deshmukh P, Preul MC, Spetzler RF, et al. Quantitative analysis of exposure of staged orbitozygomatic and retrosigmoid craniotomies for lesions of the clivus with supratentorial extension. *Neurosurgery*. 2008;**62**(5 Suppl 2):ons318–23; discussion ons23–4.
17. Siwanuwatn R, Deshmukh P, Figueiredo EG, Crawford NR, Spetzler RF, Preul MC. Quantitative analysis of the working area and angle of attack for the retrosigmoid, combined petrosal, and transcochlear approaches to the petroclival region. *J Neurosurg*. 2006;**104**(1):137–42.
18. Lemole GM, Jr., Henn JS, Zabramski JM, Spetzler RF. Modifications to the orbitozygomatic approach. Technical note. *J Neurosurg*. 2003;**99**(5):924–30.

Chapter 14

Combined Retrosigmoid and Limited Anterior Petrosectomy ("Reverse Petrosectomy")

Jamie Van Gompel

Introduction

Traditionally, lesions that connect the middle fossa or supratentorial cisterns and the posterior fossa have been addressed using approaches centered on the middle fossa with the addition of a traditional anterior petrosectomy or, alternatively, presigmoid approaches that incorporate a posterior petrosectomy (1). When global access is needed, a combined petrosal approach may be used. Surgeons who employ these approaches more frequently are well acquainted with their advantages and disadvantages, which will be covered elsewhere in this text. However, there is a less frequently utilized approach that takes advantage of the familiarity and relative ease of a retrosigmoid operation: the addition of a suprameatal boney removal, which we euphemistically call the "reverse petrosectomy." In select cases, this approach may minimize related morbidity and dissection. Further, the endoscope can be used to augment visualization – previously accomplished through boney removal, necessitated by the straight line of sight inherent to the microscope (2,3,4). Here, we describe this innovative technique, taking a detailed, component-based approach to the skull base.

The following are possible advantages of performing a retrosigmoid craniotomy with additional suprameatal bone work approaching Meckel's cave, and in select circumstances, a tentorial opening:

1. **Improved access to tumors extending above or below the tentorium.**
   This approach is ideal in cases where most of the tumor is below the tentorium and the attachment is mostly confined to the posterior fossa. If a fair amount of tumor is attached to the backside of the sigmoid sinus or the straight sinus, a presigmoid approach would be more beneficial to aid in the control of venous bleeding (5). Tumor above the tentorium can be managed when opening the tentorium; however, difficulty arises if the vascular supply originates from the superior surface of the tentorium.
2. **Improved vascular control of the tumor.** Blood supply is variable in meningiomas in the posterior fossa. However, typically the blood supply for tumors involving the tentorium or Meckel's cave comes from the arteries of the posterior trunk in the cavernous sinus, and in some circumstances, an enlarged artery can be found and embolized prior to surgery to aid in surgical removal of the tumor (6,7,8). For tumors of the petroclival fissure or the petrous apex, the attachment can be broader and the blood supply more diffuse. Some tumors, such as the commonly-found epidermoid, have little to no blood supply, which facilitates a less invasive approach to the tumor.
3. **Improved tumor access, given displacement or incorporation of the fifth cranial nerve.** Depending on the origin of the tumor, the fifth cranial nerve can be pushed up (as commonly found in vestibular schwannomas) or pushed down to run with the seventh/eighth cranial nerve complex to the petrous surface, then along the petrous face to Meckel's cave (as commonly found in petroclival meningiomas). Alternatively, the fifth cranial nerve can be incorporated in the tumor, as is seen in epidermoids. If the fifth cranial nerve is thinned and expanded on the posterior aspect of the tumor, there may not be an adequate window to facilitate debulking.
   A retrosigmoid approach can provide an improved working window.
4. **Ability to embolize the superior petrosal sinus.** The biggest challenge in approaching the petrous apex and opening the tentorium using this approach is to control venous

bleeding from the superior petrosal sinus. From both a posterior and anterior petrosectomy, the surgeon has good, open control of the superior petrosal sinus and can place clips across it if it is quite large (9). In the proposed approach, one must be accustomed to other ways of controlling venous bleeding. Expanded endonasal procedures involving injection of liquid Gelfoam into the cavernous sinus have vastly improved this approach. In order to perform this approach, one must be comfortable with pressure-injecting coagulant substances through the superior petrosal sinus toward the cavernous sinus and packing it off. Most commonly, bleeding occurs during the drilling of the petrous apex. For meningiomas resected with this approach, it is recommended to perform a preoperative angiogram to confirm the positioning of the surrounding vasculature. Theoretically, it may also be beneficial to preemptively embolize the superior petrosal sinus; however, as of this writing, an ideal case has not yet presented itself for this technique. It may also be difficult to cut through the embolic material given the awkward angles necessary in this approach.

5. **Improved visualization of tumor below the seventh/eighth cranial nerve complex.** One commonly cited limitation of the anterior petrosectomy is limited visualization below the seventh/eighth cranial nerve complex (10). However, visualization in this space is possible with some tumors. For instance, for cholesteatomas or epidermoids, an intradural petrosectomy through a transsylvian approach – especially with the assistance of an endoscope – affords a view into the posterior fossa and below the seventh/eighth cranial nerve complex. Nonetheless, this limitation still exists for vascular lesions using this approach. The retrosigmoid approach discussed here clearly allows pan-global access from cranial nerves 4 through 12 in the posterior fossa. Opening the tentorium also allows easier visualization of the course of the third nerve. The optic nerves, however, are not commonly seen using this approach.

Patient selection is key to this procedure. Commonly, this approach is used for tumors filling the clival angle that cannot be adequately accessed using an endonasal approach and that have extensive lateral extent. One must also take into account the added time at the outset of the procedure. Performing the bone work for a presigmoid approach commonly allows access to the tumor only after several hours of operative time. A retrosigmoid approach with a reverse petrosectomy can be used primarily for a mostly-intradural lesion in the posterior fossa, but with some extension above, or involvement of, the tentorium. The ideal clinical scenario includes a petrous apex-based meningioma with nearly all of the tumor located below the tentorium, with some extension above the tentorium or involving Meckel's cave (Figure 14.1). Chondrosarcomas can be targeted with this approach when there is mostly disease in the cerebellopontine angle but little clival disease. This approach is also ideal for extensive epidermoids occupying the posterior and middle fossae, especially on the left side, given the potential morbidities associated with retracting the temporal lobe (Figure 14.2).

Contraindications

There are relatively few contraindications to performing a retrosigmoid craniotomy (11). Potential contraindications include tumors of the optic nerve or tumors in the pterion, which would not be accessible via this approach. An anterior petrosectomy exists not as a stand-alone procedure independent of middle fossa craniotomies or combined petrosal approaches, but as a modular component. In a similar way, a reverse petrosectomy or suprameatal bone work (with or without a tentorial opening) is a modular component of the retrosigmoid craniotomy. However, other approaches can be considered to reach the tentorial hiatus and clival angle. A middle fossa craniotomy, the so-called Kawase approach, can be used as a stand-alone procedure to address lesions in the posterior fossa.

The bone work of the anterior petrosectomy can often be tailored. For instance, when proximal basilar control is needed for basilar aneurysms, selected petrous apex removal can be used without completely exposing the internal auditory canal (IAC) and genicular region. However, depending on the extent of tumor in the IAC, expanded bone work may be necessary; and further bone work may be necessary if the petrous carotid needs to be accessed or controlled.

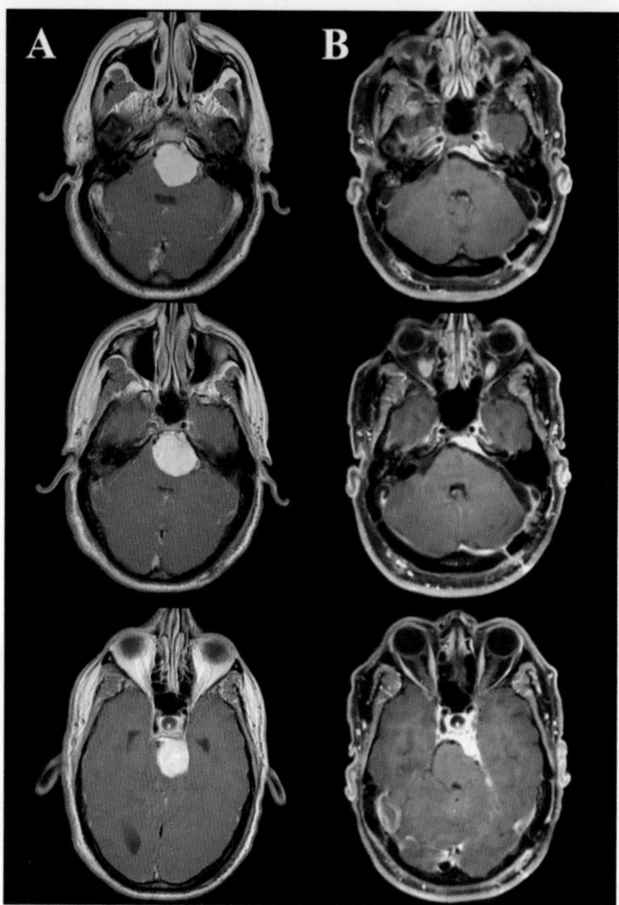

Figure 14.1 Axial MRI images acquired with T1 sequences with the addition of gadolinium of a lesion managed with a retrosigmoid craniotomy and reverse petrosectomy. (A) Preoperative images showing a large petroclival meningioma with extension into Meckel's cave. (B) Postoperative images showing residual tumor in Meckel's cave being observed currently at 3 years. The patient had a temporary fourth and sixth nerve palsy after the operation that resolved at 6 months.

Combining a frontotemporal or orbitozygomatic approach with the anterior petrosectomy can be particularly helpful. Recently, we have taken to opening the Sylvian fissure and using stereotaxis to drill out the petrous apex, a so-called intradural petrosectomy that which can lead to further extension into the posterior fossa beyond the seventh and eighth cranial nerves. Finally, the petrous apex region can be reached three ways endoscopically: first, via the paraclival route; second, with carotid mobilization; and third, using the subpetrosal route (sometimes with resection of the eustachian tube). Typically, all of these take advantage of the natural pathway created by the tumor and exploit it using endonasal procedures. Further, pathologies such as chordoma, chondrosarcoma, and cholesteatoma are often addressed this way, given the native midline extradural clival extensions.

Preoperative Workup

Preoperative planning should include a high-quality MRI with thin cuts; high-resolution images of the cranial nerves are particularly helpful. For large, high-risk meningiomas, it is recommended to perform a high-quality angiogram to better understand the arterial supply. Subtle postoperative issues commonly relate to venous insufficiency; it is beneficial to see the rate and pathway of venous drainage and to compare it to postoperative imaging, if necessary. If at all possible, preoperative embolization is very helpful if it can be achieved safely. Finally, for particularly complex cases, surgeons are strongly encouraged to present their presurgical plans to a partner, friend, or fellowship director, as a secondary perspective can offer considerations, techniques, or ideas that result in an easier or safer procedure for the patient.

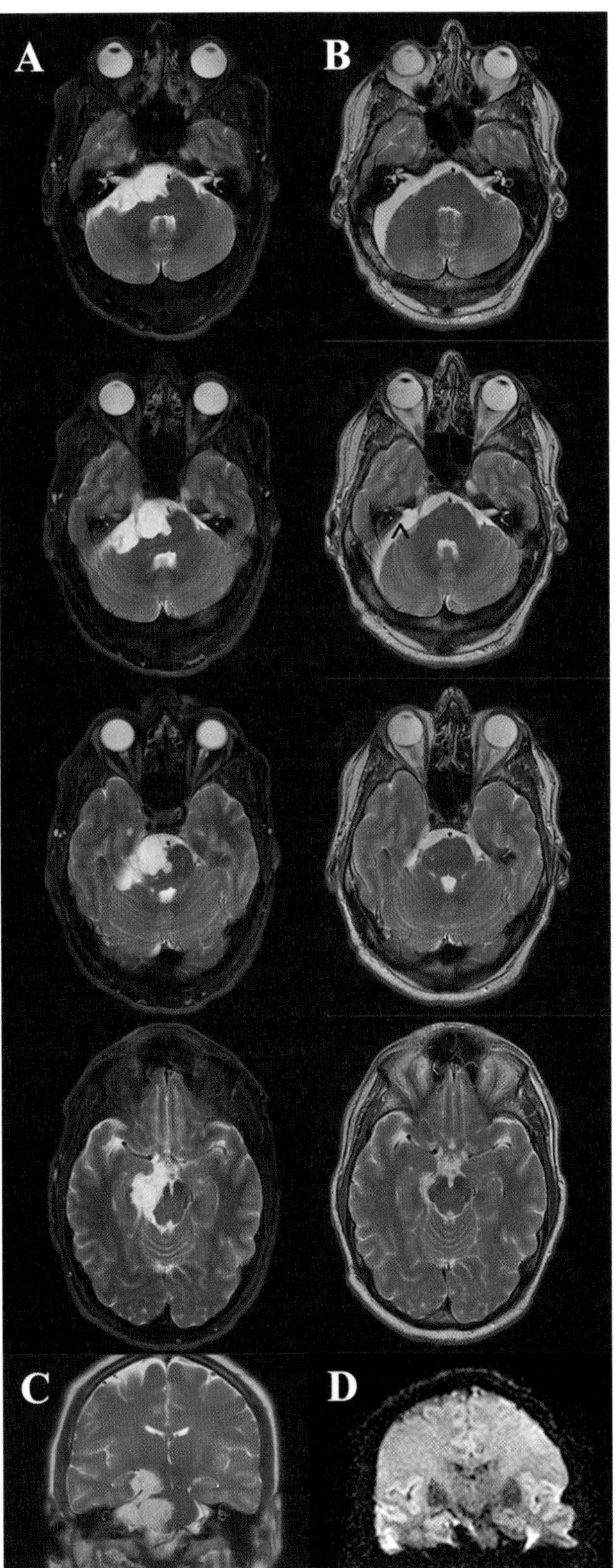

Figure 14.2 Pre- (A) and postoperative (B) T2 axial images of an epidermoid tumor removed utilizing a retrosigmoid craniotomy with reverse petrosectomy. (C) Preoperative coronal T2 image showing the extent of the tumor. (D) Postoperative coronal DWI sequence demonstrating no additional diffusion restriction on this image. The patient did well, with only a temporary third nerve palsy postoperatively that recovered by 3 months.

The patient can be positioned in either the supine or lateral decubitus position; however, considering the extreme angle necessary to look up to the tentorium and the tentorial hiatus, it is critical to ensure the patient's shoulder is rotated out of the way. Typically, the patient is placed in a lateral decubitus position but slouched forward and with the inion of the head rotated back. For more complex cases, use a stereotactic CT angiogram to aid in safe navigation of the vasculature and to offer a sense of direction; a single-view planned trajectory using the navigation can help in assessing line of sight before draping. If anticipating the use of a cranial assist endoscope, attach the fixed Mitaka arm (Karl Storz, Tuttlingen, Germany) and drape it in with the tower at the feet.

Create a curvilinear incision behind the ear and mark the midpoint by drawing a line between the inion and the zygoma. This estimates the course of the transverse sinus; however, stereotaxis can also be used. From the edge of the earlobe, measure three finger breadths behind and place a mark for the back limb of the curvilinear incision. Make the skin incision, taking care to leave down the pericranium and musculature. Create a separate, U-shaped muscle flap by cutting down on the midpoint of the mastoid, going above the transverse sinus, and continuing to midline. This flap can be moved out of the way using fishhooks with elastic bands, minimizing muscle dissection, similarly to how the muscles are handled on a far-lateral approach.

Once the muscles have been mobilized, identify the asterion and make a burr hole on the medial inferior aspect to identify the posterior fossa dura. From here, it is critical to be able to clearly see the edge of the transverse and sigmoid sinuses. The bone over the sinuses can be completely removed and the dura pulled up for better visualization; however, this should be avoided to reduce the risk of sinus thrombosis, which leads to other potential complications. Once the bone work is satisfactory, open the dura. Use the method best suited for the pathology, but opening the dura high along the transverse sinus has proven helpful. Given the length of the procedure, it is common to use pericranium to repair the dura at the end of the procedure; be mindful of this approach and during the case.

At this point, the case proceeds like any retrosigmoid craniotomy with a tumor in the posterior fossa. Access the cerebellopontine cistern adjacent to the eleventh cranial nerve to let off CSF and decompress the posterior fossa. Then, with the posterior fossa now relaxed, protect the cerebellum with Surgicel and cotton patties. Dissect the arachnoid to identify the seventh/eighth cranial nerve complex. In most tumors, the fifth nerve complex is not yet visible; however, if it is, it should also be identified and protected. Notably, neuromonitoring is critical to the success of these cases, and what is monitored varies between surgeons and institutions. The motor portion of the trigeminal nerve, portio minor, is very small, medial to the sensory branch, and can be displaced away from the rest of the nerve. Therefore, any nerve filaments that are white in color need to be preserved, as we cannot yet reliably monitor the sensory function of the trigeminal nerve, which is the majority of the fibers. Potential complications involving the fifth cranial nerve include loss of V1 function as well as anesthesia dolorosa. It is important to be very mindful of this. Commonly with large tumors, we proceed using available surgical windows to debulk the tumor and remove tumor burden from the petrous apex. Once the surgeon needs a break or a break becomes surgically necessary, the suprameatal tubercle is drilled out. While it is not necessary for an otologist to perform this step when doing limited bone work, an otologist is recommended if attempting to maximize exposure of the seventh cranial nerve without damaging the posterior semicircular canal.

Figure 14.3A (microscopic view) and Figure 14.4A (endoscopic view) demonstrate in a cadaver the intact petrous bone and the suprameatal tubercle. There is a limited view and working room. After Dandy's vein has been taken (it sometimes be preserved with epidermoids), we commonly find the cochlear aqueduct communicating to the endolymphatic sac. Using this as a landmark, the bone over the seventh/eighth nerve complex is drilled away to maximize boney removal, with care taken to avoid the posterior canal and damage to the patient's hearing. If the patient's hearing was already compromised preoperatively, drilling can be even more extensive.

The bone superior to the auditory meatus is drilled to open Meckel's cave. It is important to stay extradural during this exposure to allow the dura to absorb some of the drill heat, as well as to use extensive continuous irrigation in order to

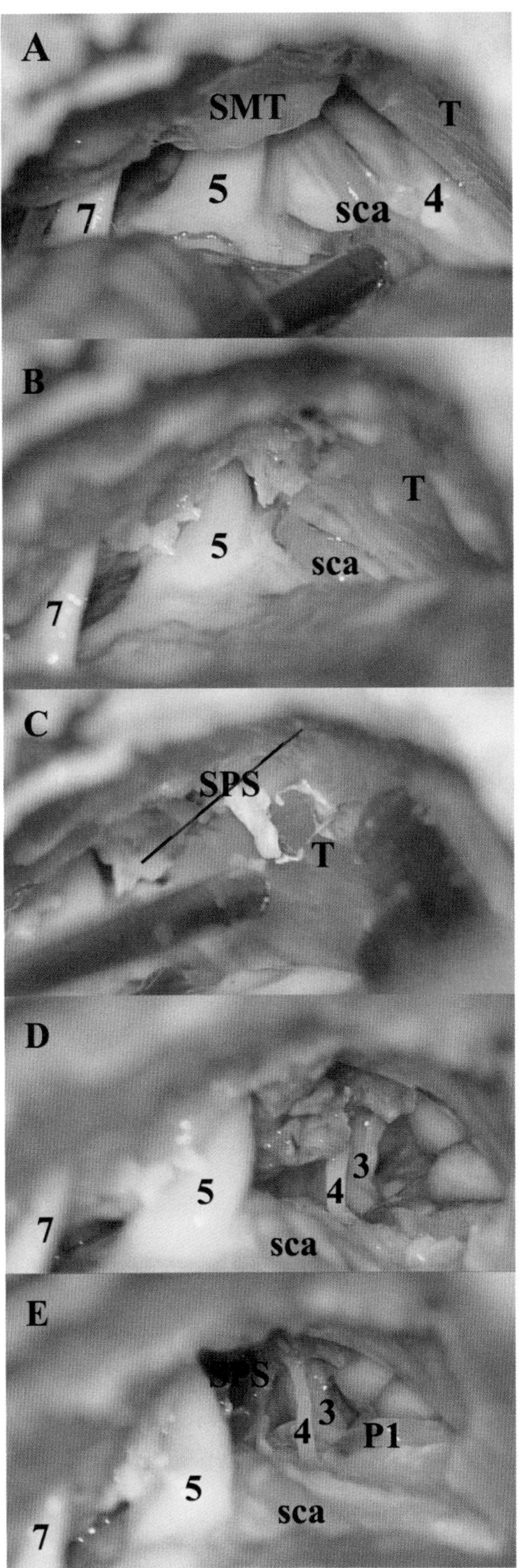

Figure 14.3 Cadaver dissection photos of the intradural portion of the approach under a microscope. (A) Exposure after

avoid injury to the fifth cranial nerve during the final boney removal. This exposure can be seen in Figures 14.3B, C, and D, and Figure 14.4B. Typically, the limitation to drilling is the bleeding that occurs from the superior petrosal sinus (SPS). This can be managed in a multitude of ways, but as stated previously, liquid embolics such as Gelfoam work well when combined with a minute or two of gentle compression. If bleeding is particularly persistent, one can inject Tisseel as done with transcavernous approaches, as the SPS essentially communicates with the posterior cavernous sinus.

Once bone work is complete, the tentorium is opened. It is critical to confirm the location of the fourth cranial nerve prior to this step. Once this is accomplished, it is recommended to open the dura at least 5 to 10 mm from the SPS, as there can be communicating veins in the supratentorial space and venous lakes that can be difficult to manage. It is helpful to leave all venous anatomy in anatomic flow as best as possible while still exposing the tentorial hiatus. Opening this space allows complete access to the third cranial nerve, P1, proximal P2, and the basal temporal lobe. Once the proximal tent is released, it self-retracts and provides increased working room, although with some tumors it may still be necessary to resect much of the attached dura. In meningiomas, it is often difficult to visualize the nerves; therefore, one may have to leave more tumor than expected. However, our current practice is to take as much tumor as is safely possible without compromising function (Figure 14.1B).

As with opening, it is important when closing to copiously wax the petrous apex air cells and the air cells of the auditory meatus. Further, if the tentorium was opened during exposure, a dural substitute can be laid supratentorially, across the opened tentorium, to avoid temporal lobe

Caption for Figure 14.3 (cont.)

dura is opened from a retrosigmoid craniotomy. Dandy's vein has been sacrificed here. Notice the limited view of 7 (here we label the seventh/eighth cranial nerve complex as 7, realizing that this is the vestibular portion of 8) and the fifth cranial nerve obstructed by the suprameatal tubercle. (B) After drilling and exposure of the base of Meckel's cave. (C) Demonstration of where a typical tentorial (T) opening is performed away from the superior petrosal sinus (SPS). (D) With the tentorium open, one can see the contents of the ambient cistern and the and third and fourth cranial nerves. (E) Additional angle showing the relationship of the third and fourth cranial nerves.

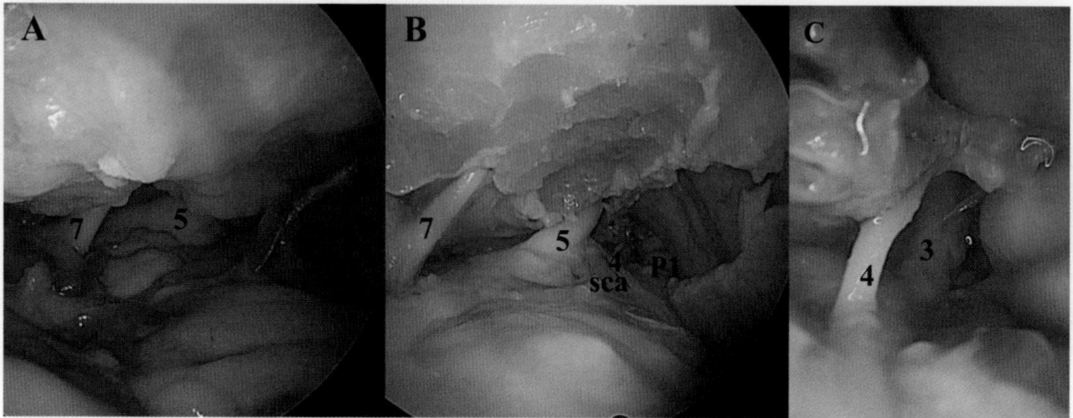

Figure 14.4 Cadaver dissection photos of the intradural portion of the approach utilizing an endoscope. (A) Exposure after dura is opened from a retrosigmoid craniotomy. Dandy's vein has not been sacrificed here. Notice the limited view of the seventh cranial nerve (here we label the seventh/eighth cranial nerve complex as 7, realizing that this is the vestibular portion of 8) and the fifth cranial nerve obstructed by the suprameatal tubercle as seen in Figure 3. (B) After drilling and exposure of the base of Meckel's cave with the dural opening. (C) An amplified view of the third and fourth cranial nerves.

herniation into the defect. Previously, when a large defect has been left behind, abdominal fat has been used for reconstruction. No matter the technique, it is critical to perform a good multi-layer closure.

One great advantage of this approach for meningiomas is the ability to work from the bottom of the tumor going up, unless there are symptoms that must be addressed using a supratentorial surgery, such as optic nerve compression. This approach typically serves as stage one in a two-stage operation for larger petroclival meningiomas. Further, little scarring is created supratentorially. However, if a second operation is anticipated, the upper portion of the tumor can be left behind to allow virgin planes for dissection.

In terms of complication avoidance, it cannot be overstated that good surgeries do not always mean great postoperative images with gross total resection. If there is no dissection plane with the brainstem, do not make one, as this can cause serious venous injury to the brainstem. If the basilar artery is encased, take care when dissecting between the basilar artery and the brainstem so as to not injure perforating vessels. If perforator injury occurs, a great surgery can still be performed and result in a terrible clinical outcome. When possible, it is advised to work from normal to abnormal anatomy, as in any surgery. This especially holds true for the basilar artery: it is safest to work from the vertebral arteries and moving up.

Postoperative Care

Typical follow-up routine calls for a three-month postoperative MRI. If performing a multi-stage operation, our current practice is to perform the second stage after the three-month MRI to allow for an adequate recovery period. Cases with a short-term return to the OR, such as in the same week, are not commonly staged in our practice. After the second stage is performed, it is common to perform repeat imaging at one year, then yearly thereafter. Of course, different pathologies warrant different follow-up strategies. With epidermoid tumors, we typically do not perform contrast imaging and instead rely on high-resolution short-spin echo images such as CISS.

Clinical Pearls

- Strategic pitfalls
  - Use the largest window between the cranial nerves to decompress the tumor as the first step.
  - Do not decompress the seventh/eighth cranial nerve complex too early; the tumor behind it needs significant room for movement, and early decompression will lead to early drying of the nerves. We recommend applying Lacri-Lube and Gelfoam to the nerves to keep them moist.
- Limitations

- This approach provides a limited view above the tentorium with potentially difficult vascular control.
- Proximal control on the PCOM and on P2 is limited.
- A steep tentorium and left-sided procedures can make the approach uncomfortable for the surgeon. There is little doubt that the presigmoid approach improves this by shortening the working distance, but it also increases working distance to the clival angle when working behind the intact bony labyrinth.
- The distance to tumor can be very long, especially in the ambient cisterns. Low-profile instruments, such as those used in endoscopic endonasal approaches, are essential.

Key Points

- The reverse petrosectomy is a useful modular addition to skull-base approaches, providing improved surgical access to tumors with significant posterior fossa involvement.
- The approach is very comfortable for surgeons, as it takes advantage of the retrosigmoid craniotomy, a commonly used approach.
- If extensive boney removal of the IAC is anticipated, consider having a neuro-otologist involved to assist.
- Preoperative vascular imaging is critical to safety with this approach.

References

1. Fujitsu K, Kitsuta Y, Takemoto Y, Matsunaga S, Tateishi K. Combined pre- and retrosigmoid approach for petroclival meningiomas with the aid of a rotatable head frame: peri-auricular three-quarter twist-rotation approach: technical note. *Skull Base*. 2004;**14**(4):209–15.
2. Rehder R, Cohen AR. Endoscope-assisted microsurgical subtemporal keyhole approach to the posterolateral suprasellar region and basal cisterns. *World Neurosurgery*. 2017 Jul **1**;103:114–21.
3. Felbaum D, Syed HR, Ryan JE, Jean WC, Anaizi A. Endoscope-assisted combined supracerebellar infratentorial and endoscopic transventricular approach to the pineal region: a technical note. *Cureus*. 2016 Mar;**8**(3).
4. Taniguchi M, Takimoto H, Yoshimine T, Shimada N, Miyao Y, Hirata M, Maruno M, Kato A, Kohmura E, Hayakawa T. Application of a rigid endoscope to the microsurgical management of 54 cerebral aneurysms: results in 48 patients. *Journal of Neurosurgery*. 1999 Aug 1;**91**(2):231–7.
5. Russell SM, Roland JT Jr., Golfinos JG. Retrolabyrinthine craniectomy: the unsung hero of skull base surgery. *Skull Base*. 2004 Feb;**14**(1):63.
6. Chotai S, Liu Y, Qi S. Review of surgical anatomy of the tumors involving cavernous sinus. *Asian Journal of Neurosurgery*. 2018 Jan;**13**(1):1.
7. Yoon N, Shah A, Couldwell WT, Kalani MY, Park MS. Preoperative embolization of skull base meningiomas: current indications, techniques, and pearls for complication avoidance. *Neurosurgical Focus*. 2018 Apr 1;**44**(4):E5.
8. Truong HQ, Sun X, Celtikci E, Borghei-Razavi H, Wang EW, Snyderman CH, Gardner PA, Fernandez-Miranda JC. Endoscopic anterior transmaxillary "transalisphenoid" approach to Meckel's cave and the middle cranial fossa: an anatomical study and clinical application. *Journal of Neurosurgery*. 2018 Feb 2;**130**(1):227–37.
9. Terasaka S, Asaoka K, Kobayashi H, Sugiyama T, Yamaguchi S. Dural opening/removal for combined petrosal approach. *Skull Base*. 2011 Mar;**21**(2):123.
10. Van Gompel JJ, Alikhani P, Youssef AS, Van Loveren HR, Boyev KP, Agazzi S. Anterior petrosectomy: consecutive series of 46 patients with attention to approach-related complications. *Journal of Neurological Surgery. Part B, Skull Base*. 2015 Sep;**76**(5):379.
11. Fernández-de Thomas RJ, De Jesus O. *Craniotomy*. InStatPearls, Jul 11, 2020. StatPearls Publishing.

Chapter 15

Combined Suboccipital Craniotomy and Neck Dissection

Michael J. Link and Daniel Price

Introduction

A combined suboccipital craniotomy and neck dissection is an approach often utilized for invasive posterior fossa skull base tumors and neck tumors. These kinds of tumors either grow from a cranial origin, invading inferiorly to neck, or vice versa (1). Management of these tumors often requires the collaboration of multiple specialties (e.g., neurosurgery, ENT, maxillofacial surgery, and plastic surgery), since the tumor can affect multiple important structures including cranial nerves, major neck vasculature, and the face (with important cosmetic implications). Patients with tumors in this location can present with various symptoms such as headache, facial pain, neck swelling, and related cranial neuropathies manifesting as hoarseness, dysphagia, and so forth (2,3,4). Preoperative evaluation of cranial nerves V, VI, VII, VIII, IX, X, XI, and XII (facial numbness, restriction of extraocular movements, facial weakness, hearing loss, dysphagia, hoarseness, sternocleidomastoid weakness, and so on), and intraoperative monitoring, as well as careful postoperative evaluation, is essential. Furthermore, these tumors often encase or invade important neurovasculature structures, such as the carotid artery or jugular vein. The intended extent of resection depends on a case-by-case analysis including the patient's age, the aggressiveness of the tumor pathology, presenting symptoms, and comorbidities.

As an illustrative example, we present below the surgical description of a case of a glomus jugulare tumor extending through the jugular foramen, with the destruction of the petrous bone.

Indications

The surgical strategy and planned extent of resection when incorporating a combined suboccipital craniotomy and neck dissection vary depending on the pathology and how invasive the lesion appears to be. The most common indication for this combined approach is a malignant neoplasm invading both the posterior fossa of the cranium and the neck, however, at times the origin of the lesion may be adjacent to structures such as the mandible. Primary examples of aggressive posterior skull base tumors invading inferiorly to the neck include chondrosarcomas, chordomas, and metastatic tumors (5). Tumors arising from the neck, invading superiorly into the posterior skull base, include glomus tumors, osteosarcomas, and sarcomas (6). This combined approach may be helpful in the surgical treatment of aggressive vascular lesions such as arteriovenous malformation (AVM) and dural arteriovenous fistula (dAVF), as well.

An ideal clinical scenario would be a tumor expanding in the neck and petrous bone and/or cerebellopontine cistern, but not further anteriorly to the middle cranial fossa, causing surrounding cranial neuropathies (V–XII), without clear evidence of metastasis, in a patient without significant comorbidities precluding surgery.

Contraindications

Given the invasiveness of the surgery, the indication of this approach for a case with other metastatic lesions should be considered carefully and on a case-by-case basis. Neoadjuvant chemotherapy or radiation treatment should be considered in a multidisciplinary fashion to minimize the risk of cerebrospinal fluid (CSF) leak and wound healing problems. In a case where the tumor invades the carotid artery significantly, tolerance of occlusion should be evaluated postoperatively since the sacrifice of the affected carotid artery can otherwise cause life-threatening sequelae. Vocal cord function and dysphagia should also be evaluated in cases where the tumor extends close to the lower cranial nerves to avoid severe airway obstruction and aspiration. Some tumors that arise in this location secrete hypertensive hormones, and adequate control should be achieved medically before surgical intervention to avoid massive intraoperative bleeding, as well as cardiac issues (7).

Preoperative Planning

CT and MRI of the head and neck with contrast are mandatory to accurately identify the extent of the tumor and to guide decision-making regarding how aggressive the surgery should be. Stereotactic navigation may be useful to help achieve safe margins. CTA, CTV, MRA, and MRV should be considered in a tumor that invades or comes close to the cerebrovasculature. A cerebral angiogram is helpful to evaluate the hypervascularity of the tumor, and preoperative embolization may also be considered in these cases if a feeding vessel can be safely occluded. As mentioned, a balloon occlusion test should be performed in cases where the tumor abuts the carotid artery. Communication with anesthesia before surgery should include preparations for a transfusion intra-operatively in the event of significant blood loss in the case of a hypervascular tumor.

Illustrative Case

This is the case of a 42-year-old woman with a year-long history of left-sided hearing loss who presented with significant tinnitus on the left side. Mild left facial weakness with a House Brackmann Grade II was noted, and an audiogram revealed no hearing on the left. MRI of the brain with and without contrast demonstrated a large, extensive, and destructive tumor involving the left temporal bone (Figure 15.1). The tumor was centered on the jugular foramen, and extended through the tympanic membrane into the external ear canal. Inferiorly, the tumor followed along the internal jugular vein. Intracranially, the cisternal component was measured to be 25 mm in length. The T2 sequence revealed multiple flow voids, indicative of a paraganglioma.

Microanatomy and Surgical Steps

Lesions in this location often involve invasion into the cerebellopontine angle (CPA) and inferior extension to the neck. Due to this, the patient may often present with hearing loss (7). In these cases, such as the example above, the authors often choose to use a translabyrinthine approach, in addition to the neck dissection. Specific operative steps for this combined approach are included as follows.

Translabyrinthine Approach

- The patient is positioned supine, and the head is positioned with Mayfield pinions with the patient's neck turned 60 degrees to the contralateral side. The patient's abdomen is also prepped for fat graft harvest for closure.
- The patient's neck and head posterior to the ear are shaved and prepped in the usual sterile fashion. A C-shaped skin incision is marked three fingerbreadths posterior to the ear. The inferior portion of the incision is incorporated with the neck incision, which runs anterior to the sternocleidomastoid muscle (SCM; and can easily be palpated).
- The skin flap is turned anteriorly to expose the mastoid process which attaches to the SCM. The SCM is sharply dissected and posteriorly mobilized from the mastoid tip.
- During the mastoidectomy the first important structure evident is the sigmoid sinus on its last segment before it joins the jugular bulb. The mastoidectomy is extended toward the mastoid tip, which is then removed by drilling the bone along the digastric ridge and the bone above the jugular bulb laterally.
- The next important structure evident is the boney canal for the vertical segment of the facial nerve. It must be drilled on its posterior aspect, and its anterior recess, which is immediately posterior to the hypotympanum.
- The facial nerve should be cautiously protected throughout the drilling process, both from direct injury and from injury due to heat. Intraoperative monitoring of the facial nerve is helpful to avoid injury.
- Just above the facial recess the chorda tympani nerve should be identified and protected.
- The semicircular canals are then skeletonized ("blue-lined").
- Complete skeletonization of the sigmoid sinus maximizes the visualization of the intracranial component of the lesion.
- Cranial nerves IX, X, and XI pass through the antero-medial aspect of the jugular foramen in

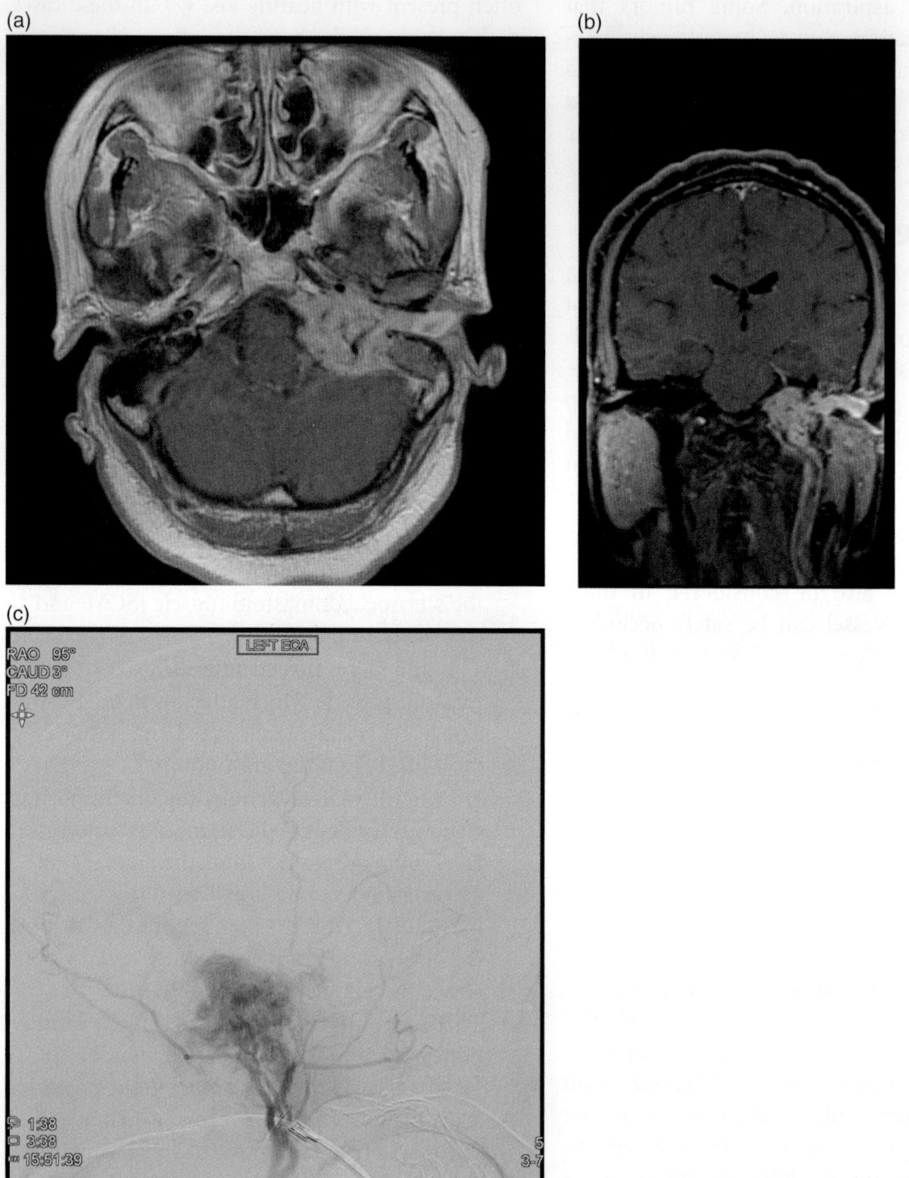

Figure 15.1 Axial MRI with contrast (a), coronal MRI with contrast (b) and cerebral angiogram (left external carotid artery injection) showing a large, extensive, vascular, and destructive tumor involving the left temporal bone

relation to the carotid artery and jugular vein. When the tumor is localized within the jugular foramen, encroachment in this area frequently jeopardizes the integrity of the lower cranial nerves, causing dysphagia which can be severe.

- A complete labyrinthectomy is then followed by identification of the internal auditory canal. Wide incision of the dura gives sufficient exposure of the CPA (Figure 15.2).
- As tumors in this area are often hypervascular, meticulous hemostasis should be obtained. Intraoperative frozen pathological investigation of the tumor may give additional clues as to how aggressive the resection should be.
- Key anatomical structures from superior to inferior of this exposure are cranial nerves of V, VI, VII, VIII, IX, X, XI, and XII. The choroid plexus arising from the Foramen of Luschka should also be identified.

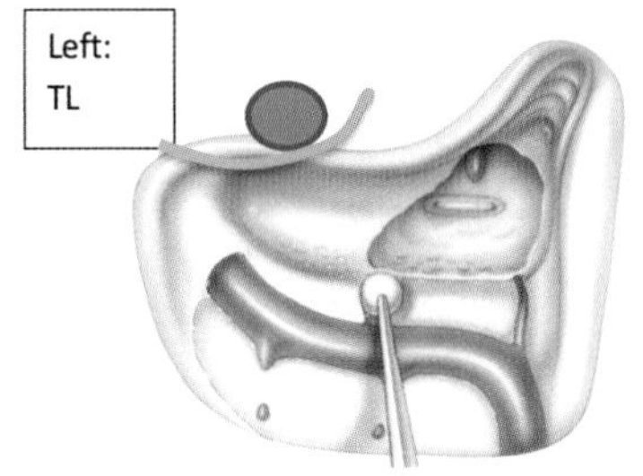

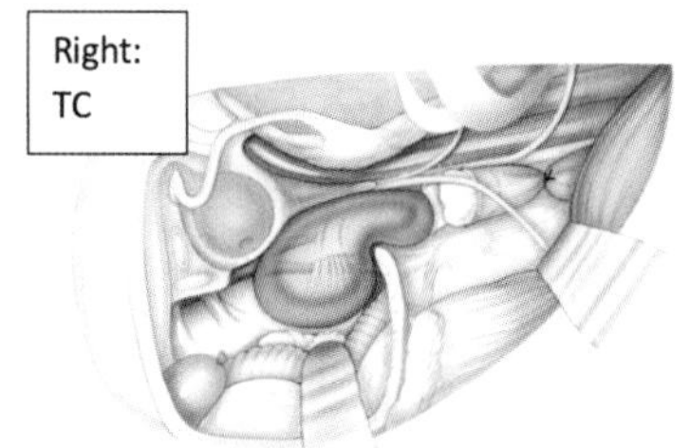

Figure 15.2 Views of the cerebollopontine angle after a left translabyrinthine approach (TL) and transcochlear approach (TC)

Neck Dissection

- A linear incision is made anterior to the SCM.
- The anterior edge of SCM is dissected, and the SCM is retracted posteriorly. The common facial vein is usually encountered at this stage, which is ligated with a 2-0 silk suture and cut to allow for wider exposure.
- The internal jugular vein (IJV) and common carotid artery (CCA) are exposed (Figure 15.3). The CCA is followed distally, and often the hypoglossal vein is encountered, which can be ligated and cut. The hypoglossal nerve is then identified running over the internal carotid artery (ICA) under the posterior belly of the digastric muscle. Vessel loops are applied to the CCA, ICA, and external carotid artery (ECA) for proximal control.
- In the case of a glomus tumor, there are usually multiple sources of blood supply from the ICA and ECA. Moving circumferentially around the tumor, feeders should be cauterized and cut. This process should be continued in a 360-degree fashion to obtain complete hemostasis.

Suboccipital Craniotomy

- A C-shaped incision is marked three fingerbreadths behind the ear.
- A skin flap is turned between the layer above the splenius capitis muscle and below the SCM. This skin flap is turned anteriorly and held in place with skin hooks on flexible bands or sutures that are attached to the drape.
- A muscle flap containing all the deeper musculature (e.g., semispinalis capitis, rectus capitis major and minor, superior oblique capitis, and longissimus capitis) is turned and reflected posteriorly.

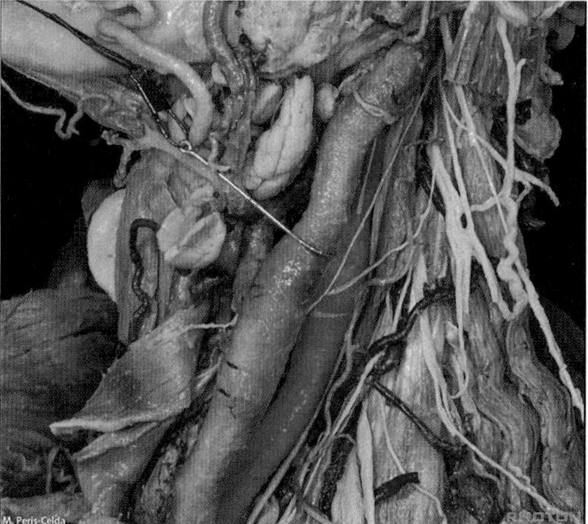

Figure 15.3 Anatomical view of the right internal jugular vien and common carotid artery

- A burr hole is made at the inferior portion of the transverse-sigmoid junction. A trough is then made just posterior to the sigmoid sinus. A cutting bar with a footplate attachment on a high-speed drill is used to turn the suboccipital craniotomy. A high-speed drill is used to expose the posterior edge of the sigmoid sinus.
- The dura is opened in a box-like fashion with its base preserved along the sigmoid sinus (Figure 15.4). A cotton pattie is used to wrap the dural flap, and this is then reflected anteriorly. The pattie is consistently irrigated throughout the case to keep the dural flap from drying out and shrinking, which increases the chances of a primary dural closure at the completion of the case (8).

Complication Avoidance

Airway and Dysphagia Management

A drain is placed in the neck incision postoperatively to avoid hematoma accumulation, which can

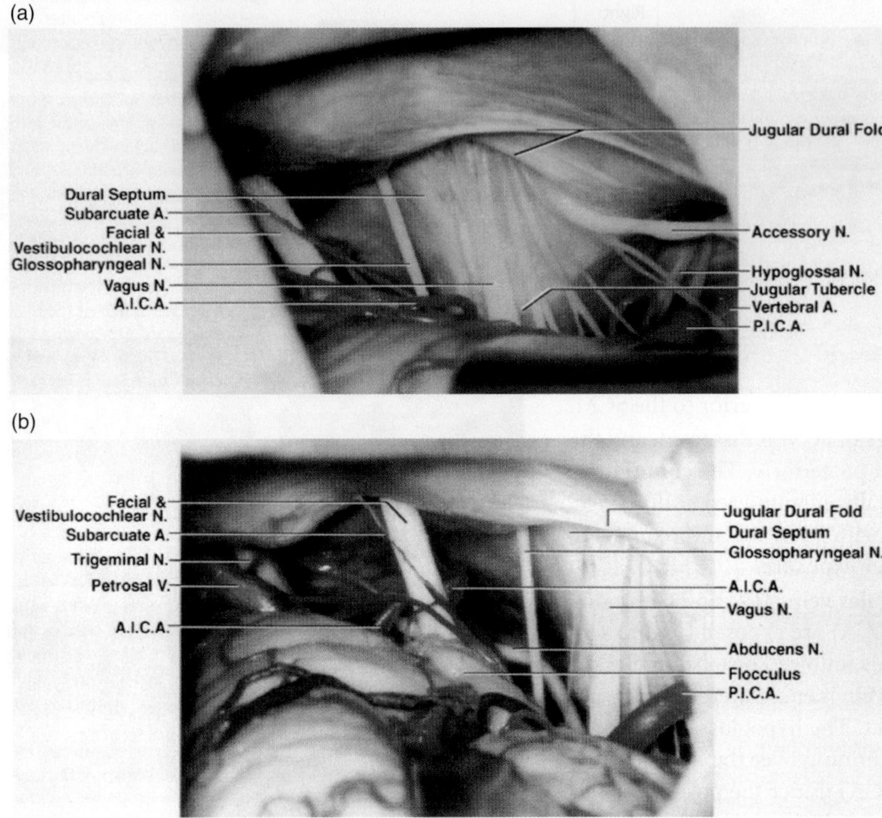

Figure 15.4 Surgical view of the lower cranial nerves (a) and facial nerve after a suboccipital craniotomy

lead to airway compromise. Due to multiple potential factors, such as preoperative vocal paralysis and perioperative lower cranial nerve deficits, swelling in the pharynx from intraoperative intubation, as well as venous obstruction (such as from the jugular vein), patients are at high risk of airway obstruction, dysphagia, and aspiration pneumonia postoperatively. There should be vigilant monitoring of airway patency in recovery, and transient tracheostomy can be a safe management option if airway obstruction is encountered. This should be discussed beforehand in multidisciplinary collaboration with ENT and anesthesiology.

CSF Leak

Watertight dural closure is sometimes unobtainable due to the destructive nature of the tumor, natural characteristics of the approach (e.g., translabyrinthine approach), and so on. Temporary lumbar drain placement can be a good option to avoid this complication, and antibiotics should be appropriately continued while the lumbar drain is inserted.

Stroke Management

Tumors often invade the carotid arteries as well as major venous structures, such as the jugular vein, and a balloon occlusion test should be considered in these cases to assess the safety of the sacrifice, if needed. Even though careful attention is paid, stroke can be encountered perioperatively due to tumor emboli migration, complications of preoperative embolization, and other unexpected reasons. If patients show any neurological change postoperatively, imaging studies such as CT or MRI should be obtained emergently. Because of the highly vascular nature of tumors in this location, the risks of postoperative antithrombotic therapy (e.g., Enoxaparin, Heparin) should be carefully considered.

Wound Dehiscence and Infection

Surgery often takes many hours, and multiple drains are often placed after surgery is completed. Postoperative antibiotics should be maintained appropriately, and good nutrition and diabetes management are necessary. Patients may require an insulin infusion if blood sugar levels are difficult to manage, particularly in the setting of high-dose perioperative steroid use.

Postoperative Considerations

Drains should be monitored for output, and removed in two or three days. Adequate perioperative antibiotics should be continued. Patients may require tube feeding or temporary tracheostomy for airway protection and dysphagia, depending on the severity of dysfunction. Postoperative rehabilitation and close follow-up should be encouraged for any cranial nerve deficits, particularly in the case of dysphagia.

Necessary Follow-Up

Follow-up imaging studies should be obtained regularly to assess for recurrence or the potential need for adjuvant chemoradiation. Typically postoperative MRI with and without contrast is obtained at three months, six months, and then yearly thereafter.

Clinical Pearls

- Extent of craniotomy, as well as the extent of neck dissection, depends on the extension of the tumor, tumor pathology, and presenting symptoms (e.g., hearing loss).
- Preoperative cerebrovasculature evaluation is crucial in cases where the tumor is close to the carotid artery or jugular vein. Preoperative angiogram, BOT, and potential embolization can contribute to safety management.
- The anesthesia service and operating room staff should be prepared for an expeditious blood transfusion if needed.
- Pre- and postoperative management of airway patency and dysphagia is essential to avoid severe morbidity and long-term sequelae.

References

1. Kumar R, Wani AA. Unusual tumors of the posterior fossa skull base. *Skull Base*. 2006 May;**16**(2):75.
2. Agarwal V, Babu R, Grier J, Adogwa O, Back A, Friedman AH, Fukushima T, Adamson C. Cerebellopontine angle meningiomas: postoperative outcomes in a modern cohort. *Neurosurgical Focus*. 2013 Dec 1;**35**(6):E10.
3. Martínez R, Vaquero J, Areitio E, Bravo G. Meningiomas of the posterior fossa. *Surgical Neurology*. 1983 Mar 1;**19**(3):237–43.
4. Meyer FB, Ebersold MJ, Reese DF. Benign tumors of the foramen magnum. *Journal of Neurosurgery*. 1984 Jul 1;**61**(1):136–42.
5. Sampson JH, Rossitch E Jr., Young JN, Lane KL, Friedman AH. Solitary eosinophilic granuloma invading the clivus of an adult: case report. *Neurosurgery*. 1992 Oct 1;**31**(4):755–7.
6. Thust SC, Yousry T. Imaging of skull base tumours. *Reports of Practical Oncology & Radiotherapy*. 2016 Jul 1;**21**(4):304–18.
7. Pacak K. Stressor-specific activation of the hypothalamic-pituitary adrenocortical axis. *Physiological Research*. 2000 Jan **1**;49:S11–18.
8. Katsuta T, Rhoton AL Jr., Matsushima T. The jugular foramen: microsurgical anatomy and operative approaches. *Neurosurgery*. 1997 Jul 1;**41**(1):149–202.

Chapter 16

Combined Petrosal Approach

Hikari Sato, Takanori Fukushima, and Allan Friedman

Introduction

Surgery of tumors of the petroclival junction and posterior cavernous sinus region is among the most difficult in neurosurgery. The deep location, complex anatomy, and involvement of multiple cranial nerves, critical blood vessels, and the brainstem present neurosurgeons with a formidable challenge to achieve radical resection with minimal morbidity. Examples of petroclival lesions include meningiomas, neurinomas, chordomas, chondrosarcomas, epidermoids, cavernomas, arteriovenous malformations (AVMs), and basilar trunk aneurysms. There are many skull base operative approaches available to approach these lesions, including the frontotemporal-transcavernous approach, middle fossa anterior petrosectomy, translabyrinthine approach, retrolabyrinthine-retrosigmoid posterior fossa approach, and the combined transpetrosal approach. The selection of the proper operative approach depends upon tumor size, extension, vascularity, adhesion, presenting symptoms, and the patient's age. The combined petrosal approach is indicated for petroclival lesions extending in front of the brainstem and dumbbell-shaped large petroclival lesions with supra- and infratentorial extension in healthy patients younger than 65 years old. In addition, this approach is utilized for posterior cerebral artery (P2) high-flow bypass in the management of basilar aneurysms unamenable to clip ligation and tumors around the posterior cavernous sinus.

Historical Background

Prior to 1970, the standard suboccipital approach to access the ventral brainstem and the clivus proved to have extremely high morbidity and mortality. The conventional approach was the retrosigmoid intradural technique, which required significant retraction of the cerebellum and the brainstem to obtain satisfactory exposure. Excessive retraction to aid in visualizing the ventral brainstem and the clivus led to cerebellar swelling and damage to the crucial bridging veins, often resulting in venous infarction or hemorrhage. For this reason, retrosigmoid approaches were considered high-risk for pathology in these regions.

In 1961, House et al. described his experience with the middle fossa approach with petrous bone drilling to expose intracanalicular acoustic neuromas (1). In 1966, Drs. Hitselberger and House described 20 patients who underwent operations between 1965 and 1966 in which the translabyrinthine approach was combined with an extended suboccipital craniotomy with ligation of the sigmoid sinus (i.e. the translabyrinthine-transsigmoid approach) (2). The development of these two techniques – the anterior petrosectomy and the posterior transmastoid approach – was crucial for the development of the current combined petrosal approach.

During the period between 1965 and 1970, there was also a dramatic evolution with advances in microsurgical techniques to neurosurgery. This rapid advance was permitted by further refinements in the free-moving or "floating" operating microscope and pneumatic drill, as well as high-speed power motor drill systems. Additionally, microsurgical instruments including pressure-adjustable tear-drop suctions, dissectors, and microscissors suitable for microsurgery with a longer and more slender design were developed to meet the needs of these approaches.

In 1973, Drs. Morrison and King in London described an extended translabyrinthine approach in which the dural opening was extended superiorly through the division of the superior petrosal sinus and the tentorium with preservation of the sigmoid sinus (3). Additionally, during this time, Dr. Malis in

New York was using a combined suboccipital retrolabyrinthine approach with the division of the sigmoid sinus but preservation of the vein of Labbé; Dr. Malis used this transsigmoid retrolabyrinthine approach for more than a decade with great success.

Starting in the late 1970s, surgeons looking for safer approaches to the ventral brainstem started to focus on combining supra- and infratentorial approaches. Around this time, a group of Japanese skull-base surgeons started to focus more on primarily extradural approaches. In 1977, Hakuba et al. reported on six cases of petroclival meningiomas treated through the combined transpetrosal approach. Dr. Hakuba, who was a research fellow with Leonard Malis, developed a combined transpetrosal approach (1977) in which he used a large subtemporal craniotomy combined with a presigmoid exposure (4). Dr. Hakuba incised the superior petrosal sinus and the tentorium in a fashion very similar to the Morrison/King procedure, exposing the petroclival region through a subtemporal approach. The most important advancement in Dr. Hakuba's method was the removal of the petrous ridge and partial labyrinthectomy to expand the combined supratentorial and infratentorial operative space. This method allowed for an extradural approach to the lateral cerebellopontine angle (CPA), the ventral brainstem, and the base of the temporal lobe. Dr. Hakuba's transpetrosal approach (with a partial labyrinthectomy) preserved the sigmoid sinus. Although a partial labyrinthectomy carries the risk of hearing loss, Dr. Hakuba reported preservation of at least partial hearing in his series (5, 6)

Dr. Fukushima further defined and developed the combined transpetrosal approach to treat large petroclival lesions (7). His approach involves the combination of an extended middle fossa anterior petrosal "rhomboid" resection combined with a true labyrinth-sparing retrolabyrinthine mastoidectomy (8), resulting in preservation of the sigmoid sinus and of hearing. This primarily extradural combined retrolabyrinthine and rhomboid middle fossa approach allows for extensive exposure of the CPA, the clivus anterior to the brainstem, and the posterolateral cavernous sinus. In this method, dissection and preservation of cranial nerves III through XII, the basilar artery and its ipsilateral branches, and the lateral brainstem is possible.

In the 1980s to 1990s, a number of investigators reported the application of this combined petrosal approach; however, the majority did not describe precise microanatomical construction of the middle fossa rhomboid space or skeletonization of the labyrinth and common crus. As was described by Dr. Hakuba, other investigators, and several textbooks, a presigmoid-to-subtemporal dural incision was made in a Y-shape. Dr. Fukushima made it clear that a posterior incision along the transverse sinus should not be performed, as it risks injury to the vein of Labbé. Dr. Fukushima advocated for a precise retrolabyrinthine presigmoid exposure and more complete anterior petrosectomy with full drilling of the described "rhomboid" area and the petrous ridge. Dr. Fukushima's petrosal dural incision is curvilinear, consisting of a presigmoid incision and double ligation of the superior petrosal sinus 10 mm anterior to the sinodural angle and a subtemporal incision along the superior petrosal sinus, without a posterior incision. The subtemporal dural incision is more basilar, at the tentorial attachment, so that the temporal lobe is not exposed and is protected by the overlying dura mater (9). This protects the temporal lobe, decreases edema and swelling, and minimizes any risk of damaging the vein of Labbé, which could cause a large venous infarct and significant neurological deficit (10, 11).

Operative Technique

Step 1: Head Positioning and Skin Incision

A lumbar cerebral spinal fluid (CSF) drainage catheter is placed to allow CSF drainage to decrease intracranial pressure, allowing the brain to fall away from the skull base. Monitoring electrodes are placed. Auditory brainstem response (ABR) monitoring is important to help preserve the patient's hearing function. Facial nerve monitoring is useful for the identification of the geniculate ganglion in the middle cranial fossa and for guiding exposure of the internal auditory and fallopian canals. Three-dimensional volumetric computer navigation should be available to help define the key intraoperative landmarks and for intraoperative assessment of the extent of the tumor resection.

The patient is placed in the Fukushima lateral position, and the head is supported with three-point pin fixation (Figure 16.1A–D).

The important points of the Fukushima lateral position are that the patient's head is placed in the straight lateral and vertex down position with the sagittal suture parallel to the floor and the neck moderately flexed (Figure 16.1A). The body is placed obliquely on the table. The head is kept horizontal and elevated away from the lower shoulder, with the vertex tilted down to avoid venous congestion and injury to the brachial plexus. The face is slightly turned toward the floor to make the posterior border of the body of the mastoid the highest point in the surgical field. The patient's back is placed at the edge of the table, and the head is positioned as close to the surgeon as possible. The upper shoulder and arm are held in an arm holder, and the superior shoulder is rotated forward 45 degrees. An axillary pillow is placed. The patient's hips are placed in the middle of the table and rotated gently backward to facilitate the harvesting of abdominal fat. The lower leg is flexed 90 degrees and the straightened upper leg is separated from the lower leg with ample padding (Figure 16.1A). One pin on the rocker arm portion of the Mayfield head holder is placed on the inion, and the second pin is placed on the upper portion of the mastoid on the side opposite the surgery. The single pin of the Mayfield head holder is placed on the ipsilateral frontal bone just behind the patient's hairline. The body of the Mayfield head holder is rotated out 45 degrees (Figure 16.1C, D). The abdominal wall is prepared so that fat and fascia can be harvested at

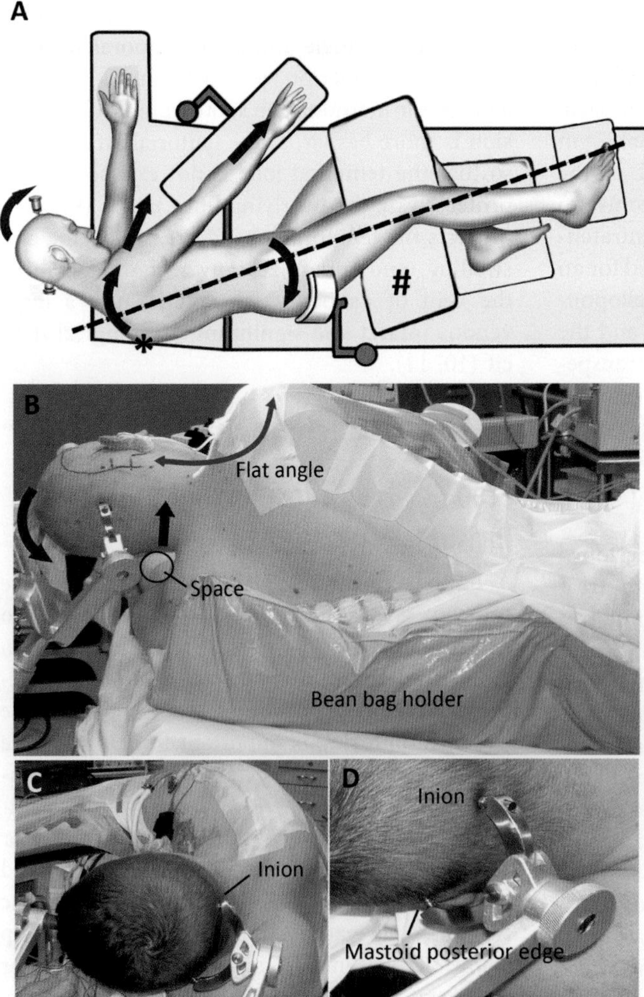

Figure 16.1 Fukushima lateral position and Mayfield headclamp application

(A) The shoulder and back are placed at the far edge of the table on the surgeon's side (*). The upper shoulder and arm are held with an arm holder with the body three-fourths lateral prone and 45-degree anterior and caudal to craniocervical axis. The axilla is padded. The hip is placed in the middle of the table and twisted gently backward for the possible harvest of abdominal fat. The lower leg is flexed 90-degree and the upper leg overlays using a big, soft pillow (#). The dashed black line shows the oblique lying of the body. Blue arrows indicate the direction of flexion and angulation.

The exact location of Mayfield pins: the upper one is placed on the inion, and the other is placed onto the mastoid posterior edge (B–D). The opposing one pin is placed in the midfrontal region inside the hairline, fixing the head obliquely (A, B).

The Mayfield arm is turned 45 degrees out toward the vertex (B, D). The head is flexed moderately and kept horizontal, with the vertex slightly pointed down and elevated up from the lower shoulder (A, B).

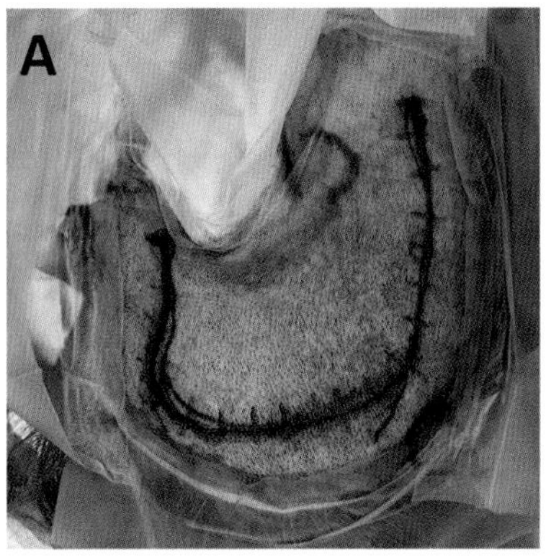

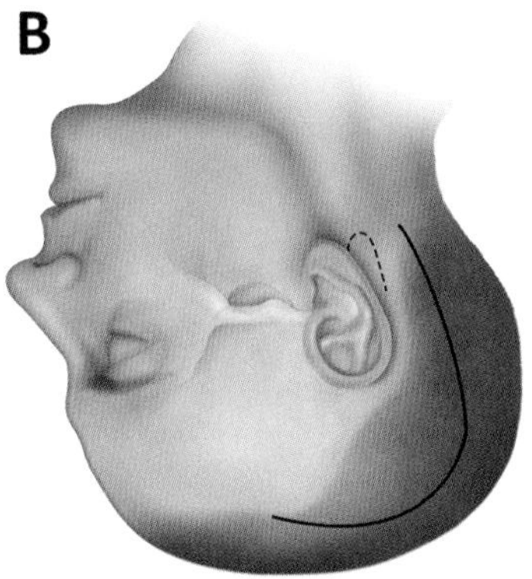

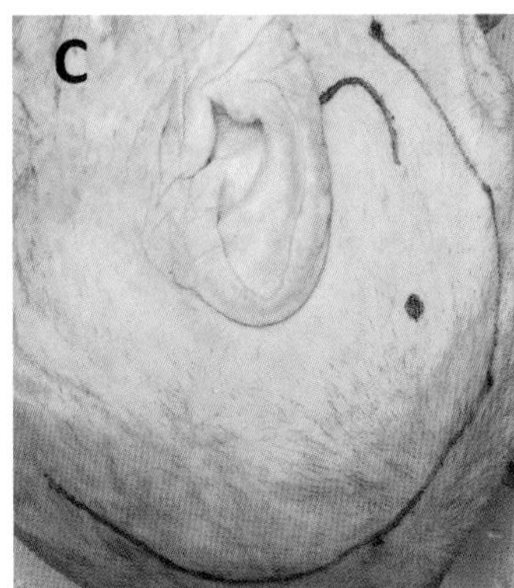

Figure 16.2 Possible skin incisions (Rt)

(A) "Chef hat" incision to dissect the superior temporal artery (STA) parietal branch
(B) Postauricular L-shaped incision
(C) Postauricular C-shaped incision (anatomical specimen)

the end of the case, if needed to close the surgical dead space. The skin can be incised in a large "C" shape extending from the temporal line at the patient's hairline back to a point 2.5 cm behind the mastoid tip. More commonly in our practice, we use a sagging U-shaped incision that begins in front of the ear at the zygomatic arch, proceeds superiorly along the patient's hairline to a point approximately 1 cm above the temporal line, and then curves back to a point 7 cm above the external auditory canal. The incision continues back to a point 2.5 cm behind the asterion and then inferiorly behind the mastoid tip (Figure 16.2).

Dissection of Long and Wide STA-Attached Vascularized Galeo-Fascial-Pericranial Flap

The skin and the subcutaneous tissue are elevated using a sharp dissection technique. The parietal-temporal fascia, the galea, and the superficial temporal artery (STA) are left attached to the skull. The pericranium is contiguous with the fascia of the temporal muscle and the sternocleidomastoid muscles (SCM). The skin around the flap is undermined for ~2–3 cm. The pericranium is cut as far under the intact skin as possible and elevated as a vascularized flap along with the temporal-parietal fascia, temporal muscle fascia, and parietal branch of the superficial temporal artery (Figure 16.3A). This STA parietal branch-enhanced vascularized galeo-fascial-pericranial (GFP) flap is sharply elevated from the temporal muscle and SCM. The STA frontal branch is preserved to maintain blood flow through the STA and to avoid surgical wound dehiscence, and preserving the fascia over the suprazygomatic area preserves the branch of the facial nerve to the frontalis muscle. A thin portion of SCM and temporal muscle is usually elevated together with the fascia. The pedicle attachment of this vascularized GFP flap needs to be kept as wide as possible; the length of the pedicle will be trimmed at closure. This long and wide vascularized GFP flap is crucial for promoting satisfactory healing and for preventing CSF leakage and infection (Figure 16.3B). In our practice, we prefer to have the wide, vascularized pedicle attached to the frontotemporal base to protect the STA parietal branch.

Step 3: Temporal and Suboccipital Muscle Elevation and Outer Bony Landmarks

The temporal muscle is reflected anteroinferiorly. The suboccipital muscles are elevated off of the mastoid and the superior and inferior nuchal lines as one block and retracted posteriorly and inferiorly with multiple blunt hooks. Bony landmarks are noted (Figure 16.4).

The suboccipital muscles are arranged in three layers. The first layer of the suboccipital muscles, composed of the sternocleidomastoid muscle (SCM) and the trapezius muscle, is attached to

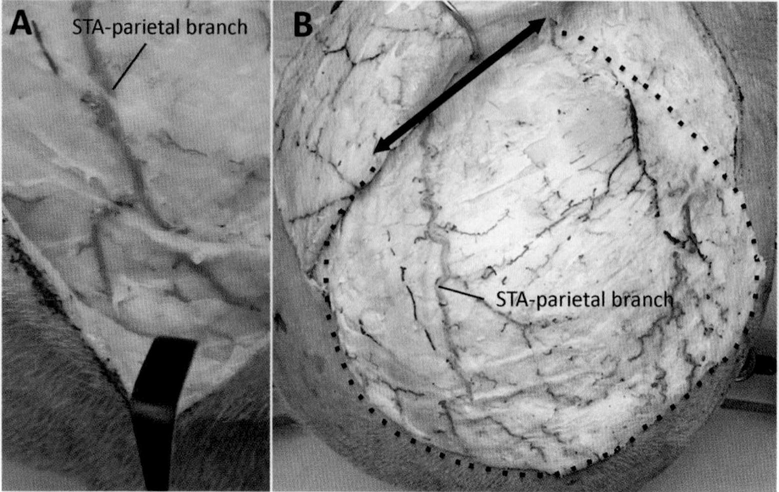

Figure 16.3 Dissection and elevation of superficial temporal artery (STA) attached vascularized galeo-fascial-pericranial (GFP) flap

(A) Meticulous dissection of the STA parietal branch in a cadaver under an operating microscope. The posterior margin of the skin incision is retracted with a flat blade army-navy retractor and undermined approximately 2–3 cm to harvest a long and wide pericranial flap.

(B) The galeo-fascial-pericranial flap is elevated from the undermined deep end with a No. 15 blade knife and a periosteal elevator. The parietal branch of the STA is included in the flap and the frontal branch of the STA is preserved with the skin flap.

Arrow: Wide pedicle of GFP flap

Broken line: Wide and large vascularized GFP flap

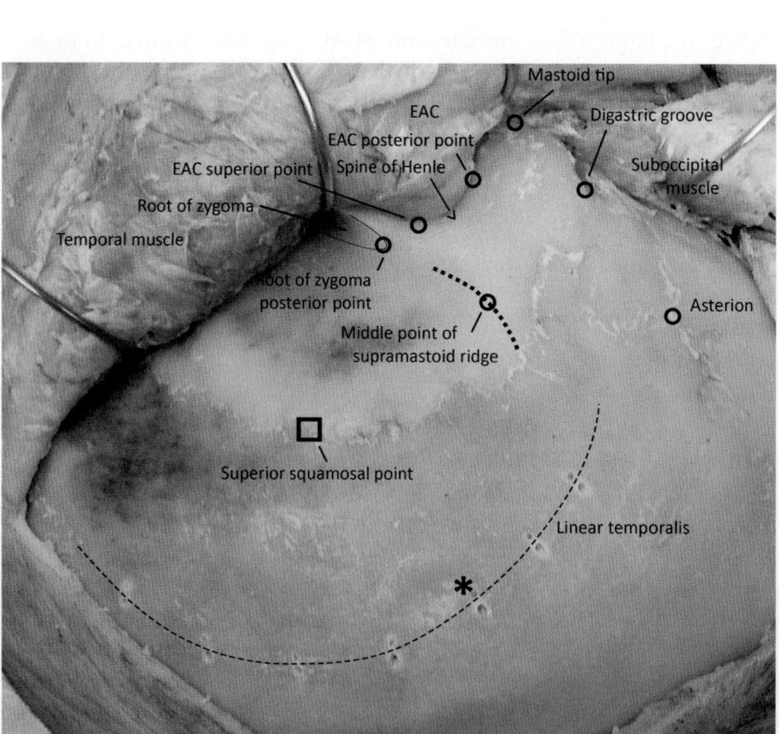

Figure 16.4 Muscle elevation and the key bony landmarks

Dissect the temporal muscle and the suboccipital muscles cleanly.

Small circles and the spine of Henle arrow indicate the boundary of mastoid drilling (outer mastoid triangle).

*: Multiple pair holes are used to suture securely the edge of temporal muscle along the linea temporalis at closure.
□: Superior squamosal point
Dashed line: Linea temporalis
Dotted line: Supramastoid ridge or crest
Curved line: Root of zygoma
EAC: External auditory canal

the superior nuchal line. The second layer consists of the splenius and longissimus capitis muscles and is separated from the deep layer by the deep cervical fascia, which encases the occipital artery (OA) and is contiguous with the styloid diaphragm.

A thick fat pad and venous plexus lie between the second and third layers. The third layer consists of the superior oblique muscle and the rectus capitis posterior major and minor muscles that are attached to the inferior nuchal line. In this procedure, it is not necessary to identify the suboccipital triangle, consisting of the rectus capitis posterior major, obliquus capitis superior, and obliquus capitis inferior muscles, or the vertebral artery contained within it.

Step 4: Mastoidectomy and L-Shaped Middle and Posterior Fossa Bone Flap Craniotomy

For the combined petrosal approach, begin by performing a mastoidectomy. The surgeon should have a good grasp of the anatomy of structures in and adjacent to the mastoid. The mastoidectomy commences with drilling of the outer triangle marked by the asterion, the root of the zygoma, and the mastoid tip. Superficial drilling is carried out with a 6-mm cutting burr and a 5-mm extra-coarse diamond burr (Figure 16.4, 16.5B, 16.6A). Air cells are drilled out, and the transverse and sigmoid sinuses are skeletonized. Bone is carefully removed from the sinodural angle and from the inferior surface of the posterior temporal dura (temporal tegmen). Note that the dura is generally robust over the superior segment of the sigmoid sinus, but as the surgeon works in a superior-to-inferior direction, the dura over the sigmoid sinus and jugular bulb may be extremely thin (Figure 16.6A–C). Here, the bone should be very thin prior to being extirpated from the dura. We suggest using a 4- or 5-mm coarse diamond burr to completely skeletonize the sigmoid sinus and the jugular bulb. In principle, all cortical bone should be removed from the sigmoid sinus, but if the surgeon encounters a particularly thin wall of the inferior sigmoid sinus, a very thin layer of bone may be left in place in order to avoid venous sinus injury.

Approximately 15 mm deep into the spine of Henle, the surgeon will encounter the mastoid antrum. The antrum is a large air cell that contains the short crus of the incus. Posteriorly in the antrum, the hard bone surrounding the lateral semicircular canal is identified and skeletonized (Figures 16.5B, 16.6B). The lateral semicircular canal is a good landmark for the fallopian canal, which runs just anterior to it. While the bone around the fallopian canal is thinned, we do not recommend exposing the facial nerve for this approach in a clinical case. The presigmoid bone is removed with the eggshell technique, exposing the dura of the posterior fossa. The endolymphatic sac is seen as a triangular thickening of the posterior fossa dura. The apex of the triangular sac points to the posterior semicircular canal, which runs perpendicular to the lateral semicircular canal. The superior semicircular canal protrudes into the temporal tegmentum. The center of the superior semicircular canal is marked by the subarcuate artery. Removal of the bone deep to the posterior semicircular canal adjacent to the posterior fossa dura improves the surgeon's visualization of the lateral cerebellopontine angle.

The path of the fallopian canal is variable. The only two places in which the seventh nerve can be consistently located are anterior to the lateral semicircular canal and at the stylomastoid foramen. The bone overlying the tympanic segment of the facial nerve lies immediately anterior to the lateral semicircular canal. The stylomastoid foramen can be found by following the digastric groove anteriorly. Here, the nerve is not distinct, as it is covered by fibrous tissue as it exits the stylomastoid foramen. The course of the seventh nerve between these two points may vary as the nerve is "pushed" by adjacent air cells. For the combined petrosal approach, it is not important to completely skeletonize the facial nerve. The fallopian canal, which lies 12–15 mm deep to the lateral-most edge of the external auditory canal, can be found by removing the retrofacial air cells. The jugular bulb is encountered in the space inferior to the posterior semicircular canal. Care must be taken, as the wall of the jugular bulb is often very thin. The relationship between the jugular bulb and the inferior posterior semicircular canal varies, so drilling in this space must be done delicately with a 3-mm coarse diamond burr. If a small rent is made in the jugular bulb, the hole should be covered with a small piece of Gelfoam or muscle, which should be held in place until the bleeding stops. At this stage, the surgeon should be able to visualize the inferior middle fossa dura; the presigmoid dura; a small strip of retrosigmoid dura; the sigmoid sinus and lateral-most aspect of the transverse sinus; the sinodural angle; the superior petrosal sinus in the sinodural angle; the lateral, superior, and posterior semicircular canals; and the fallopian canal. To maximize exposure, the posterior lateral bone overlying the labyrinth should be skeletonized using a 1- to 2-mm diamond burr. As the bone is removed, the blue line of the superior and posterior semicircular canals can be seen (the line is brown in cadavers).

Step 5: One-Piece L-Shaped Temporo-occipital and Suboccipital Craniotomy

After the mastoidectomy is complete, a groove is drilled along the floor of the middle fossa in line

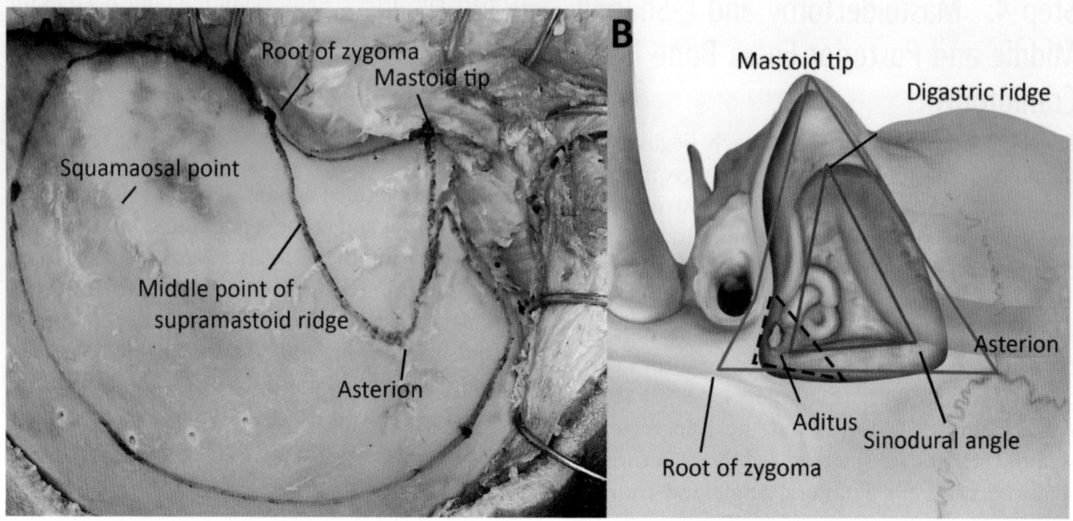

Figure 16.5 Mastoid drilling: Outer and inner mastoid triangle

(A) The outline of mastoid drilling and L-shape craniotomy
(B) Blue and red triangles indicate outer and inner triangles, respectively.

The outer triangle (blue line) consists of the asterion, root of zygoma as the posterior point, and the mastoid tip. The line between the root of zygoma and mastoid tip is slightly curved in the initial drilling. The line from the root of zygoma to asterion shown also curves upward through the midpoint of the supramastoid ridge to secure a wider working space in the mastoidectomy (5A).

The inner triangle (red line) consists of the sinodural angle, aditus and digastric ridge, and shows the corridors for the presigmoid approach.

MacEwen's triangle or mastoid fossa (dashed line) indicates the location of the mastoid antrum. The external auditory canal (EAC) and the superior and the posterior limits of the EAC are important landmarks. It is important not to disrupt the EAC fascial wall.

with the root of the zygoma using a 4-mm coarse diamond burr. This groove is extended superiorly along the posterior border of the elevated temporal muscle out to the pterion. A second groove is drilled extending from the inferior aspect of the mastoid tip and extending posterior through the occipital bone at the inferior edge of the exposure. It is difficult to use a craniotome at the base of the skull; thus the groove is drilled using a 4-mm coarse diamond burr. The bone is eggshelled, and the thin bone shell is removed using a small curette. At least two burr holes are made along the superior line of the proposed bone flap using a 5-mm extra-coarse diamond burr. One of the burr holes is made 1.5 cm above the squamous suture. The second hole is made 2 cm behind the asterion (Figure 16.7A). The asterion marks the junction between the parietal mastoid, occipital mastoid, and lambdoid sutures. The asterion is within 1 cm of the transverse-sigmoid junction. If the surgeon finds that the dura is particularly stuck to the bone, additional burr holes should be made to separate the dura from the bone prior to connecting the holes with a craniotome. Using a small L-shaped dissection, separate the transverse sinus from the overlying bone. The inferior bony groove is connected to the burr hole over the transverse sinus. Using a drill with a router attachment, a cut is made between the two burr holes, and then anteriorly to the superior-most aspect of the anterior bony groove. The bone flap is carefully raised, and meticulous hemostasis of the underlining dura is attained. Small V-shaped holes are made superior to the linea temporalis in order to fix the temporal muscle to the bone at the end of the operation (Figures 16.4, 16.5A, 16.7A).

Step 6: Middle Fossa Extradural Dissection and Drilling of the Rhomboid Space

The dura of the middle fossa is elevated from the underlying bone and held in place using two rigid 2-mm retractors. The subtemporal dura is gradually elevated from the floor of the middle fossa with the help of lumbar CSF drainage, with attempts made to preserve the integrity of the dura. The superior semicircular canal lying in close proximity to the arcuate eminence has already been identified. The inner plate of the

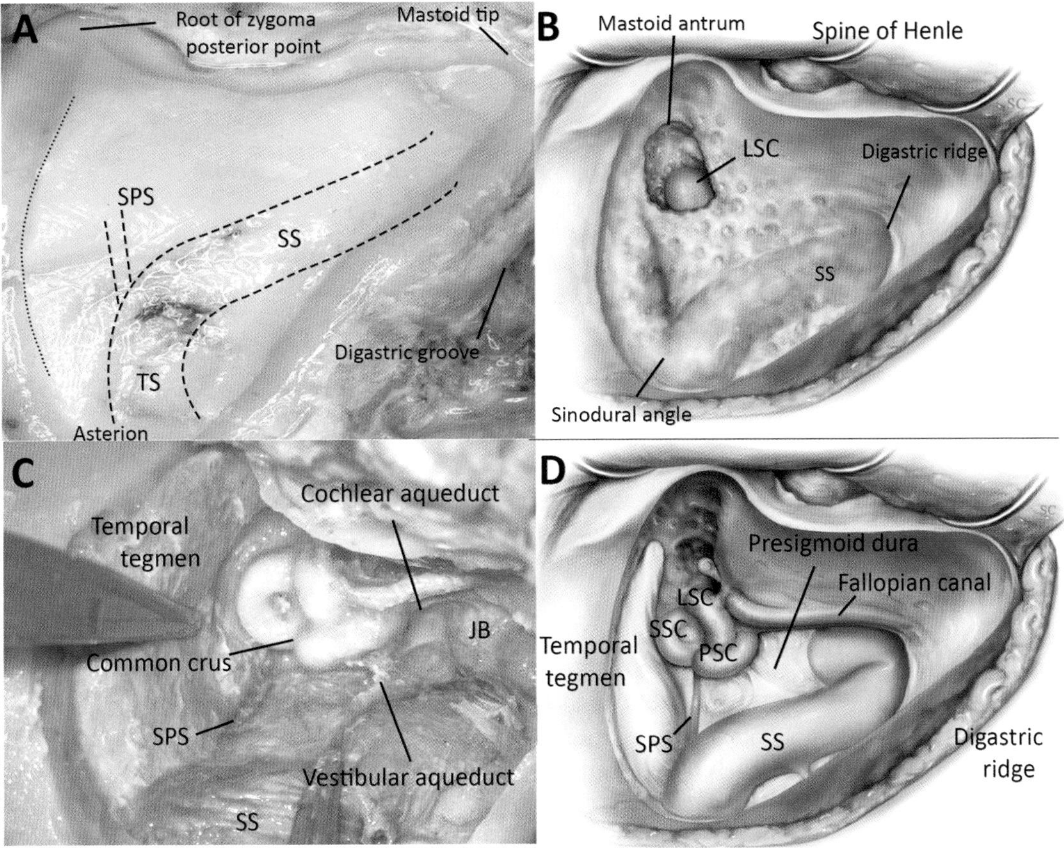

Figure 16.6 Mastoidectomy

(A) Initial groove drilling along the mastoid outer triangle.
Dashed and dotted lines show presumable limits of the temporal tegmen and venous sinus.
(B) The mastoid antrum cavity is the most important key to finding the lateral semicircular canal (LSC). Compact yellow bone is seen inside the mastoid antrum.
(C, D) Skeletonization of the labyrinths, temporal tegmen, and presigmoid dura
JB: jugular bulb
SPS: superior petrosal sinus
SS: sigmoid sinus
TS: transverse sinus

floor of the middle fossa is drilled flat so that the surgeon's vision is unobstructed by bony protrusions. Take care not to enter the middle ear or drill down the arcuate eminence. The foramen spinosum (FS) is often hidden by a bony protuberance. The easiest way to find the FS is to follow the middle meningeal artery proximally. The bony overhang hiding the FS can then be drilled flat using a diamond drill. The middle meningeal artery is then coagulated and cut. The foramen ovale is seen medial and anterior to the FS. The dura propria is sharply separated from the mandibular nerve. The surgeon will often encounter venous bleeding at this stage, which should be controlled using hemostatic agents. Using bipolar cautery to stop the bleeding poses the risk of producing facial dysesthesias from injury to the mandibular nerve, so is discouraged. There is almost always an emissary vein running along the superior aspect of the mandibular nerve that connects the pterygoid plexus with the cavernous sinus. After separating the dura propria from the mandibular nerve, the greater superficial petrosal nerve (GSPN) can be seen running alongside a branch of the middle meningeal artery in a groove along the floor of the middle fossa. The nerve originates from the facial hiatus and passes underneath the mandibular nerve. The GSPN is usually attached to the dura; it can be separated from the dura using

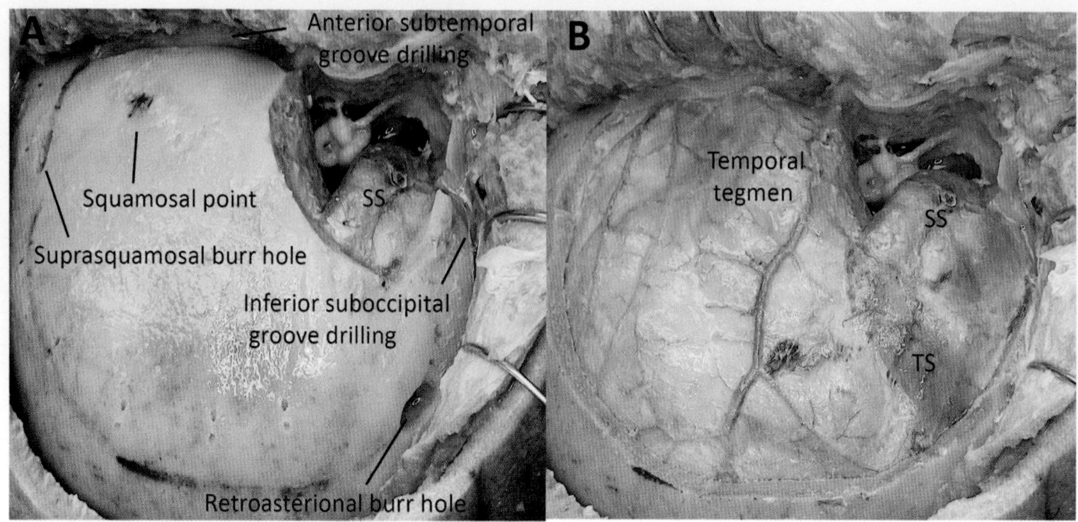

Figure 16.7 L-shaped petrosal craniotomy

(A) Location of burr holes and groove drillings
(B) After L-shaped petrosal craniotomy

a No. 11 blade knife. Traction on the GSPN can injure the geniculate ganglion and the facial nerve. The geniculate ganglion can be identified using 0.3 mA of electrical stimulation. With the mandibular nerve and Gasserian ganglion freed from the dura propria, the posterior surface of the petrous bone medial to the GSPN is exposed. These structures can be displaced anteriorly by the surgeon, exposing the tip of the petrous bone. The rhomboid fossa is defined by the greater superficial petrosal nerve laterally, the Gasserian ganglion anteriorly, and the arcuate eminence posteriorly (Figure 16.8A–C).

The carotid artery runs in the carotid canal of the petrous bone, just underneath the GSPN. The cochlea sits in the corner, between the arcuate eminence and the GSPN. This is the only structure in this petrous exposure that is not exactly defined by the more superficial landmarks. The posterior margin of the petrous ridge is marked by a groove that contains the middle portion of the superior petrosal sinus. The surgeon must free the dura from this ridge. Retractors can be advanced beyond this ridge to support the inferior temporal dura and completely expose the rhomboid space. Drilling along the petrous ridge between the arcuate eminence in the mandibular nerve will expose the dura lining the porus acousticus. It is safest to expose the internal auditory canal medially away from the cochlea and the superior semicircular canal. The internal auditory canal is found by bisecting the angle between the GSPN and the arcuate eminence. The cortical and cancellous bone over the rhomboid area is removed. Like the semicircular canals, the cochlea is surrounded by a hard, bony shell and lies medial to the genu of the carotid artery. While the IAC can be exposed for 270 degrees medially at the porous acousticus as the surgeon drills laterally, care must be taken not to drill into the superior semicircular canal or the cochlea, which flank the lateral most aspect of the internal auditory canal at the fundus. Drilling the bone anterior to the internal auditory canal and lateral to the cochlea and GSPN will reveal the posterior fossa dura. This dura can be exposed all the way down to the inferior petrosal sinus, which marks the junction between the petrous bone and the clivus. Drilling laterally under the GSPN will open the carotid canal and expose the carotid artery, which is surrounded by a venous plexus. Drilling then continues posterior to the internal auditory canal and anterior to the superior semicircular canal, further exposing the posterior fossa dura. It may be necessary to remove bone from the lateral border of the foramen ovale to further mobilize the mandibular nerve in order to expose the tip of the petrous bone. It is important to remove this tip in order to optimize exposure of petroclival meningiomas or lesions within the posterior cavernous sinus.

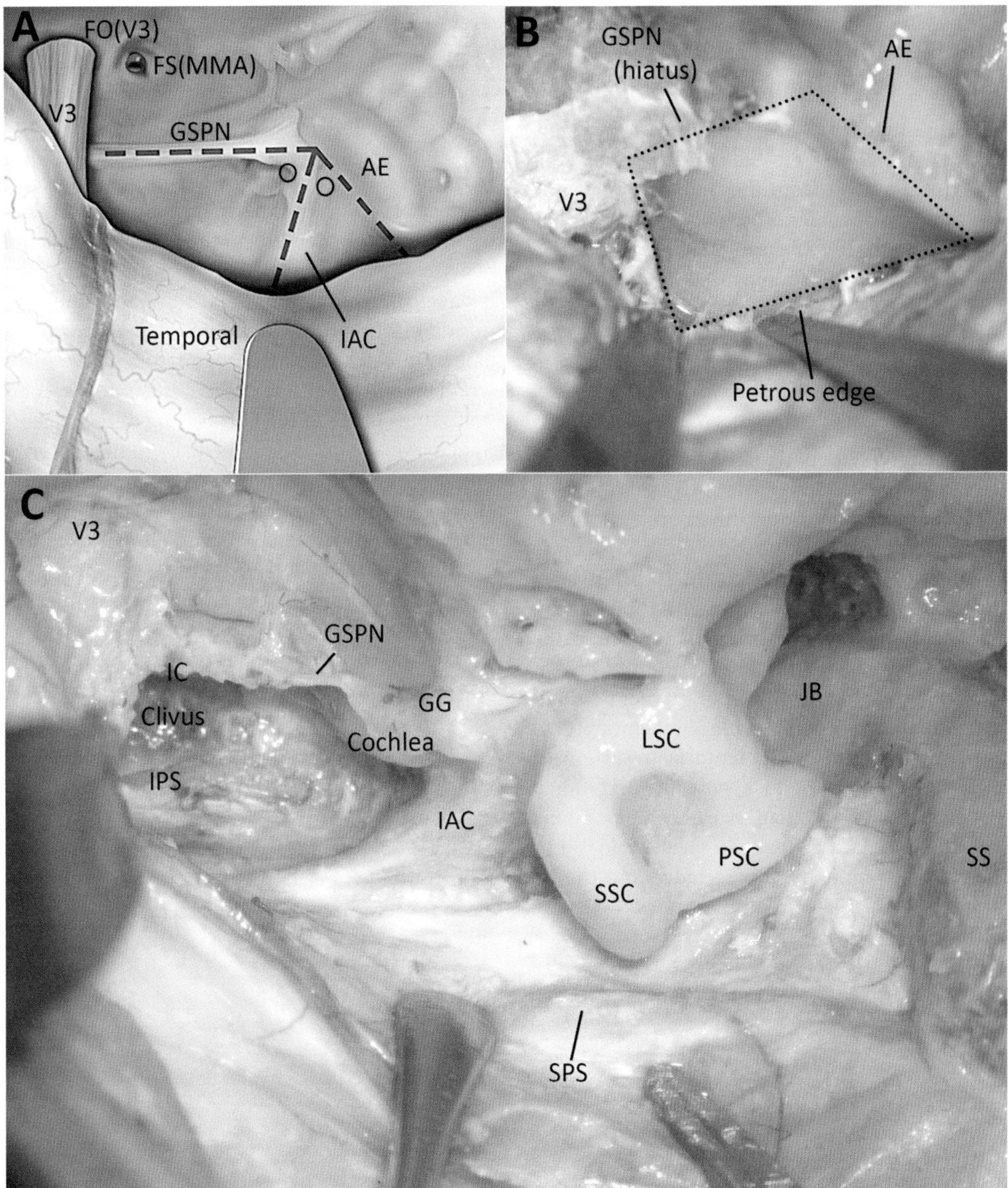

Figure 16.8 Dissection of the middle fossa rhomboid area

(A) Initial subtemporal dura elevation and identification of foramen spinosum (FS) and foramen ovale (FO). A pair of 2mm tip rigid extradural spatulas facilitate subtemporal dissection.
(B) The rhomboid construct (dashed line) consists of the greater superficial petrosal nerve (GSPN), the third branch of the trigeminal nerve (V3), arcuate eminence (AE), and petrous edge.
(C) Whole view after dissection of middle fossa rhomboid area
GG: geniculate ganglion, IC: internal carotid artery, IPS: inferior petrosal sinus, JB: jugular bulb, PSC: posterior semicircular canal, SPS: superior petrosal sinus, SS: sigmoid sinus, SSC: superior semicircular canal

Step 7: Presigmoid Dural Incision, Subtemporal Dural Incision, and Tentorium Resection

The conventional L-shaped dural incision (Figure 16.9A) crosses over the superior petrosal sinus (SPS) 10 mm away from the sinodural angle and then gently curves anteriorly along the subtemporal dura close to the SPS (Figure 16.9B).

The incision should approach the SPS at least 10 mm anterior to the junction of the superior petrosal sinus and the sigmoid transverse sinus genu in order to preserve drainage to the vein of Labbé. The opening is made in such a way that dural flaps can be reapproximated at the end of the procedure. A second incision is made through the subtemporal dura. Posteriorly, this incision meets the presigmoid dural incision. Anteriorly, the incision is continued parallel to the SPS up to the superior end of the trigeminal fibrous ring. This incision is made as far medially as possible in order to provide a dural flap that protects the temporal lobe during the long intradural dissection (Figure 16.9A, B). For larger petroclival meningiomas with wide attachment to the petroclival dura or for tentorial resection, it is crucially important to expose the trigeminal root in order to devascularize the meningioma and to create a wider surgical field (12). The petrosal vein is usually occluded and can be cut in cases of large petroclival tumors.

The presigmoid dura is opened from the jugular bulb to the SPS. A 2-mm tapered brain spatula is placed on the dorsal lateral surface of the cerebellum, exposing the undersurface of the tentorium. The tentorium is cut medial to the SPS ligation. Using a second 2-mm spatula, the temporal lobe is supported away from the superior surface of the tentorium. An incision is then made in the tentorium, ending in the posterior incisura. This maneuver is especially helpful in cases of petroclival meningiomas that traverse the tentorium and obscure the anatomy of the brainstem, superior cerebellar artery, and fifth and fourth cranial nerves. For a tentorial resection, a second incision is made in the fibrous ring of the trigeminal nerve and extending medially to the entrance of the fourth cranial nerve into the tentorium. When possible, the tentorium cerebelli is obliquely cut approximately 10 mm along the course of the trochlear nerve, opening the trochlear canal. This allows for the anterior tentorium cut to be made even more anteriorly while the integrity of the trochlear nerve is preserved. This cut is especially important when operating on large petroclival meningiomas in that the incision disrupts the blood supply to the meningioma coming from the cavernous carotid artery (Figure 16.10A–E).

Step 8: Intradural Dissection

The combined petrosal approach allows the surgeon to view the anterior brainstem, the associated

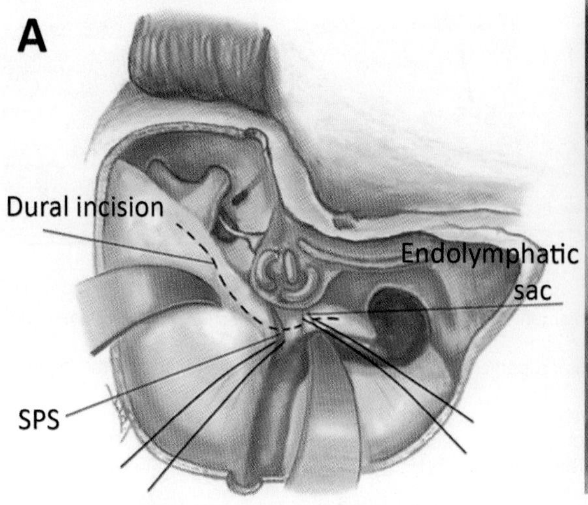

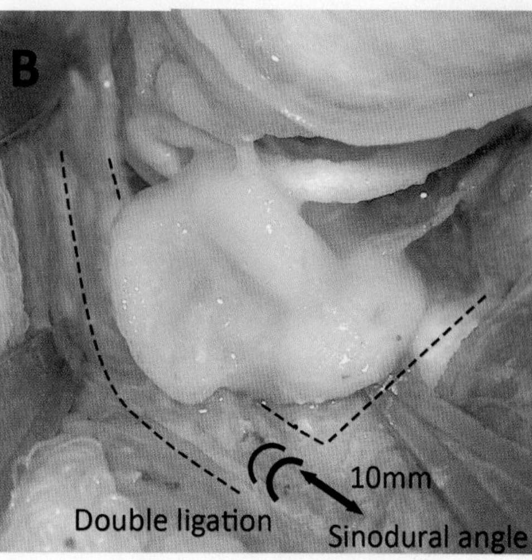

Figure 16.9 Subtemporal and presigmoid curve linear dural incision

(A) L-shaped curvilinear dural incision
(B) L-shaped dural incision along SPS parallel incision
SPS double ligation (black semicircle) 10 mm away from the sinodural angle.

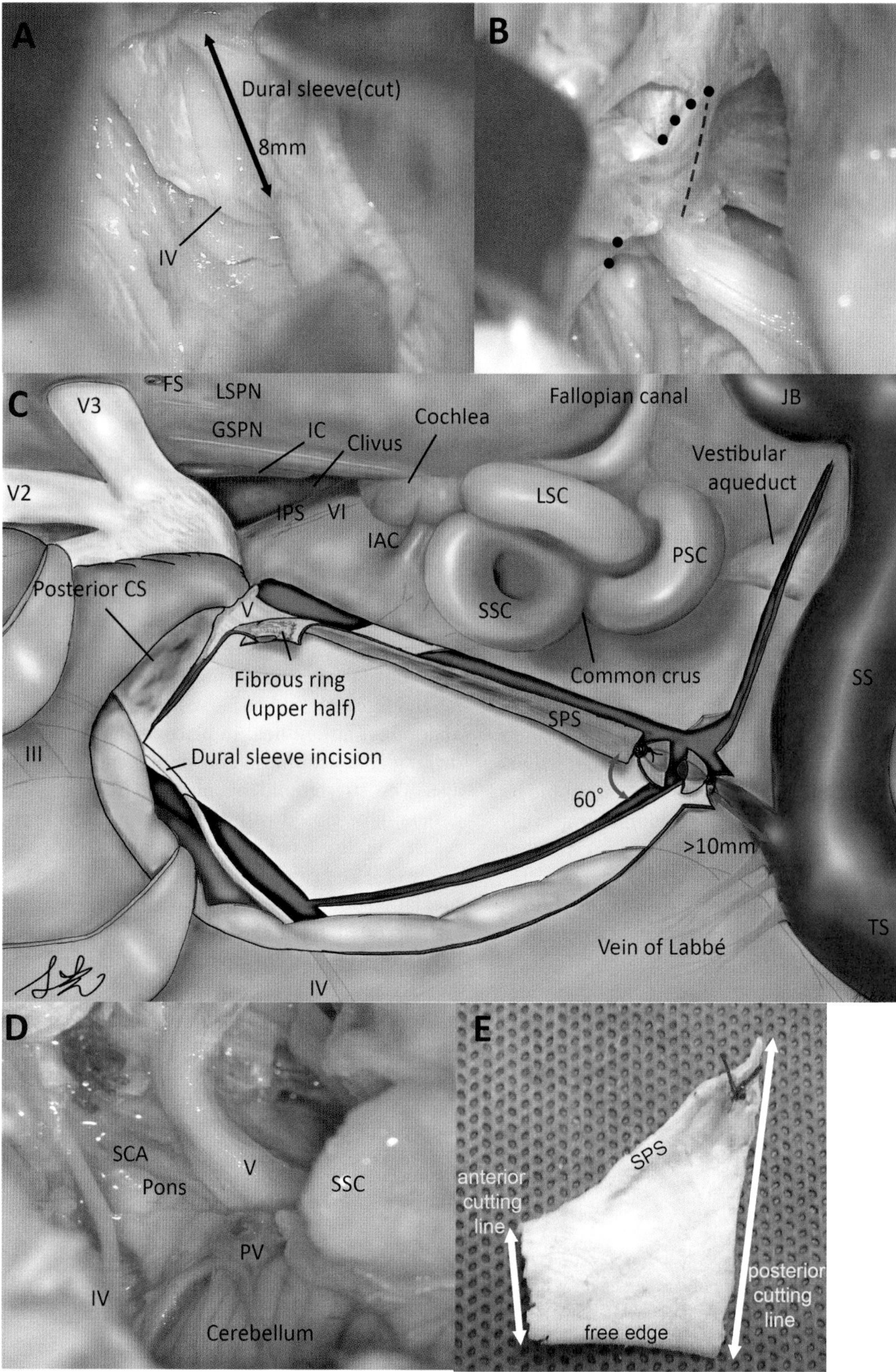

Figure 16.10 Tentorial resection (Rt)

(A) Dural sleeve cutting along the fourth nerve (continued overleaf)

neurovascular structures under the temporal lobe, and the structures inferior to the seventh and eighth nerves from in front of the cerebellum. In most cases, a lumbar drain will have been placed during the preparation for surgery. As the dissections often require several hours of surgery, the release of CSF reduces the incidence of inferior temporal or anterior cerebellar contusion.

Incising the arachnoid of the lateral ambient cistern exposes the trochlear nerve and superior cerebellar artery as they pass around the lateral pons. The tentorium is removed from the roof of Meckel's cave to expose the trigeminal nerve and Gasserian ganglion. Bleeding from the superior petrosal sinus and veins within the roof of Meckel's cave is controlled with absorbable hemostatic agents and sutures. Cautery is used sparingly to minimize the risk of postoperative dysesthesias in the trigeminal distribution. The trigeminal nerve can be followed from the Gasserian ganglion up to its entrance into the pons. The abducens nerve may be buried in a petroclival meningioma. It is easiest to find the nerve as it exits from the underside of the pons, close to the branching of the anterior inferior cerebellar artery from the basilar artery. The abducens nerve enters Dorello's canal through the inferior petrosal sinus. For this reason, coagulation around the inferior petrosal sinus should be performed with caution. The oculomotor nerve is seen passing between the superior cerebellar artery and the P1 segment of the posterior cerebral artery. The internal carotid, anterior choroidal, and posterior communicating arteries and perforators can easily be seen with minimal retraction of the temporal pole. In the lateral pontomesencephalic and perimesencephalic cisterns, the upper portion of the basilar artery, the superior cerebellar artery, and the posterior cerebral arteries can be identified. The oculomotor nerve is followed to its entrance into the dura. The oculomotor tunnel can be opened for a length of 6–7 mm, increasing the mobility of the third cranial nerve. Cutting open the tunnel for more than 7 mm runs the risk of injuring the trochlear nerve as it passes over the oculomotor nerve.

By supporting the petrous surface of the cerebellum posteriorly, the arachnoid of the lateral pontine and medullary cisterns can be seen. Opening the cisterns allows the surgeon to identify the lower cranial nerves entering the jugular foramen as well as the seventh and eighth cranial nerves. The vertebral artery is seen passing in front of the lower cranial nerves, and the mid basilar trunk is seen anterior to the pons. The origin of the posterior inferior cerebellar and anterior inferior cerebellar arteries can be identified. The origin of the anterior inferior cerebellar artery from the basilar artery is usually seen in the vicinity of the emergence of the abducens nerve from the pontomedullary junction. (Figure 16.11A, B)

Step 9: Reconstruction and Closure

Completely watertight closure of the dura is not possible following resection of the tentorium and opening of the trigeminal fibrous ring. Abdominal fat and fascia should be harvested. Small pieces of abdominal fat are held in place in the rhomboid drilling area with fibrin glue to prevent CSF leakage. The presigmoid opening in the dura can generally be closed with the aid of a fascia graft. A fascia graft is fixed by a microplate-bridge technique (13) and can be sutured meticulously to the medial edge of the infratemporal dura. Strips of fat harvested from the abdomen close the gap between the inferior temporal dura and the resected tentorium. The mastoid antrum is closed with fascia in order to prevent spinal fluid from leaking through the eustachian tube. The large, vascularized GFP flap is placed to provide vascularized tissue as a barrier, and abdominal fat is used to fill the remaining dead space to prevent CSF leakage. This graft is fixed to the bony skull

Caption for Figure 16.10 (cont.)

(B) Resection of the upper half of the trigeminal fibrous ring and anterior tentorial portion of the cavernous sinus. Dashed line and dotted line indicate the lateral border of fibrous ring and tentorium incision line, respectively.

(C) Illustration of tentorium incision. Binary 2 color circles indicate stumps.

(D) Intradural exposure after tentorial resection

(E) Rhomboid shape excised tentorium provides wider operative space.

III: oculomotor nerve; IV: trochlear nerve; V: trigeminal nerve (V2: Second branch of trigeminal nerve/maxillary nerve); VI: abducens nerve; VII: facial nerve; VIII: auditory nerve; IX: glossopharyngeal nerve; X: vagus nerve; XI: accessory nerve; LSPN: lessor superficial petrosal nerve; AICA: anterior inferior cerebellar artery ; SCA: superior cerebellar artery; Posterior CS: posterior cavernous sinus; PV: petrosal vein; End

base with titanium microplates and sewn to the temporal dura (Figure 16.12). The craniotomy plate is fixed in place using titanium mesh and calcium phosphate or calcium carbonate bone cement to serve as a cranioplasty over the area where the mastoid was drilled. The temporal muscle is sutured into place through holes made above the temporal line. The wound is then closed in layers. CSF is allowed to drain through a lumbar drain for generally the next three days to allow for healing.

Clinical Cases

From 1980 to 2017 (over the course of 37 years), the authors performed the combined petrosal approach in 259 cases (Table 16.1).

Two hundred and fifteen patients with petroclival meningiomas constituted the largest proportion. There were 13 large or extensive giant chordoma cases included. These large or giant lesions often

Table 16.1

Combined Petrosal Approach	
PC meningiomas	215
Chordomas	13
Giant neurinomas	8
Giant epidermoids	7
Giant cell tumors	2
Malignant tumors	7
Dural AVMs	7
	259 case

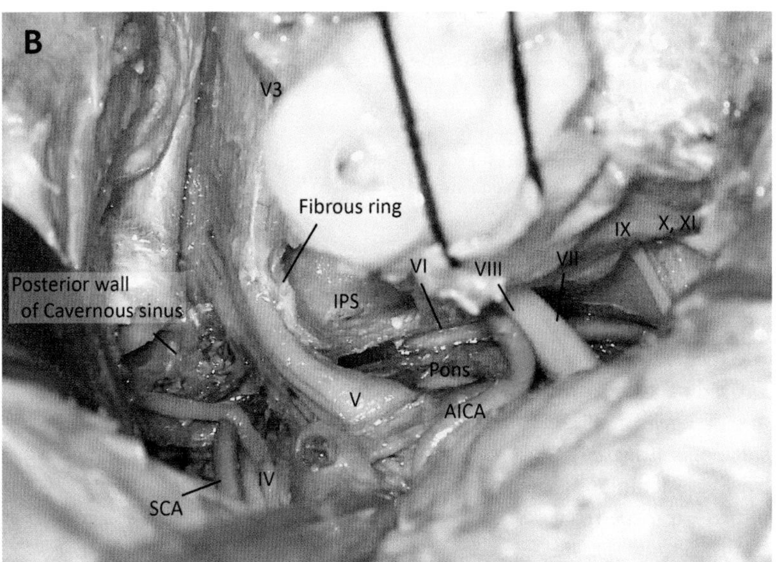

Figure 16.11 Intradural exposure

(A) Illustration of entire intradural exposure
(B) Rt combined petrosal intradural microanatomy with head specimen
SCA: superior cerebellar artery

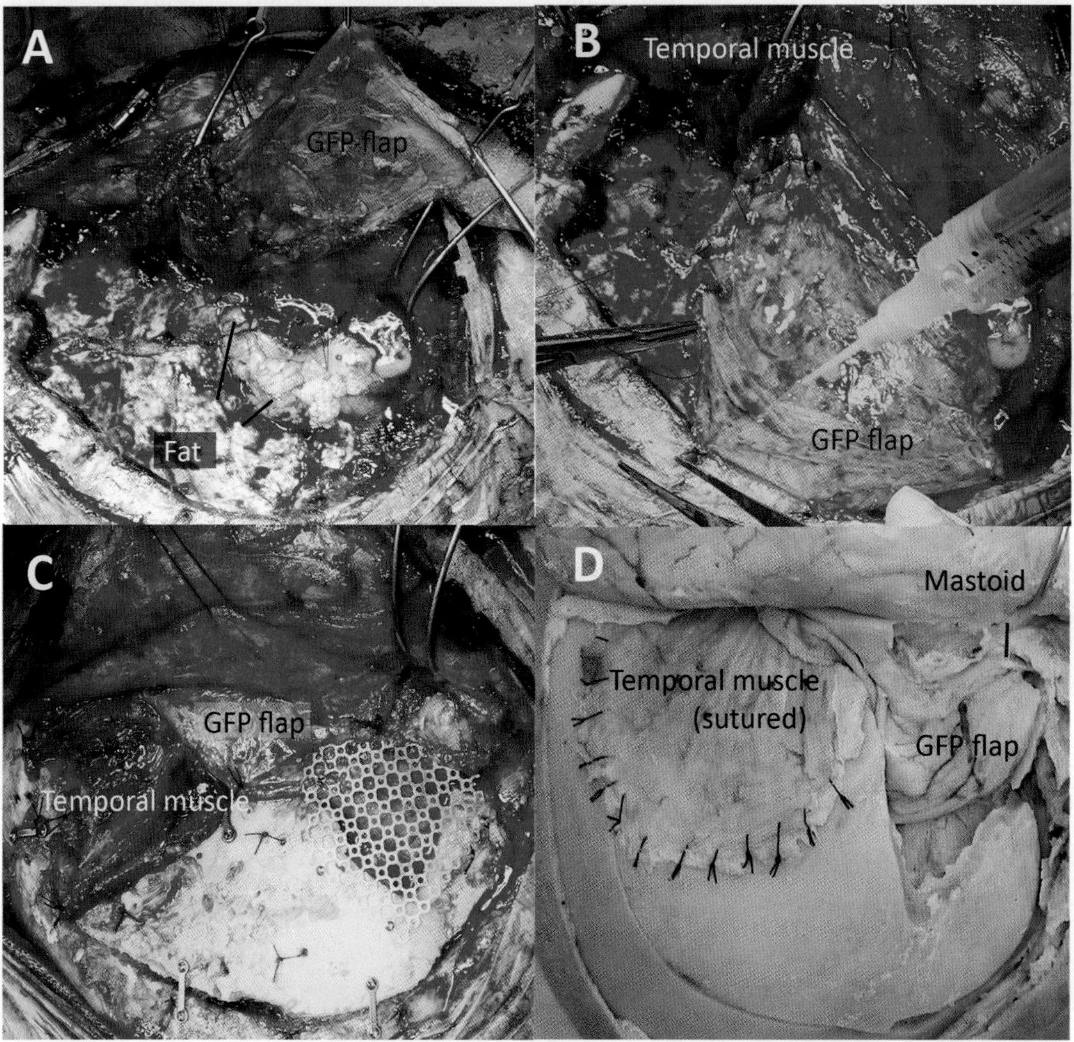

Figure 16.12 Reconstruction and closure

(A) Abdominal fat grafting into the petrous apex and the mastoid cavity
(B) Vascularized GFP flap covers and fixes tightly abdominal fat grafts with sutures and fibrin glue.
(C) Large cranioplasty of L-shaped bone flap and titanium mesh to reconstruct the mastoid bone defect.
(D) Temporal muscle is sutured securely using 2-0 non-absorbable stitches to the bone hole along the linear temporalis.

involve the supratentorial and infratentorial spaces. Because of the magnitude of the combined skull base exposure and the prolonged operative time, we restricted this single-stage procedure to healthy patients younger than 65 years of age. In older patients, we performed a two-stage operation.

Case 1 involves a right petroclival meningioma (Figure 16.13A). The combined transpetrosal approach was used to expose the tumor. The tumor was adhered to cranial nerves IV, V, VII, and VIII, but was detached using microdissection techniques at high magnification (Figure 16.13C, D). Postoperative imaging demonstrated a complete resection of the meningioma (Figure 16.13B). Other representative cases are shown in Figure 16.14. The combined transpetrosal approach is particularly useful for huge petroclival lesions and, in such cases, makes for a good postoperative result.

We highly suggest the following text: *Fukushima Manual of Skull Base Dissection* (14).

Key Points

- Harvest of a vascularized GFP flap is essential for closure, along with a fat graft.

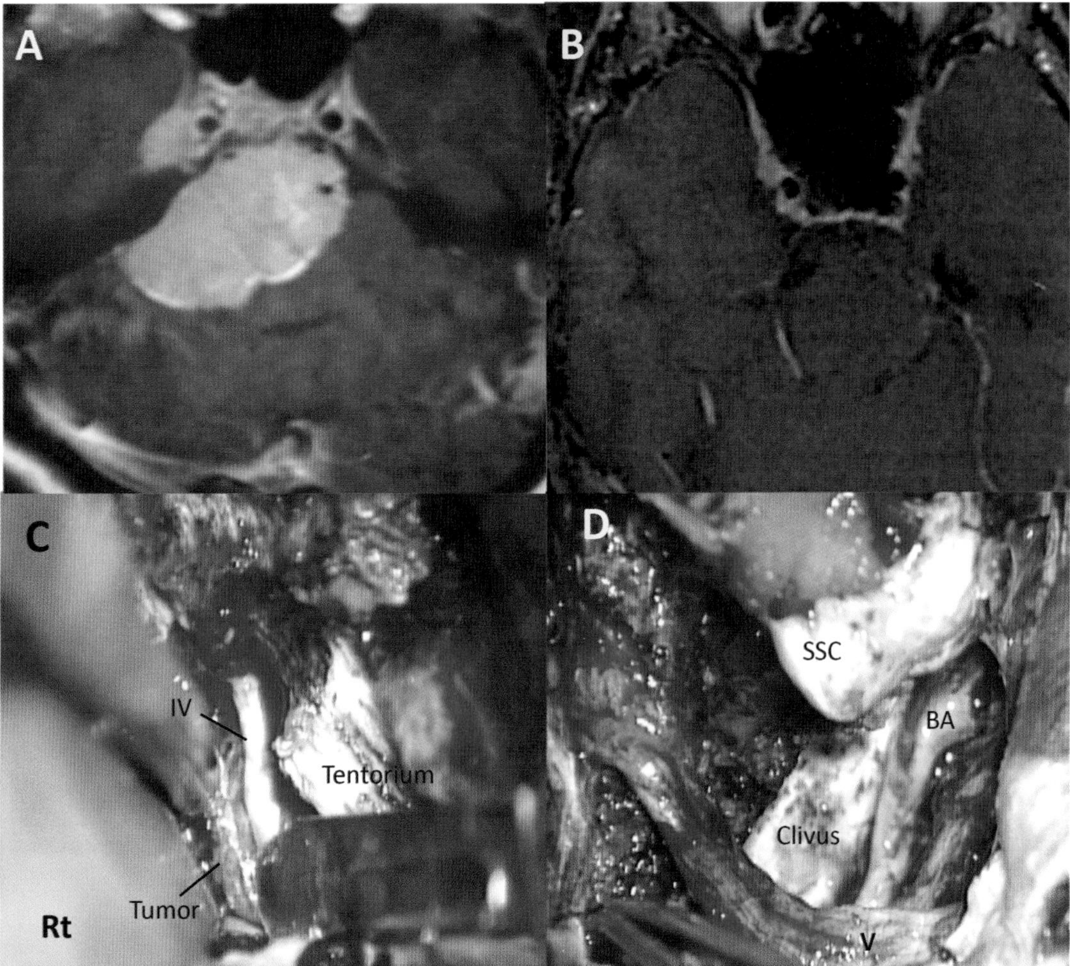

Figure 16.13 Clinical case 1

(A) Right petroclival meningioma (preoperative contrast-enhanced MRI)
(B) Postoperative MRI
(C) Intraoperative view. The fourth cranial nerve was engulfed in the tumor.
(D) The clivus and BA were revealed after total resection.

- It is important to maximally skeletonize the semicircular canals.
- The petrous ridge and apex must be completely resected.
- Care must be taken with the tentorial incision, including SPS ligation.

References

1. House WF. Surgical exposure of the internal auditory canal and its contents through the middle, cranial fossa. *The Laryngoscope*. 1961;**71**:1363–85.
2. Hitselberger WE, House WF. A combined approach to the cerebellopontine angle. A suboccipital-petrosal approach. *Archives of Otolaryngology*. 1966;**84**(3):267–85.
3. Morrison AW, King TT. Experiences with a translabyrinthine-transtentorial approach to the cerebellopontine angle. Technical note. *J Neurosurg*. 1973;**38**(3):382–90.
4. Hakuba A, Nishimura S, Tanaka K, Kishi H, Nakamura T. Clivus meningioma: six cases of total removal. *Neurologia Medico-Chirurgica*. 1977;**17** (1 Pt 1):63–77.
5. Hakuba A, Nishimura S. Total removal of clivus meningiomas and the operative results. *Neurologia Medico-Chirurgica*. 1981;**21** (1):59–73.
6. Hakuba A, Nishimura S, Jang BJ. A combined retroauricular and preauricular transpetrosal-transtentorial approach to clivus

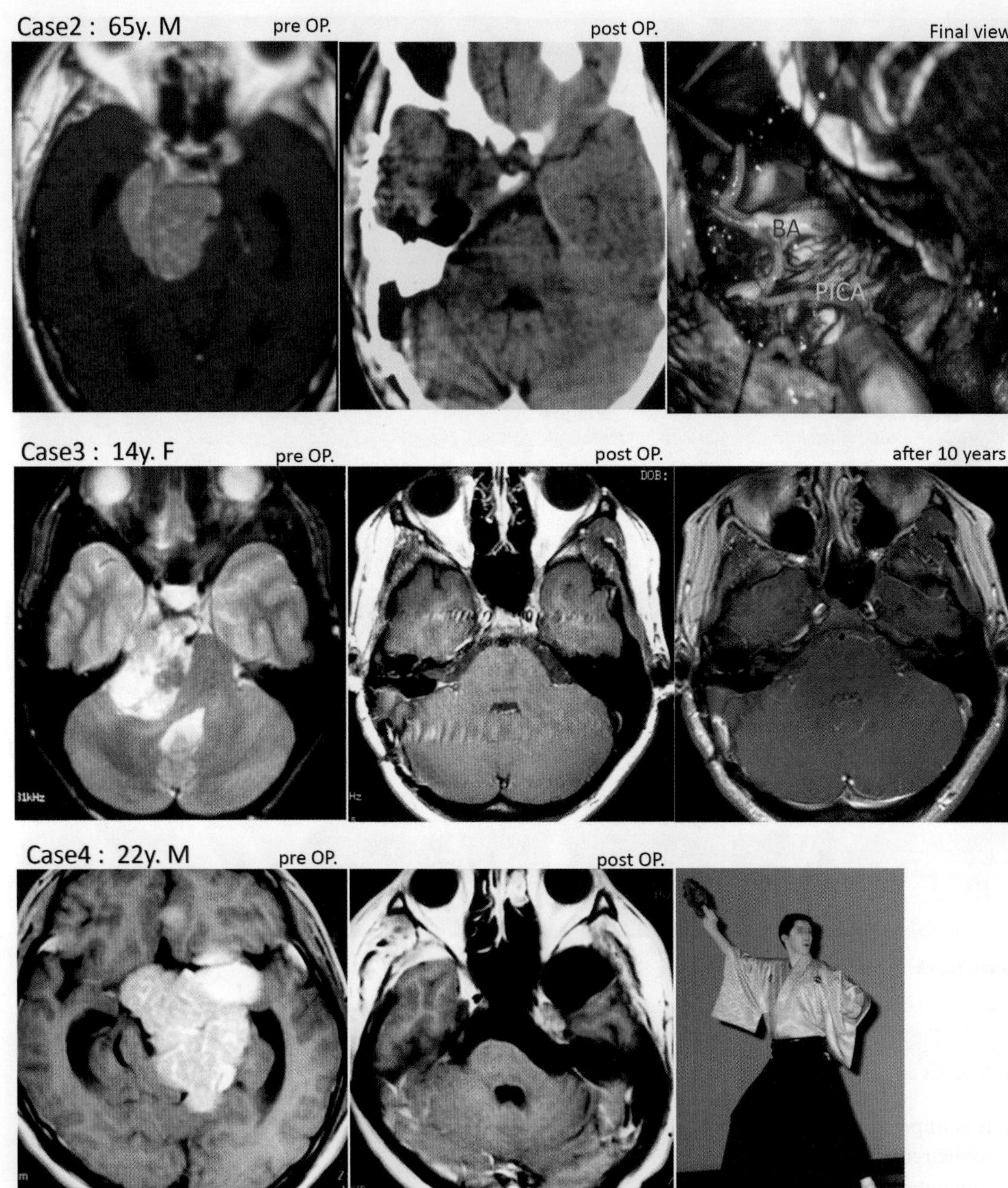

Figure 16.14 Clinical cases 2–4

Case 2: 65-year-old male, right dumbbell-shaped petroclival meningioma
Preop, postop images, and intraoperative final view after total resection
Case 3: 14-year-old female with a right petroclival meningioma with complete resection
Preop, postop MRI images, and MRI after 10 years
Case 4: 22-year-old male with a left petroclival giant size meningioma, who presented with severe ataxia
Preop, postop MRI images, and the photo after discharge. At follow-up, the patient was neurologically intact.

meningiomas. *Surgical Neurology*. 1988;**30**(2):108–16.

7. Grossi PM, Nonaka Y, Watanabe K, Fukushima T. The history of the combined supra- and infratentorial approach to the petroclival region. *Neurosurgical Focus*. 2012;**33**(2):E8.

8. Day JD, Fukushima T, Giannotta SL. Microanatomical study of the extradural middle

fossa approach to the petroclival and posterior cavernous sinus region: description of the rhomboid construct. *Neurosurgery*. 1994;**34**(6):1009–16; discussion 16.

9. Fukushima T. Combined supra- and infra-parapetrosal approach for petroclival lesions. *Surgery of Cranial Base Tumors*. 1993;**39**:661–9.
10. Couldwell WT, Fukushima T, Giannotta SL, Weiss MH. Petroclival meningiomas: surgical experience in 109 cases. *J Neurosurg*. 1996;**84**(1):20–8.
11. Little KM, Friedman AH, Sampson JH, Wanibuchi M, Fukushima T. Surgical management of petroclival meningiomas: defining resection goals based on risk of neurological morbidity and tumor recurrence rates in 137 patients. *Neurosurgery*. 2005;**56**(3):546–59; discussion 559.
12. Kusumi M, Fukushima T, Mehta AI, Aliabadi H, Nonaka Y, Friedman AH, et al. Tentorial detachment technique in the combined petrosal approach for petroclival meningiomas. *J Neurosurg*. 2012;**116**(3):566–73.
13. Kusumi M, Fukushima T, Aliabadi H, Mehta AI, Noro S, Rosen CL, et al. Microplate-bridge technique for watertight dural closures in the combined petrosal approach. *Neurosurgery*. 2012;**70**(2 Suppl Operative):264–9.
14. Fukushima TN. *Fukushima Manual of Skull Base Dissection* 3rd ed. AF-Neuro Video.

Chapter 17

Combined Keyhole Paramedian Supracerebellar-Transtentorial Approach

Steven Carr, Amit Goyal, and Charlie Teo

Introduction

Deep intracranial skull base regions are notoriously difficult to access without approach- or retraction-related morbidity. In the modern neurosurgical era, skull base neurosurgery has seen an emphasis on avoiding manipulation or harm to normal brain structures by taking advantage of cisternal corridors and more safely traversing structures without neurological function; for example, strategic bony drilling or dural openings. Lesions within the posterior mediobasal temporal lobe can be reached with several different approaches, each with a unique set of associated trade-offs. The first reported use of the supracerebellar-transtentorial (SCTT) approach to this region is generally credited to Drs. Voigt and Yasargil in 1976, who employed a tentorial opening during a supracerebellar infratentorial approach to successfully resect a cavernous malformation within the medial parahippocampal gyrus (16). This was essentially a modification of the well-used supracerebellar infratentorial approach and incorporated a supracerebellar opening of the tentorium in order to access the supratentorial compartment from a posterior fossa exposure. This exposure is a good example of how strategically combining intracranial compartments using keyhole techniques can provide access that would otherwise require an approach involving potentially unnecessary brain transgression or significant brain retraction.

Indications

The first consideration facing the surgeon is the anatomical location of the lesion of interest. This approach has been used successfully in accessing the mediobasal temporal lobe and has the benefit of avoiding the optic radiations and inferior fronto-occipital fasciculus (IFOF). The mediobasal temporal lobe is divided into three segments: anterior, middle, and posterior (2,14). Most authors agree that the posterior aspect of the mediobasal temporal lobe is the most reliably accessible. However, some argue that this approach can be used to access lesions in the middle and even anterior aspects of the mediobasal temporal lobe (14). Access to the pulvinar can also be accomplished using this approach (Akiyama et al. 2017), as well as to the atrium of the lateral ventricle (7,8). Lastly and perhaps most intuitively, the SCTT approach can be used to remove lesions arising from the tentorium itself (1,11,12).

The second consideration for the surgeon is the type of lesion being addressed. Several types of lesions, both intra- and extra-axial, have been surgically addressed using the SCTT approach. Intra-axial lesions such as primary brain tumors (13), cavernous malformations (3,10), and arteriovenous malformations (AVMs; 4,6) have been removed successfully. When addressing intra-axial lesions through this approach, frameless neuronavigation becomes very important for locating lesions and planning safe brain transgression sites. Several authors have advocated for utilizing the collateral sulcus when possible (7,8). One group reported even addressing epilepsy due to hippocampal sclerosis using this approach (6,14).

Extra-axial lesions such as tentorial meningiomas (1,11,12), epidermoids (5), and aneurysms (4) can be reached and addressed, as well. Tentorial meningiomas with superior projection can be particularly well resected because this approach gives the surgeon a dry view of the base of the tumor (i.e., the tentorium from below) allowing for an early view of the dural attachment and the opportunity for early devascularization via electrocautery.

Contraindications

While the SCTT approach has its strengths, it also has its limitations. This approach employs a long, narrow corridor and relies on appropriate regional anatomy to access lesions. Firstly, patients with obese habitus or inability to rotate their head due to cervical or other range of motion-limiting pathology can be difficult to position in the three-quarters prone position, and the associated risks from selecting the sitting position are not inconsequential; thus, patient selection with regard to positioning options is important. Second, in addressing vascular lesions such as cerebral aneurysms, the ability to obtain early proximal control (or find feeder arteries early, in the case of AVMs) can be limited. Third, a tentorium situated with a steep inclination may make visualization challenging (9), and we recommend surgeons use the endoscope to expand visualization in this case. Lastly, given the deep, narrow corridor and important neurovascular structures necessarily encountered with this approach, a solid knowledge base and comfort with the complex anatomy of the region is requisite. This approach is best utilized by experienced surgeons.

Other surgical approaches to this region have their own array of risks and benefits. The supratentorial transtemporal route can give access to the posterior medial temporal lobe; however, this requires traversing the supratentorial cortex, which could cause language dysfunction on the dominant hemisphere or damage to the optic radiations, causing visual field disturbances. The other common route to reach this region is the occipital interhemispheric route; however, this requires significant retraction of the exposed overlying occipital lobe, which can cause injury to the visual cortex or optic radiations, as well. While we would propose that keyhole principles decrease the likelihood of some of these problems, these undesirable risks still remain.

Surgical Technique

The patient is positioned in a lateral decubitus position in three-pin fixation, with the head turned toward the floor in gentle flexion to elevate the suboccipital region. Care should be taken to ensure that the ipsilateral shoulder is out of the surgeon's working space. Neuronavigation should be registered and can be used to assist in the planning of the incision from just over the expected location of the transverse sinus to just above the base of the occiput, two fingerbreadths lateral to the midline (see Figure 17.1A–B). Recall that the transverse sinus is generally along an imaginary line between the inion and the zygomatic arch, or immediately beneath the superior nuchal line at the site of muscle attachment to the occipital bone.

A single burr hole should be made at the superior extent of the exposure just on the edge of the transverse sinus, and a small suboccipital keyhole craniotomy is made with the side-cutting osteotome. If the blue transverse sinus is not appreciated, use a fluted burr to gradually work superiorly to expose the edge of the sinus. We use a V-shaped dural opening hinged superiorly at the edge of the transverse sinus (see Figure 17.1E) and reflect the leaflet superiorly. Using a small craniotomy and dural opening helps prevent outward herniation of the cerebellum.

A cottonoid is placed over the superior surface of the cerebellum, and a careful supracerebellar approach is made using bipolar coagulation, subsequent division of bridging veins, and drainage of CSF from the opening of the supracerebellar and quadrigeminal cisterns (see Figure 17.1C). Exercising patience at this stage is paramount; we find that slow removal of cisternal CSF gives excellent cerebellar brain relaxation, which allows for adequate exposure. Rarely is a lumbar drain necessary.

The navigation wand is used to ensure appropriate trajectory. The tentorium is coagulated with bipolar electrocautery and opened sharply, and a window is resected (see Figure 17.1D). This gives access to the supratentorial compartment. Using navigation, dissect the lesion and remove it using standard keyhole microsurgical techniques. It can be very helpful to use 0- and 30-degree endoscopes to see adjacent structures, such as the trochlear nerve near the incisura; to improve visualization around any corners; and, under microscopy after resection, to inspect for residual tumor or bleeding. Achieve hemostasis, perform a watertight dural closure (see Figure 17.1E), reaffix the bone flap, and perform a standard closure (see Figure 17.1F).

Complication Avoidance

Complications arising from the SCTT approach are largely those associated with a posterior fossa exposure and those that can be encountered in any deep brain region. Posterior fossa exposures can be fraught with CSF leaks and headaches, and

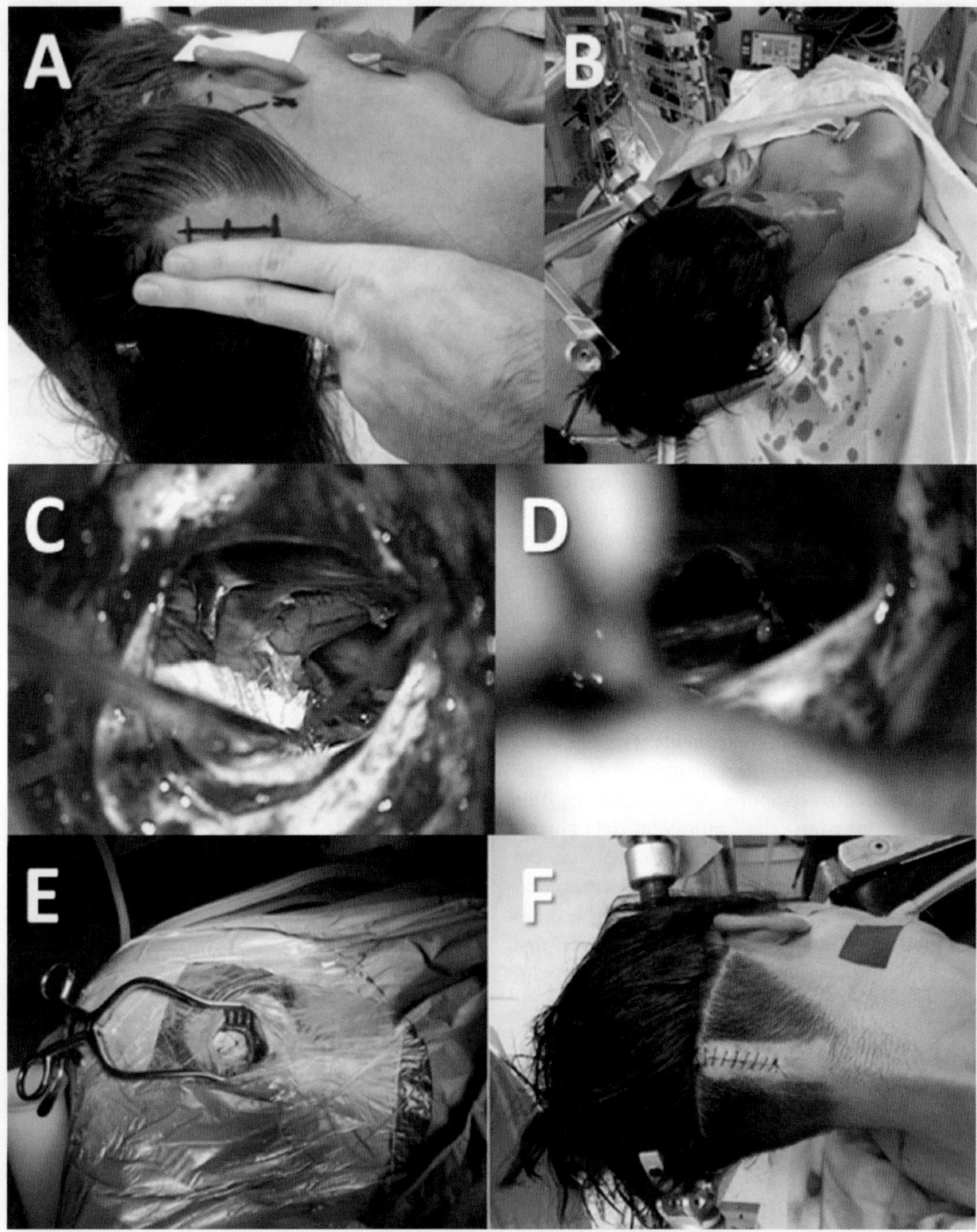

Figure 17.1 Steps of the SCTT approach

(A) Location of paramedian incision
(B) Three-quarter prone positioning
(C) View of the supracerebellar corridor
(D) View of the tentorial opening
(E) Dural closure
(F) Skin closure

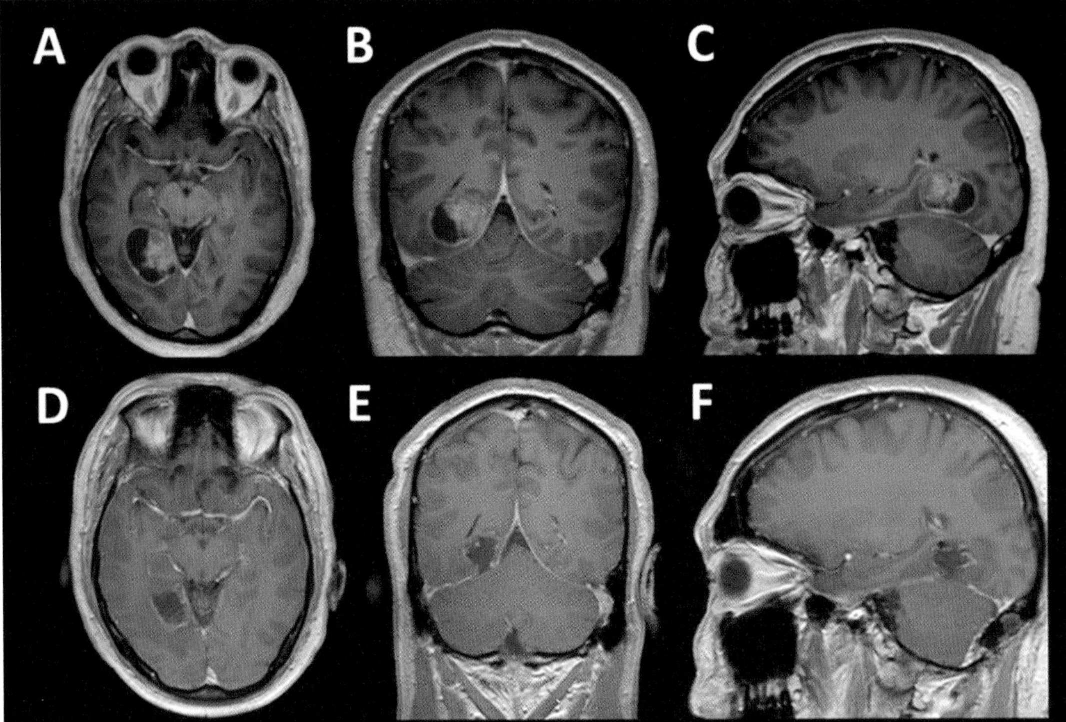

Figure 17.2 Pre- and postoperative MRI of Illustrative case

(A, B, C) Preoperative T1 post-contrast axial, coronal, sagittal
(D, E, F) Postoperative T1 post-contrast axial, coronal, sagittal

watertight dural closure (see Figure 17.1E) with cranial reconstruction (autologous cranioplasty) should be performed to avoid these problems. We use a running 4–0 Nurolon suture for dural closure and a running 3–0 nylon suture for skin closure (see Figure 17.1F). Given the surgical location, vessel injury (causing venous or arterial bleeding and/or strokes from the deep cerebral veins or posterior cerebral artery) is a concern. The surgeon should be aware of what vessels are likely to be situated on the other side of the tentorium being opened from below and study preoperative imaging carefully to understand an individual patient's vascular anatomy (see Figure 17.1D). Some surgeons prefer to perform this approach with the patient in the sitting or semi-sitting position; however, we feel this puts an unnecessary fatigue burden on the surgeon and puts the patient at risk of venous embolism.

The surgical corridor from a keyhole paramedian suboccipital craniotomy can feel intimidatingly narrow at first. However, familiarity with endoscopic assistance can expand the field of view significantly and can help the surgeon look around corners to avoid injuries (15). The bone edge of the craniotomy can be beveled to allow a greater angle to the microscopic view and can always be enlarged, if necessary. Further, it is important to note that patient drainage of CSF in the supracerebellar space is necessary for relaxation of the cerebellum. Lastly, the tentorium can be resected more generously to allow for a greater view of the supratentorial space. (Figure 17.2)

Key Points

- The SCTT approach can be used to access the posterior mediobasal regions with low risk to the optic radiations and eloquent cortex.
- A keyhole paramedian suboccipital craniotomy with a tentorial opening is sufficient to address lesions, and endoscopic assistance is recommended.
- A solid knowledge of and comfort with the supracerebellar-infratentorial approach and the relevant anatomy is requisite to utilize the SCTT approach.

References

1. Ansari SF, Young RL, Bohnstedt BN, Cohen-Gadol AA. The extended supracerebellar transtentorial approach for resection of medial tentorial meningiomas. *Surg Neurol Int* 2014;**5**:35.
2. Campero A, Troccoli G, Martins C et al. Microsurgical approaches to the medial temporal region: an anatomical study. *Neurosurgery* 2006;**59**: ons279–308.
3. Choudhri O, Davies J, Lawton MT. The supracerebellar-transtentorial approach to vascular lesions in the inferomedial temporal lobe: 3-dimensional operative video. *Oper Neurosurg* 2017;**13**(4):536.
4. de Oliveira JG, Parraga RG, Chaddad-Neto F, Ribas GC, de Oliveira EPL. Supracerebellar transtentorial approach – resection of the tentorium instead of an opening – to provide broad exposure of the mediobasal temporal lobe: anatomical aspects and surgical applications. *J Neurosurg* 2012;**116**:764–72.
5. Goel A, Shah A. Lateral supracerebellar transtentorial approach to a middle fossa epidermoid tumor. *J Clin Neurosci* 2010;**17** (3):372–3.
6. Harput MV, Ture U. The paramedian supracerebellar-transtentorial approach to remove a posterior fusiform gyrus arteriovenous malformation. *Neurosurg Focus* 2017;**43** (Suppl 1):V7
7. Izci Y, Seckin H, Ates O, Baskaya MK. Supracerebellar transtentorial transcollateral sulcus approach to the atrium of the lateral ventricle: microsurgical anatomy and surgical technique in cadaveric dissections. *Surg Neurol* 2009;**72** (5):509–14.
8. Jeelani Y, Gokoglu A, Anor T, Al-Mefty O, Cohen AR. Transtentorial transcollateral sulcus approach to the ventricular atrium: an endoscope-assisted anatomical study. *J Neurosurg* 2017;**126**:1246–52.
9. Jittapiromsak P, Deshmukh P, Nakaji P, Spetzler RF, Preul MC. Comparative analysis of posterior approaches to the medial temporal region: supracerebellar transtentorial versus occipital transtentorial. *Neurosurgery* 2009;**64**(3 Suppl):ons35–42.
10. Kalani MYS, Lei T, Martirosyan NL, Oppenlander ME, Spetzler RF, Nakaji P. Endoscope-assisted supracerebellar transtentorial approach to the posterior medial temporal lobe for resection of cavernous malformation. *Neurosurg Focus* 2016;**40**(Suppl 1):v18.
11. Manilha R, Harput VM, Ture U. The paramedian supracerebellar-transtentorial approach for a tentorial incisura meningioma: 3-dimensional operative video. *Oper Neurosurg* 2018;**15**(1):102.
12. Robert T, Weil AG, Obaid S, Al-Jehani H, Bojanowski MW. Supracerebellar transtentorial removal of a large tentorial tumor. *Neurosurg Focus* 2016;**40**(Suppl 1):V12.
13. Swanson KI, Cikla U, Uluc K, Baskaya MK. Supracerebellar transtentorial approach to the tentorial incisura and beyond. *Neurosurg Focus* 2016;**40**(Suppl 1):V11.
14. Ture U, Harput MV, Kaya AH et al. The paramedian supracerebellar-transtentorial approach to the entire length of the mediobasal temporal region: an anatomical and clinical study. *J Neurosurg* 2012;**116**:773–91.
15. Villanueva P, Louis RG, Cutler AR et al. Endoscopic and gravity-assisted resection of medial temporo-occipital lesions through a supracerebellar transtentorial approach: technical notes with case illustrations. *Oper Neurosurg* 2015;**11**(4):475–483.
16. Voigt K, Yasargil MG. Cerebral cavernous haemangiomas or cavernomas. Incidence, pathology, localization, diagnosis, clinical features and treatment. Review of the literature and report of an unusual case. *Neurochirurgia* 1976;**19** (2):59–68.

Chapter 18

Combined Multi-portal "Pull-Through" Keyhole Craniotomy

Robert G. Briggs, Andrew K. Conner, Ali H. Palejwala, Panayiotis Pelargos, Griffin Ernst, Kyle P. O'Connor, Chad A. Glenn, and Michael E. Sughrue

Introduction

The "pull-through" technique is an extensive, dual-keyhole craniotomy approach that was developed in part to achieve maximal resection of large gliomas extending between the temporal and occipital poles. The surgical treatment of these lesions is made complex by the variability and complex nature of the neuroanatomic structures in this region. Eloquent cortical and subcortical structures may be infiltrated or shifted as a result of the tumor. In either hemisphere, involvement of motor, sensory, and visual pathways is common. In the dominant hemisphere, white matter pathways related to speech (e.g., the superior longitudinal fasciculus, inferior longitudinal fasciculus, and the inferior fronto-occipital fasciculus) may be disrupted (1, 2). In the non-dominant hemisphere, these same fasciculi are frequently associated with the development of neglect when they are damaged or disrupted (3–5).

The "pull-through" technique is tailored to the minimum exposure trajectories needed for accessing the tumor. Briefly, it involves creating an occipital and temporal keyhole craniotomy, performing occipital and temporal lobectomies, and then connecting the two approaches as needed for tumor removal. This technique was developed for two purposes. First, the procedure minimizes the amount of bone work necessary to remove these tumors by first performing temporal and occipital lobectomies, allowing for surgical access of the remaining tumor without requiring a large craniotomy. The ideal tumors for this approach are gliomas involving the temporal and occipital lobes. Given the infiltrating nature of these tumors (6), patients often undergo awake brain mapping during the procedure (7). For those who routinely perform this type of surgery, it is common knowledge that patients are only able to tolerate awake mapping for a finite period of time. By minimizing the time spent obtaining access to these large tumors, the surgeon is able to maximize the time spent mapping critical brain functions before the patient tires. Second, performing occipital and temporal lobectomies creates the dead space necessary for the neurosurgeon to work posteriorly from pole-to-pole between the two bone flaps, connecting the lobectomy sites and achieving maximal surgical resection of these tumors with the minimum craniotomy size. Working from front to back or back to front allows the surgeon to work nearly parallel to the regional white matter tracts mentioned previously.

Indications

As discussed previously, the use of this surgical approach is limited to patients presenting with large temporal-occipital gliomas, typically extending between the temporal and occipital poles. Figure 18.1 demonstrates two different tumors on T1- and T2-weighted MRI. The patients presenting with these were ideal candidates to undergo the "pull-through" technique.

Contraindications

Elective removal of giant occipital-temporal gliomas is contraindicated when patients present with significant medical comorbidities, including significant heart and lung disease and/or uncontrolled diabetes mellitus.

Alternative Approaches

Surgical alternatives to this approach include a large fronto-temporal-based craniotomy with

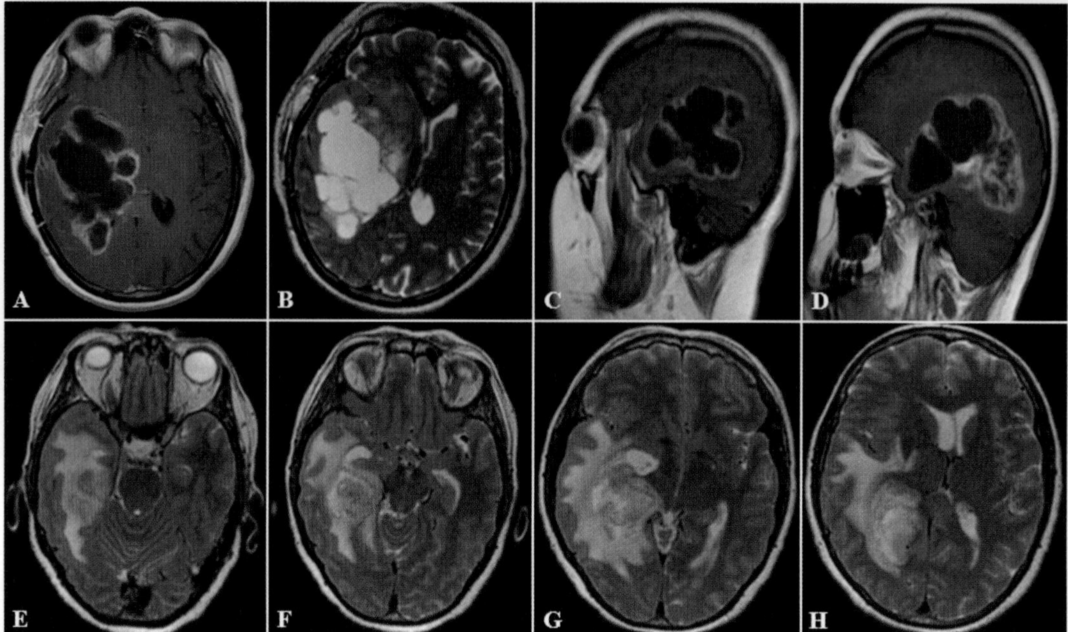

Figure 18.1 Preoperative MRI scans of two patients (A-D, E-F) who were ideal candidates to undergo pull-through surgery. (A-B) A 50-year-old woman who presented with glioblastoma shown on gadolinium-enhanced T1-weighted and T2-weighted axial magnetic resonance imaging (MRI). (C-D) Sagittal T1-weighted images from the same patient reveal the extent of the tumor from the temporal to the occipital pole. (E-H) A 60-year-old man who presented with glioblastoma. The T2-weighted axial slices are oriented from most inferior to most superior, revealing the extent of T2-hyperintensity the temporal lobe to the occipital lobe.

occipital extension. This type of approach necessitates a significant amount of brain exposure and dural defect repair. Other variations on this technique involve large two-site craniotomies that expose the occipital midline, including the posterior sagittal sinus, and larger exposure of the temporal lobe. Staging the temporal and occipital approaches is also a consideration that may benefit the surgeon, given that large resections of this type can be physically and mentally demanding.

Preoperative Planning

The following should be obtained prior to surgery:

- An updated history and neurologic exam
- Baseline metabolic and blood labs, including anticoagulation studies
- Electrocardiogram and chest x-ray to evaluate the patient's cardiopulmonary status
- Preoperative, contrast-enhanced anatomic MRI scan
- Preoperative diffusion-weighted MRI scan to perform DTI-based white matter fiber tractography

The diffusion-weighted MR imaging is critical to determine the position of the superior longitudinal fasciculus relative to the inferior longitudinal fasciculus during the procedure. This allows the neurosurgeon to preserve the connections of the superior longitudinal fasciculus in the postero-lateral temporal lobe, while excising the tumor posteriorly along the length of the inferior longitudinal fasciculus.

Surgical Technique

The "pull-through" technique can be roughly divided into five stages: 1) creation of a keyhole craniotomy centered over the temporal lobe, 2) creation of a keyhole craniotomy centered over the occipital lobe, 3) a temporal lobectomy, 4) an occipital lobectomy, and 5) excision of any remaining tumor along the path of the inferior longitudinal fasciculus to connect the lobectomy sites. Each step of this operation is described as follows.

Positioning

Patients are positioned laterally with 10 degrees of coronal head tilt to facilitate brain relaxation near

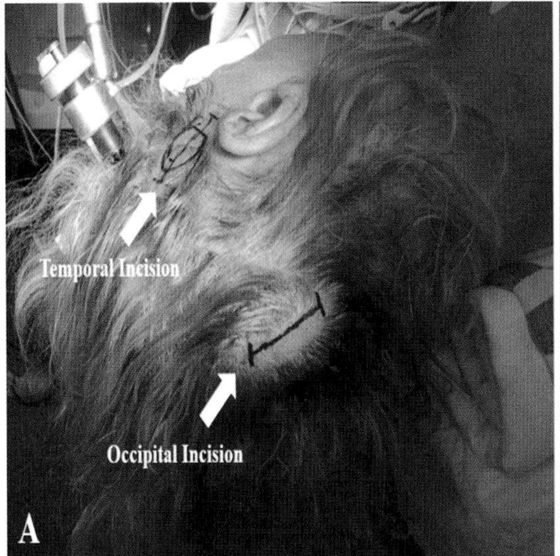

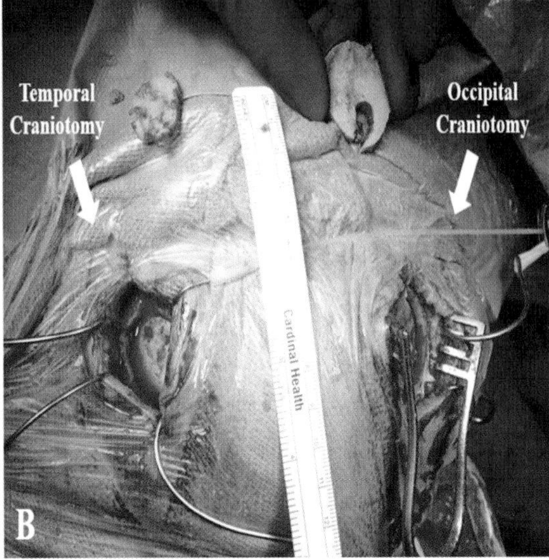

Figure 18.2 Patient positioning for the pull-through technique. (A) The patient is positioned laterally with 10 degrees of coronal head tilt to allow the brain to fall away from the skull base by gravity. Prior to the operation, the patient's hair is shaved, and the planned incisions identifying the locations of the temporal and occipital keyhole craniotomies are drawn on the skin with a marking pen. (B) Completion of the two keyhole craniotomies. Both craniotomies are cut before beginning the intracranial work. The skin is retracted using scalp hooks, and the dura is clearly visible at both craniotomy sites. The temporal craniotomy should measure approximately 3 centimeters in diameter, while the occipital craniotomy should measure 2 centimeters in diameter (see the ruler in (B)).

the skull base. Care should be taken when pinning the patient's head with the Mayfield to prevent compromising the occipital operative site due to pin position. We recommend placing the posterior Mayfield pins in the sagittal plane slightly off of midline, given that the occipital keyhole craniotomy is placed near midline. An example of how to position patients for the pull-through technique is shown in Figure 18.2A.

Temporal Keyhole

The temporal keyhole craniotomy is planned over the postero-superior aspect of the boundary between tumor and cortex with the aid of image guidance (8). We typically ensure that the superior edge of the craniotomy allows for adequate exposure of the inferior-most aspect of the operculum. The inferior edge of the craniotomy should expose the center of the middle temporal gyrus in most cases. However, the anterior and superior aspects of the temporal lobe adjacent to the Sylvian fissure are not entirely exposed; instead, they rest under the bone flap edge of the craniotomy. The angles made with the anterior aspect of the craniotomy site allow the neurosurgeon to reach the anterior part of the superior temporal gyrus and front of the Sylvian fissure without complication, while respecting the limits of the perisylvian fibers coursing within the superior longitudinal fasciculus into the posterior temporal lobe. The relationships between these structures relative to the site of the temporal craniotomy are shown in Figure 18.3.

After planning the craniotomy, a linear incision of approximately 5 centimeters is made in the coronal plane. The scalp is retracted with the aid of multiple scalp hooks attached to flexible bands, and a single, small burr hole is made at the bottom of the field with a round cutting drill bit. The craniotomy is completed with a craniotome, and should be approximately 3 centimeters in diameter. The temporal lobectomy is then performed with a surgical microscope to allow for increased light and visualization through the opening. Figure 18.2 demonstrates the planned incision (Figure 18.2A) and resulting temporal keyhole craniotomy (Figure 18.2B).

Temporal Lobectomy

The most important risk factor associated with temporal keyhole lobectomy involves the posterior disconnection that must occur between the tumor, cortex, and speech pathways in the posterior

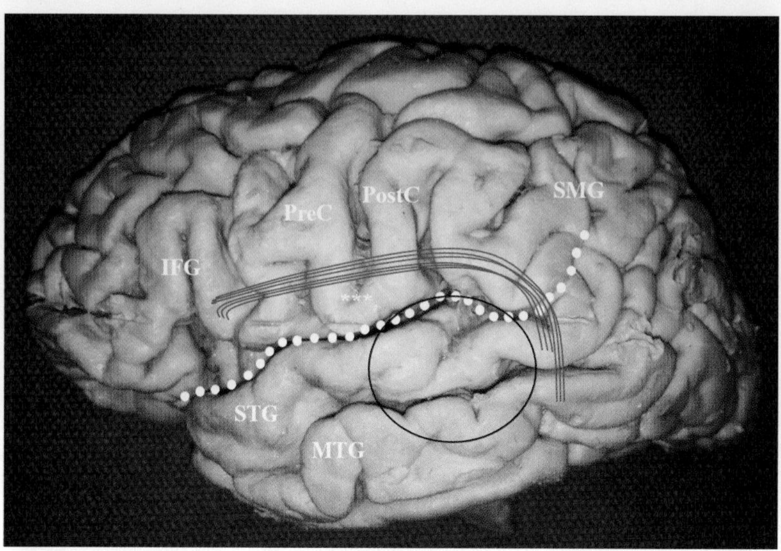

Figure 18.3 Relationship between the sulci, gyri, and superior longitudinal fasciculus (blue streamlines) relative to the temporal keyhole craniotomy (black oval). The Sylvian fissure is delineated by the line of white circles. The position of the temporal craniotomy should be anterior to the perisylvian fibers of the superior longitudinal fasciculus (blue). The craniotomy should reveal the posterior aspects of the superior temporal gyrus (STG) and middle temporal gyrus (MTG). The operculum (***) is located superior to the temporal craniotomy site. IFG = inferior frontal gyrus, PreC = pre-central gyrus, PostC = post-central gyrus, SMG = supramarginal gyrus, STG = superior temporal gyrus, MTG = middle temporal gyrus.

temporal lobe (8,9). To prevent damaging these networks, the lobectomy is performed as an L-shaped dissection, anterior to the superior longitudinal fasciculus. Awake cortical mapping followed by subcortical mapping is performed to identify the critical language areas present within the posterior temporal lobe. For cases involving the non-dominant temporal lobe, awake line-bisection and target cancelation tasks are performed to map visuospatial function (10).

The patient remains awake as subcortical dissection is performed. During this part of the operation, the patient is instructed to perform a double task; one that tests two different modalities in two different functional systems (e.g., having the patient complete a naming task while moving the contralateral arm or leg) (11). This is done continuously until the disconnection to the temporal horn is complete. Dissection is then continued below the subinsular region, while avoiding the inferior fronto-occipital fasciculus (12). The inferior fronto-occipital fasciculus can be identified with subcortical mapping using DTI integrated with image guidance; however, its location can also be confirmed with stimulation if needed.

The posterior and superior disconnections are made first, separating eloquent white matter tracts and cortex from the tumor. The dissection is continued medially into the temporal horn, as the tracts are revealed laterally. The anterior temporal vein is coagulated and transected. Once this maneuver is complete, the anterior temporal lobe contents can be reflected posteriorly and removed en bloc. The hippocampus and amygdala can then be resected using the subpial technique. However, this part of the procedure can be tailored based on the preference of the surgeon. We typically resect these structures even in the absence of tumor involvement based on studies that have reported reduced incidence of postoperative seizures with the use of this practice (13). Care must be taken, though, to avoid transgressing the pial border in this region to prevent disturbance of the choroidal arteries and surrounding structures.

The posterior disconnection is complete after 1) entering the ventricle, 2) continuing the cut to the front of the middle fossa, and 3) removing the superior temporal gyrus from anterior-to-posterior. The hippocampus is preserved as a temporary landmark to help define the location of the basal ganglia superiorly, but is usually removed following completion of the lobectomy.

Occipital Keyhole

The occipital keyhole craniotomy is planned over the antero-superior aspect of the cortical boundary between the tumor and cortex with the aid of image guidance (14). We always ensure that the superior edge of the craniotomy allows for adequate exposure of the trajectory planned toward the pineal region. In addition, the inferior edge of the craniotomy should expose the posterior-most aspect of the angular gyrus. This typically ensures

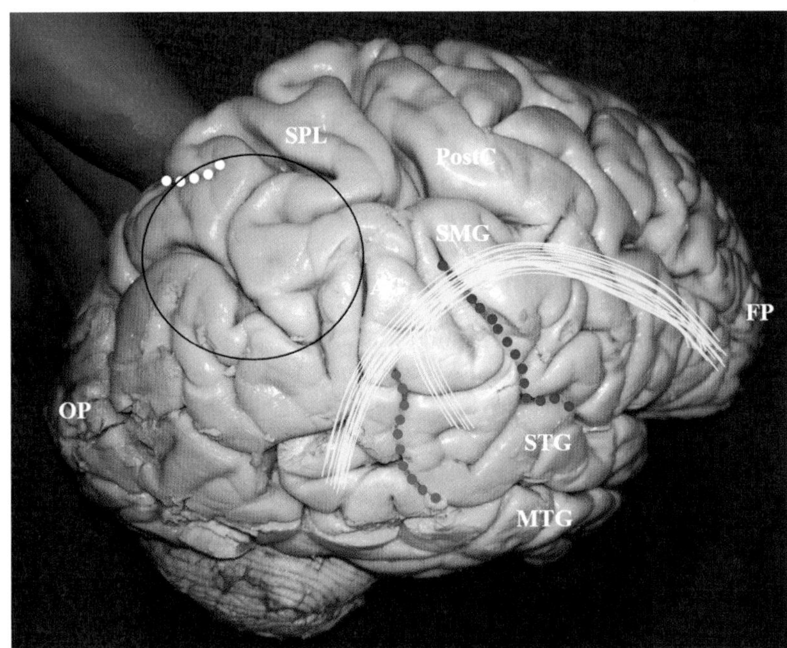

Figure 18.4 Relationship between the sulci, gyri, and superior longitudinal fasciculus (yellow streamlines) relative to the occipital keyhole craniotomy (black oval). The Sylvian fissure and superior temporal sulcus are delineated by lines of red and blue dots, respectively. The parieto-occipital sulcus is delineated by a line of white dots. The position of the occipital craniotomy should be posterior to the perisylvian fibers of the superior longitudinal fasciculus (yellow). The craniotomy should reveal the posterior aspects of the angular gyrus on its inferior border. FP = frontal pole, PostC = post-central gyrus, SMG = supramarginal gyrus, AG = angular gyrus, STG = superior temporal gyrus, MTG = middle temporal gyrus, SPL = superior parietal lobule, OP = occipital pole.

that the superior longitudinal fasciculus and inferior fronto-occipital fasciculus lie just underneath the anterior and inferior borders of the craniotomy, respectively. The relationships between these structures relative to the site of the occipital craniotomy are shown in Figure 18.4.

Once the craniotomy is planned, a linear incision of approximately 5 centimeters is made in the coronal plane. Note that the medial border of the superior longitudinal fasciculus defines the boundary of the lateral incision. The scalp is then retracted with the aid of multiple scalp hooks attached to flexible bands, and a single small burr hole is made at the bottom of the field with a round cutting drill bit. The craniotomy is finished with a craniotome and should be approximately 2 centimeters in diameter once completed. Figure 18.2 demonstrates the planned occipital incision (Figure 18.2A) and resulting occipital keyhole craniotomy (Figure 18.2B) in one patient undergoing the pull-through technique.

Occipital Lobectomy

In contrast to the temporal lobectomy, the most important risk factor when performing the occipital keyhole lobectomy involves the anterior disconnection between the occipital tumor, occipital cortex, and the adjacent speech and visuospatial pathways at the boundary of the temporal, parietal, and occipital lobes (9,14). Important landmarks to consider when beginning this part of the operation include the parieto-occipital sulcus which forms the superior border of the occipital lobe, as well as the posterior aspect of the angular gyrus, which constitutes its anterior border. Awake cortical mapping followed by subcortical mapping is carried out, and the patient is again instructed to perform a double task in order to identify and preserve any functionally eloquent portions of cortex (11).

Two different subcortical disconnections are made. The anterior dissection is performed first with a trajectory planned posterior to the superior longitudinal fasciculus. The first disconnection is complete after reaching the occipital horn, and the dissection is then extended medially to end within the pineal region where the falx cerebri can be visualized. A second infero-lateral dissection is then performed adjacent to the inferior fronto-occipital fasciculus, which delimits the antero-lateral disconnection border. The inferior disconnection is complete once the tentorium cerebelli is visualized. During both dissections, the superior longitudinal fasciculus and inferior fronto-occipital fasciculus are identified with subcortical mapping using DTI integrated with image guidance. In each case, the dissections are initiated at the superior and lateral margins of the craniotomy and are continued medially and inferiorly until the falx and tentorium are identified without exposing the posterior superior sagittal sinus.

Pull-Through (Connecting the Lobectomy Sites)

The "pull-through" approach is based on the idea that gliomas which extend from the temporal pole to the occipital pole are following the path of the inferior longitudinal fasciculus, and that the resection should conform to this white matter tract and its principle connections as closely as possible. Tractographic and anatomic work demonstrate that the inferior longitudinal fasciculus courses deep to the superior longitudinal fasciculus (15–18), with connections in the occipital pole, including the cuneus and lingual gyrus, the ventral occipital stream, and to parts of the medial, lateral, and polar regions of the temporal lobe (14, 16–19). These connections and the relationship between the superior and inferior longitudinal fasciculi are shown in Figure 18.5.

Because of this relationship, we view the working angle as an attempt to remain medial to the fibers of the superior longitudinal fasciculus. Adopting these principles, the remaining tumor between the two craniotomies sites can be removed following completion of the lobectomies by working underneath the superior longitudinal fasciculus complex. In our own experience, we have found it is usually easiest to finish resecting the tumor from the occipital side. During the pull-through stage, the superior longitudinal fasciculus can be identified with subcortical mapping using DTI integrated with image guidance. This allows for the preservation of the connections of the superior longitudinal fasciculus to the temporal and lateral occipital lobes (16, 17). Following complete tumor resection, a light can usually be shone through the craniotomy sites (Figure 18.6).

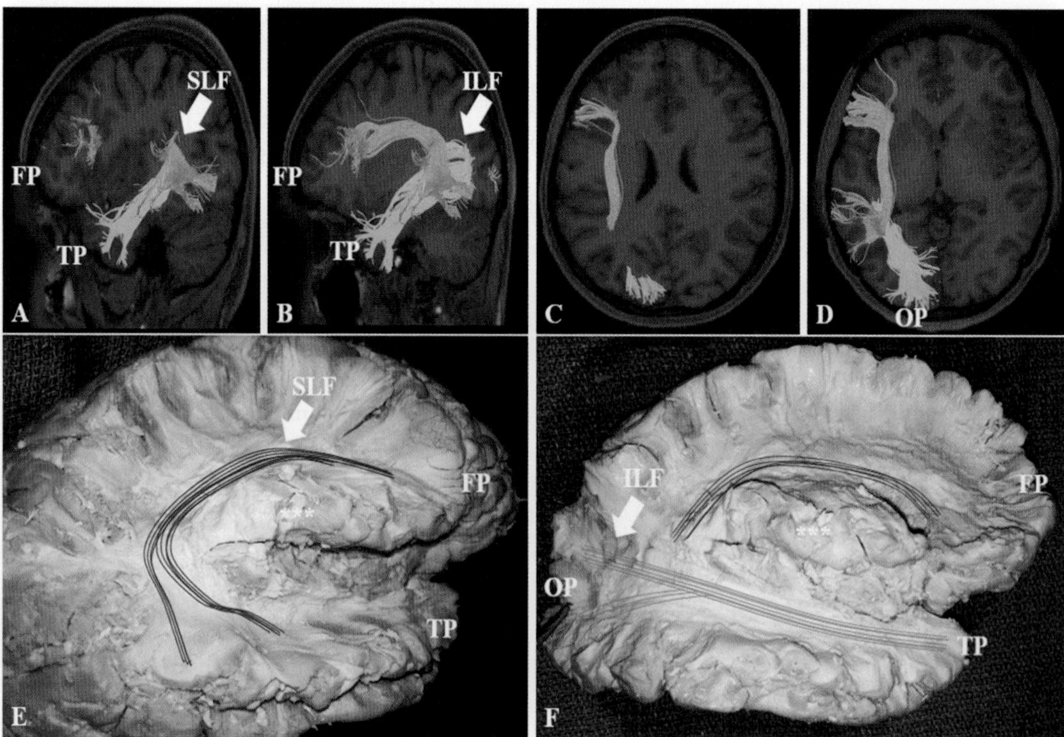

Figure 18.5 Relationship of the superior longitudinal fasciculus (pink streamlines) relative to the inferior longitudinal fasciculus (green streamlines). The superior longitudinal fasciculus connects aspects of the frontal, parietal, temporal, and occipital lobes. (A-B) Tractographic representation of the fibers of the superior longitudinal fasciculus (pink) on sagittal T1-weighted MRI slices. These fibers course under the sensorimotor strip before curving 90 degrees inferiorly at the level of the inferior parietal lobule to terminate in the posterior aspects of the superior and middle temporal gyri. (C-D) Tractographic representation of the fibers of the inferior longitudinal fasciculus (green) on axial T1-weighted MRI slices. These fibers course deep to the superior longitudinal fasciculus to terminate in polar parts of the temporal and occipital lobes. (E-F) White matter dissection images in a right cerebral hemisphere showing the relationship of the superior and inferior longitudinal fasciculi. Deep dissection after identifying the extent of the SLF revealed the ILF.

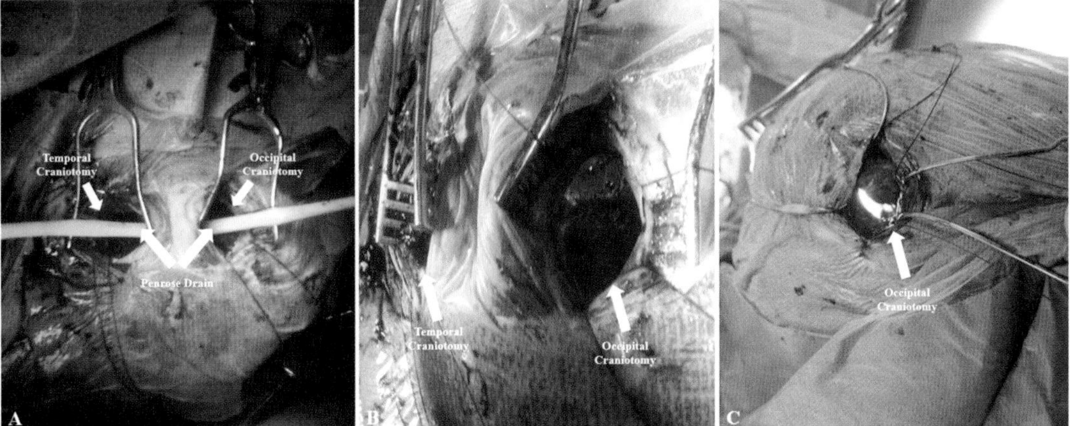

Figure 18.6 Completed pull-through technique. (A) A Penrose drain is shown passing through the temporal and occipital craniotomies after the tumor remaining between lobectomy sites is resected. (B-C) Light can also be shone through one craniotomy site (in this case, the temporal craniotomy) to confirm the connection of the lobectomies.

Complication Avoidance

Temporal Lobectomy

Given the small nature of the craniotomy carried out over the temporal lobe, it is possible to have some hesitation regarding the identification of standard anatomical landmarks, such as the Sylvian fissure. This is due to the posterior position of the craniotomy, and the fact that in many cases the fissure is displaced or compressed due to the bulk of the tumor. One must carefully identify the superior temporal gyrus to prevent entering the frontal operculum inadvertently. One technique to facilitate identification of the Sylvian fissure, beyond confirming with image guidance, is to angle the microscope anteriorly to look underneath the bone flap to identify the sphenoid wing. This structure is a consistent landmark that can be used to identify the proximal Sylvian fissure. The fissure can then be easily traced along its course to the exposure provided by the craniotomy. Further complication avoidance is aided in using a sub-pial dissection technique at the medial temporal operculum to avoid damaging the middle cerebral artery (20, 21). While performing the amygdala-hippocampectomy, a sub-pial dissection is crucial for two reasons: 1) to avoid damage to the anterior choroidal artery as well as crus cerebri, and 2) to identify the medial sub-pial border in this region. Large tumors tend to displace the medial temporal lobe, and without proper care to respect the medial sub-pial boundary, one may either leave the tumor behind if too lateral or possibly injure the brainstem if too medial.

Occipital Lobectomy

Two technical maneuvers should be utilized when performing the occipital lobectomy to avoid unnecessary complications: 1) early identification, coagulation, and division of bridging veins, and 2) early identification of the parieto-occipital sulcus. Further avoidance of the superior longitudinal fasciculus is aided by the early identification and preservation of this sulcus.

Postoperative Considerations

The following should be completed after surgery:

- Updated and regular neurologic exams to assess for new or changing neurologic deficits
- Routine postoperative labs, including chemistry and blood panels
- A postoperative, contrast-enhanced anatomic MRI scan, typically within 48 hours, to assess for residual tumor
- Planning for a two-week follow-up visit at the point of discharge to examine wound sites and re-evaluate the patient's clinical condition

The postoperative MRI scans for two patients having undergone the pull-through technique are shown in Figures 18.7 and 18.8.

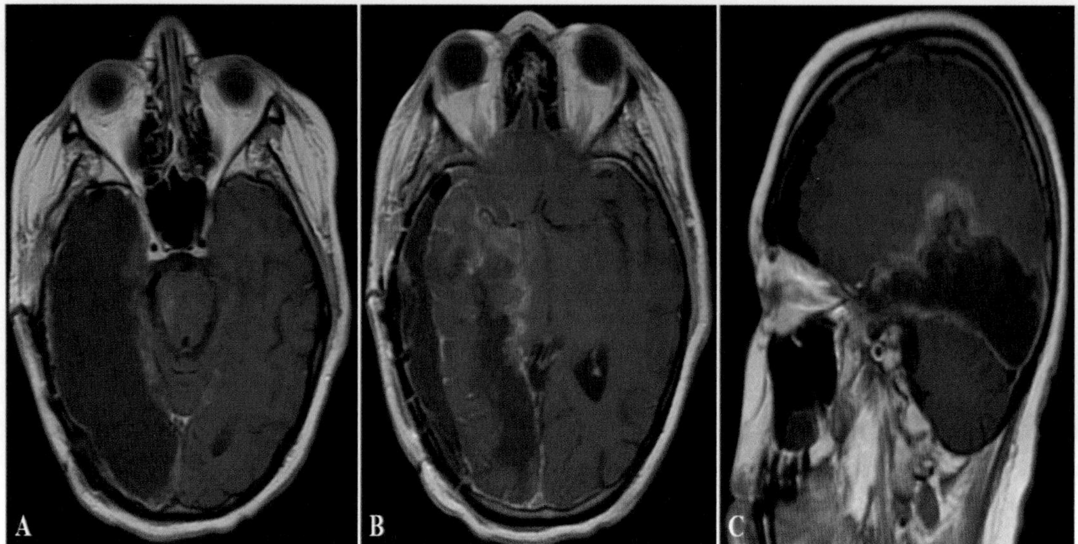

Figure 18.7 Postoperative MRI scan of the first patient presented in Figure 18.1. (A-B) Axial and (C) sagittal contrast-enhanced, T1-weighted MRI slices reveal the extent of resection, the dead space between the temporal and occipital poles, as well as the remaining temporal tissue (Panel B) preserved by resecting the tumor along the length of the inferior longitudinal fasciculus.

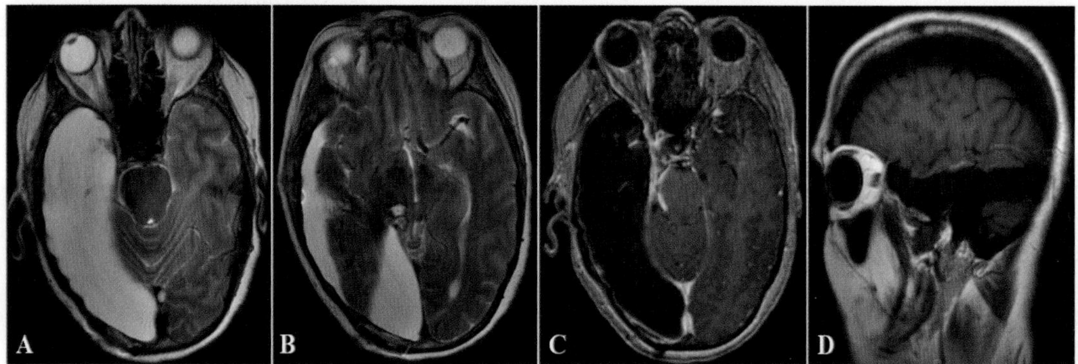

Figure 18.8 Postoperative MRI scan of the second patient presented in Figure 18.1. (A-C) Axial T1-and T2-weighted MRI slices reveal the extent of resection between the occipital and temporal lobes. Note the remaining temporal tissue (Panel B) preserved by resecting the tumor along the length of the inferior longitudinal fasciculus. (D) A sagittal contrast-enhanced, T1-weighted MRI slice reveals the extent of resection from the temporal pole to the occipital pole.

Clinical Pearls

The "pull-through" technique, while limited in scope, is a procedure that serves two fundamental purposes: 1) to make possible the resection of large temporal-occipital gliomas using a minimally invasive approach and 2) to preserve the connections of the superior longitudinal fasciculus and inferior fronto-occipital fasciculus whenever possible.

Key Points

- The multi-portal "pull-through" keyhole technique was designed for the removal of large gliomas extending between the temporal and occipital poles.
- The approach involves five critical steps: 1) construction of a temporal keyhole, 2) construction of an occipital keyhole, 3) a temporal lobectomy, 4) an occipital lobectomy, and 5) excision of the remaining tumor along the pathway of the inferior longitudinal fasciculus.
- The technique seeks to preserve the connections of the superior longitudinal fasciculus and inferior fronto-occipital fasciculus whenever possible.

References

1. Ivanova MV, Isaev DY, Dragoy OV, Akinina YS, Petrushevskiy AG, Fedina ON, et al. Diffusion-tensor imaging of major white matter tracts and their role in language processing in aphasia. *Cortex* 2016; **85**: 165–81.
2. Chang EF, Raygor KP, Berger MS. Contemporary model of language organization: an overview for neurosurgeons. *Journal of Neurosurgery* 2015; **122** (2): 250–61.
3. Toba MN, Migliaccio R, Batrancourt B, Bourlon C, Duret C, Pradat-Diehl P, et al. Common brain networks for distinct deficits in visual neglect. A combined structural and tractography MRI approach. *Neuropsychologia* 2018; **115**: 167–78.
4. Vaessen MJ, Saj A, Lovblad KO, Gschwind M, Vuilleumier P. Structural white-matter connections mediating distinct behavioral components of spatial neglect in right brain-damaged patients. *Cortex* 2016; **77**: 54–68.
5. Urbanski M, Thiebaut de Schotten M, Rodrigo S, Catani M, Oppenheim C, Touze E, et al. Brain networks of spatial awareness: evidence from diffusion tensor imaging tractography. *Journal of Neurology, Neurosurgery, and Psychiatry* 2008; **79** (5): 598–601.
6. Ferrer VP, Moura Neto V, Mentlein R. Glioma infiltration and extracellular matrix: key players and modulators. *Glia* 2018.
7. Hervey-Jumper SL, Li J, Lau D, Molinaro AM, Perry DW, Meng L, et al. Awake craniotomy to maximize glioma resection: methods and technical nuances over a 27-year period. *Journal of Neurosurgery* 2015; **123**(2): 325–39.
8. Conner AK, Burks JD, Baker CM, Smitherman AD, Pryor DP, Glenn CA, et al. Method for temporal keyhole lobectomies in resection of low- and high-grade gliomas. *Journal of Neurosurgery* 2018; **128**(5): 1388–95.
9. Glenn C, Conner AK, Rahimi M, Briggs RG, Baker C, Sughrue M. Common disconnections in glioma surgery: an anatomic description. *Cureus* 2017; **9**(10): e1778.
10. Charras P, Herbet G, Deverdun J, de Champfleur NM, Duffau H, Bartolomeo P, et al. Functional reorganization of the attentional networks in low-grade glioma patients: a longitudinal study. *Cortex* 2015; **63**: 27–41.
11. Mandonnet E, Sarubbo S, Duffau H. Proposal of an optimized strategy for intraoperative testing of speech and language during awake mapping. *Neurosurgical Review* 2017; **40**(1): 29–35.
12. Martino J, Vergani F, Robles SG, Duffau H. New insights into the anatomic dissection of the temporal stem with special emphasis on the inferior fronto-occipital fasciculus: implications in surgical approach to left mesiotemporal and temporoinsular structures. *Neurosurgery* 2010; **66** (3 Suppl Operative): 4–12.
13. Ghareeb F, Duffau H. Intractable epilepsy in paralimbic Word Health Organization Grade II gliomas: should the hippocampus be resected when not invaded by the tumor? *Journal of Neurosurgery* 2012; **116**(6): 1226–34.
14. Conner AK, Baker CM, Briggs RG, Burks JD, Glenn CA, Smitherman AD, et al. A technique for resecting occipital pole gliomas using a keyhole lobectomy. *World Neurosurgery* 2017; **106**: 707–14.
15. Mori S, Kaufmann WE, Davatzikos C, Stieltjes B, Amodei L, Fredericksen K, et al. Imaging cortical association tracts in the human brain using diffusion-tensor-based axonal tracking. *Magnetic Resonance in Medicine* 2002; **47**(2): 215–23.
16. Baker CM, Burks JD, Briggs RG, Conner AK, Glenn CA, Sali G, et al. A connectomic atlas of the human cerebrum. Chapter 1: introduction, methods, and significance. *Operative Neurosurgery* 2018; **15**(Suppl 1): s1–9.
17. Conner AK, Briggs RG, Rahimi M, Sali G, Baker CM, Burks JD, et al. A connectomic atlas of the human cerebrum. Chapter 10: tractographic description of the superior longitudinal fasciculus. *Operative Neurosurgery* 2018; **15**(Suppl 1): s407–22.
18. Sali G, Briggs RG, Conner AK, Rahimi M, Baker CM, Burks JD, et al. A connectomic atlas of the human cerebrum. Chapter 11: tractographic description of the inferior longitudinal fasciculus. *Operative Neurosurgery* 2018; **15**(Suppl 1): s423–8.
19. Baker CM, Burks JD, Briggs RG, Stafford J, Conner AK, Glenn CA, et al. A connectomic atlas of the human cerebrum. Chapter 9: the occipital lobe. *Operative Neurosurgery* 2018; **15**(Suppl 1): S372–406.
20. Duffau H. A new concept of diffuse (low-grade) glioma surgery. *Advances and Technical Standards in Neurosurgery* 2012; **38**: 3–27.
21. Hebb AO, Yang T, Silbergeld DL. The sub-pial resection technique for intrinsic tumor surgery. *Surgical Neurology International* 2011; **2**: 180.

Chapter 19

Combined Keyhole Craniotomies for Multifocal or Multiple Lesions

Abigail Funari, Murray Echt, and Vijay Agarwal

Introduction

The management of solitary symptomatic brain metastasis with surgical resection is well established with class-one evidence (1). Even in the presence of systemic disease, aggressive surgical treatment and adjuvant therapy of metastatic brain tumors have been shown to prolong survival in patients with a solitary lesion (2). The prognosis of neurologically symptomatic patients with two or more lesions is less clear, with aggressive management often leading to patient survival well beyond estimates (3,4). Recent data advocates that with proper selection of patients with multiple brain lesions can obtain a survival benefit and increased quality of life after surgical resection (5,6). Multiple keyhole craniotomies for simultaneous resection of multifocal lesions is a relatively new approach utilized to reduce morbidity and extend survival (7). Select patients with multifocal or multicentric glioblastomas can also benefit from aggressive resection utilizing this strategy. This approach results in a survival benefit comparable with that of patients undergoing surgery for a single lesion without an associated increase in postoperative morbidity (8,9). These findings indicate that it is necessary to question the conventional wisdom of a minimal role for surgical treatment in multifocal lesions, especially in light of the advent of minimally invasive ("keyhole") techniques that allow for decreased surgical morbidity and decreased patient recovery time, and in light of improved adjuvant cancer treatments with increased life expectancies (10-13).

Currently, performing multiple sequential craniotomies in one surgical sitting is not as common as one would think, as many surgeons fear that performing multiple craniotomies places the patient at an increased risk for complications and exposes the patient to prolonged anesthesia. In a study on the postoperative survival of patients with multiple brain metastases, multiple craniotomies were not associated with an increased complication rate per craniotomy or with higher 30-day mortality rates (12). Patients undergoing multiple craniotomies, however, do have a higher *cumulative* probability of developing a complication, with a complication rate of about 4–7% per individual craniotomy (7,13). This should be compared, however, with the rate of complication in the surgical treatment of brain metastases utilizing a single craniotomy, which one study found to be as high as 12% (14). In addition, patients undergoing multiple craniotomies are not necessarily exposed to extended anesthesia times relative to those undergoing single craniotomies. The median operative time reported for multiple craniotomies in a single session is 2.4 hours, compared to 3 hours for single metastatic resections (7). In general, neither the presence of multiple lesions nor the need for multiple craniotomies should be a major deterrent to resecting more than one lesion in a single surgical sitting.

Indications

The goal of using multiple keyhole craniotomies for multifocal lesions is to resect 1) any symptomatic tumors, 2) tumors with significant edema or mass effect, 3) tumors that are resistant to chemotherapy and radiation, and/or 4) lesions larger than 2 cm, whenever accessible. Surgery is generally performed in order to improve quality of life rather than to achieve disease control and/or to cure (6). If a surgical resection of one lesion is deemed necessary, the authors also advocate resection of any other lesions within the same operative corridor that can be accessed safely.

Patient selection remains crucial to achieving the optimal surgical benefits without imparting undue risk. We recommend selecting candidates with intermediate to excellent preoperative condition, with a Karnofski Performance Status (KPS) greater than 70. A cutoff age of 70 years is suggested, with exceptions for older patients in extremely good neurologic condition (15). Patients with limited or controlled systemic cancer and brain lesions that are in non-eloquent cortex are excellent surgical candidates; however, even patients in whom all lesions cannot be removed may be considered surgical candidates under certain circumstances, including if one or two lesions are life-threatening or highly symptomatic (13). Given the success rate of stereotactic radiosurgery for brain metastatic disease, even patients with numerous brain lesions can lead extended lives with good quality. Numerous factors have been correlated with poor patient survival, including the presence of active systemic disease, poor neurological status, extensive number of brain tumors, the time between the development of the primary tumor and metastasis to the brain, and tumor histology (16).

Patients with multifocal glioblastoma often have independent lesions that are located too far apart to allow for resection using a single craniotomy. The extent of resection has been shown to best predict survival in patients with glioblastoma regardless of age, KPS score, or subsequent treatment modalities, with gross total resection being associated with significantly improved survival (17-19). For this reason, multiple craniotomies may be indicated in this patient population.

An ideal clinical scenario is exemplified by a 71-year-old female with a history of breast cancer, with good systemic disease control, treated surgically at our institution for multiple brain metastases. The patient originally presented two years prior with invasive ductal carcinoma. A left breast lumpectomy was performed in February 2017, followed by radiation therapy. The systemic disease was well controlled with adjuvant chemotherapy. Work-up for a fall incidentally revealed an ~4.5 cm right frontal lobe cystic lesion with significant vasogenic edema and a 2.8 cm midline heterogeneously enhancing cerebellar lesion (Figures 19.1 and 19.2). The patient was found to have weakness in the left arm and leg (rated 4 out of 5 in strength). After extensive discussion of the risks and benefits with the patient, she underwent two successful keyhole craniotomies in the same surgical sitting to remove both large brain metastases (Figures 19.3 and 19.4). There were no intraoperative or postoperative complications, and a gross total resection was achieved for both lesions (Figures 19.5 and 19.6). Her left-sided weakness resolved postoperatively.

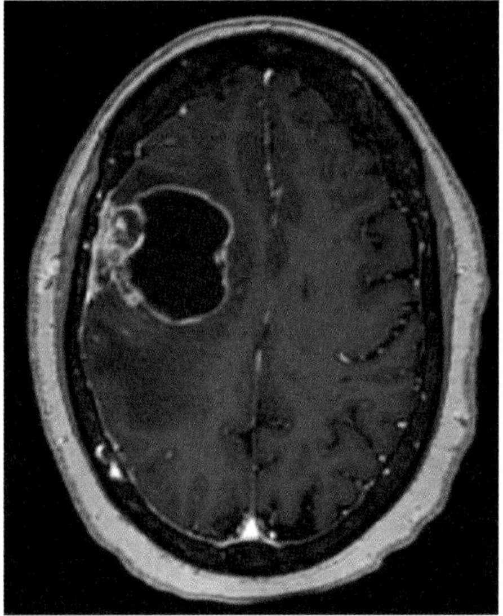

Figure 19.1 Preoperative axial MRI brain with contrast showing an ~4.5 cm right frontal lobe cystic lesion with significant vasogenic edema

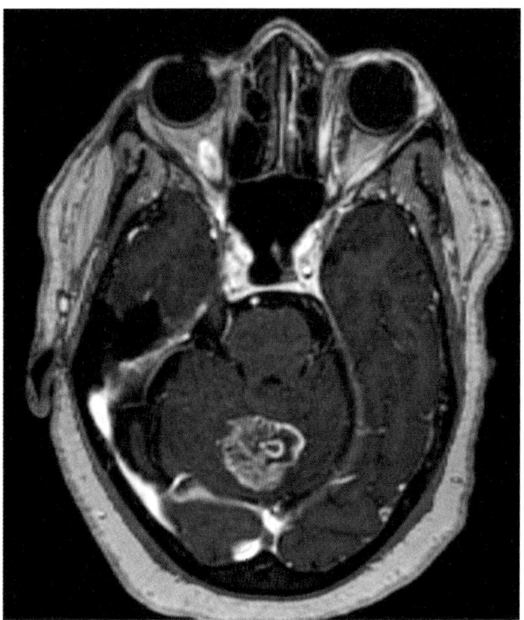

Figure 19.2 Preoperative axial MRI brain with contrast showing a 2.8 cm midline heterogeneously enhancing cerebellar lesion

Contraindications

Contraindications to this approach primarily include patients with a poor overall prognosis. Specifically, this includes patients who are not expected to survive for longer than three months

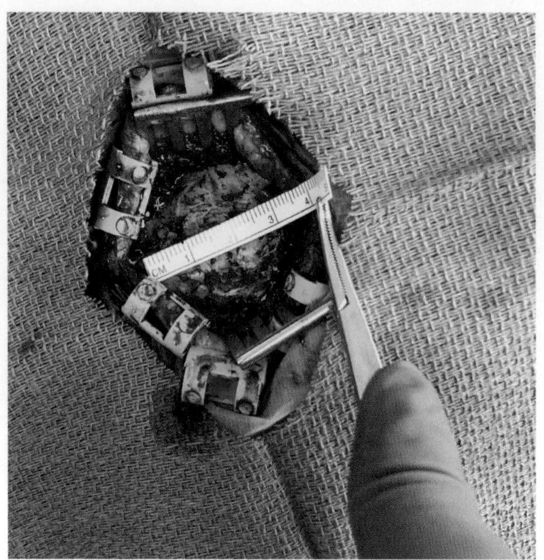

Figure 19.3 Skin incision length for the right frontal keyhole craniotomy

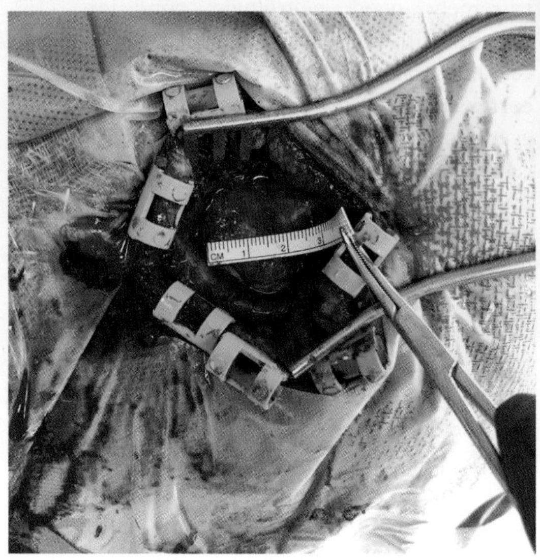

Figure 19.4 Keyhole craniotomy size for the midline cerebellar lesion

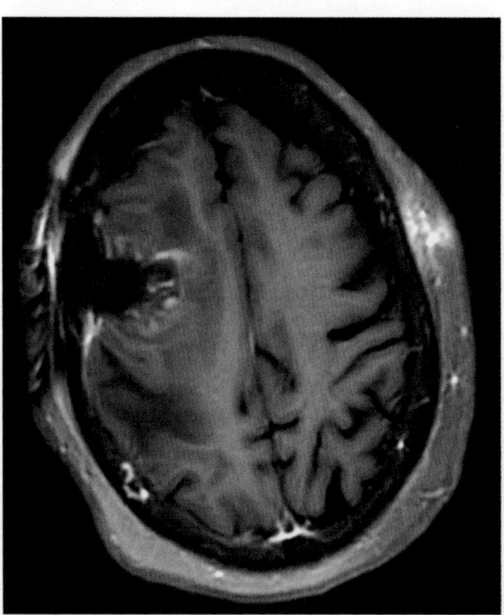

Figure 19.5 Postoperative axial brain with contrast showing a gross total resection of the right frontal cystic lesion

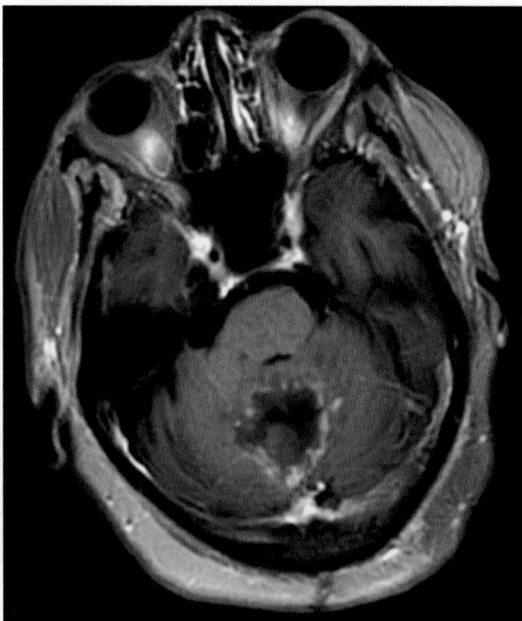

Figure 19.6 Postoperative axial brain with contrast showing a gross total resection of the midline cerebellar lesion

due to their systemic cancer or patients who have four or more metastases (12,13). However, in our experience, patients with more than four metastases can still have improved survival with this approach, depending on their clinical status and systemic disease control. This decision must be made on a case-by-case basis. This approach is also not advised for multiple difficult-to-access lesions, such as deep-seated lesions or those that involve eloquent cortex. Alternative strategies include resection of dominant or symptomatic lesions with radiation treatment reserved for the remaining lesions, radiation alone or with medical treatment, or supportive care alone.

Preoperative Planning

Preoperative evaluation includes discussion with a multidisciplinary tumor board consisting of at least a radiation oncologist, a medical oncologist, and the surgeon to determine optimal peri- and postoperative therapy for the patient. Suggested preoperative imaging includes a contrast-enhanced MRI containing image guidance sequences (e.g., MP-RAGE) and diffusion tensor imaging (DTI) with white matter tractography for deep-seated tumors. Using DTI tractography, the corticospinal tract, superior longitudinal fasciculus, arcuate fasciculus, inferior fronto-occipital fasciculus, and optic pathways, among others, can be included or merged into image guidance for operative planning and resection (20). Awake-mapping may be employed in any patient where tumor involves, or is near, eloquent portions of the brain (21).

Surgical Technique

The surgical technique for multiple keyhole craniotomies involves the fundamental principles of keyhole surgery. Frameless stereotactic navigation should be used to plan each craniotomy such that surgery proceeds along the long axis of the tumor while avoiding major white matter tracts (10). When possible, the patient should be placed in a position that allows multiple craniotomy incisions to be included in the same operative field. In cases where more than one tumor will be approached in a single patient position, extra care should be taken to pad pressure points and secure the patient with straps and tape to allow for maximal rotation of the bed. Repositioning and subsequent re-prepping and re-draping of the patient may be required; this does not usually significantly increase the risk of infection or operative time compared with staging the individual procedures. Planned craniotomy size and incision length depend on the tumor location. For cortically based tumors, the craniotomy is tailored to expose only the extent of the tumor surface. For tumors located deep to the cortical surface, the maximal craniotomy size is typically 2.0–2.5 cm. Deeply seated tumors are readily accessible through a 2-cm craniotomy, whereas larger and/or more superficial tumors greater than 2 cm in diameter may require a slightly larger craniotomy tailored to the individual tumor and planned with the assistance of stereotactic navigation.

It is also essential to incorporate endoscopic assistance in these cases. Use of the endoscope is crucial to inspecting the tumor bed to ensure complete tumor removal or when working behind brain structures to access deep intracranial spaces. Use of the endoscope precludes the use of larger craniotomies and allows for complete visualization of the tumor margins with clearer detail. Endoscopes also allow for the removal of multiple lesions from a single surgical corridor, allowing for access around difficult angles that would otherwise only be achieved by an additional craniotomy. Often, an endoscope is used at or near the end of the case to inspect for residual tumors that would otherwise have been missed with the use of a microscope alone. At our institution, a planned keyhole craniotomy setup includes an endoscopic tower with a camera and monitor in the operating room, and the endoscope and angled instruments are prepared in an unopened sterile pack, ready for use.

Complication Avoidance

To avoid complications with this approach, important points to consider include maximizing working angles and extending the operative reach within the smaller craniotomy flap. This may be accomplished with frequent microscope adjustments, by maintaining a low-profile operative field by limiting the number of fixed retractors, and by using the space created by the tumor itself. Increasing space within a keyhole approach may be achieved by intraoperative CSF drainage (e.g., through the cerebellopontine cistern, foramen magnum, carotid cistern, Liliequist membrane, etc.), drainage of cystic tumor structures, debulking of the tumor, or during removal of exposed non-eloquent brain, if necessary (e.g., the gyrus rectus), depending on the location and type of lesion and the depth required for resection. When two or more lesions are within the same compartment, we often observe that resection of the second lesion is aided by the extra space conferred by removal of the other mass, and oftentimes from brain relaxation. Significant brain shift upon the surgical approach is generally avoided in a keyhole compared with a more traditional open craniotomy, allowing for more accurate use of frameless stereotactic navigation. The decreased brain swelling also makes the preservation and protection of normal brain parenchyma easier. Inspection with an endoscope, typically toward the end of the tumor resection, can help in avoiding leaving behind unseen residual tumor; it can also allow for decreased retraction of the brain to access tumor remnants that are difficult to reach.

Postoperative Considerations

For patients determined to be suitable candidates for multiple craniotomies in a single surgical setting, current treatment paradigms include, first, resection of all lesions when feasible, followed by postoperative radiotherapy and concomitant chemotherapy, depending on tumor type (8). Patients should undergo a Gd-enhanced MRI of the brain shortly following surgery to determine the extent of tumor resection (8). A Gd-enhanced MRI may be performed every two to three months during follow-up to assess for early recurrence or new brain metastasis, or sooner if the patient shows signs of neurological deterioration or is newly symptomatic (8).

It has been well established that the extent of resection of glioblastoma correlates with overall patient survival (8,17-19,22). It has been suggested that the same concept applies to multiple brain metastases (7,13). Postoperative adjuvant radiotherapy has also been shown to significantly increase survival (23-24), and adjuvant postoperative whole-brain radiation therapy (WBRT) or stereotactic radiosurgery (SRS) has been reported to significantly reduce intracranial recurrence and early death (7). WBRT was formerly the gold standard for patients with cranial metastases; however, multiple studies recommend using limited-field radiation, with an increasing prevalence of postoperative SRS to the surgical cavity. SRS avoids unnecessary radiation to a healthy brain and, generally, is used as an adjuvant therapy for metastases greater than 1.5–2 cm in size (12,25-31). As in all cases, the selection of postoperative adjuvant therapy should be done in a multidisciplinary fashion and on a case-by-case basis; there are reported cases where surgery alone, followed by surveillance instead is the most appropriate course of action (25).

Postoperative considerations should be made based on the type of primary tumor identified. Of the common primary tumors associated with brain metastases, melanoma, kidney, and colon cancers are considered to be the most radioresistant (32,33).

In terms of conventional chemotherapy, brain metastases offer a unique challenge, due to the inability of many agents to cross the blood-brain barrier. However, chemotherapy is and should be used when appropriate to help control systemic disease and to extend overall survival (12,25). Immunotherapeutic agents such as nivolumab (Opdivo) and pembrolizumab (Keytruda) have also significantly enhanced the field of oncology in non-neurological primary sites, and they should be used appropriately for primary cancers such as those of the lung.

Clinical Pearls

The cumulative significant advances in systemic control of various non-neurological cancers further necessitate aggressive control of large or symptomatic brain metastasis, such as the control afforded by multiple craniotomies for multifocal disease. While the need for multiple craniotomies should not be a deterrent to surgery, it is important to understand that not all patients will benefit from the surgical removal of multiple brain metastases, and that the decision should be made on a case-by-case basis and in a multidisciplinary fashion. Numerous factors should be carefully considered when developing an overall treatment plan, including patient preference and overall health, in order to appropriately select patients whose quality of life will ultimately be improved (15). Poor outcomes for multiple craniotomies for multifocal lesions may be associated with patients with four or more brain metastases or those who have a life expectancy of less than three months (12).

Key Points

- Many patients with multiple or multifocal brain lesions may benefit from aggressive surgical management, often leading to survival well beyond estimates.
- Patients undergoing multiple craniotomies in a single surgical setting should be appropriately counseled on the overall risk and the long-term treatment plan, which may include radiotherapy, chemotherapy, and/or immunotherapy.

- With proper patient selection and reliance on the principles of keyhole techniques, significant improvement in survival and quality of life can be achieved.
- In cases where more than one lesion will be approached in a single operative sitting via a single operative corridor, extra care should be taken in padding and securing the patient to the operative bed.
- If required, reposition and re-prep the patient, as this does not add significantly more risk or time compared with staging the procedures.
- It has been suggested that the extent of resection of all brain metastases correlates well with patient survival.

References

1. Patchell RA, Tibbs PA, Walsh JW, Dempsey RJ, Maruyama Y, Kryscio RJ, Markesbery WR, Macdonald JS, Young B (1990) A randomized trial of surgery in the treatment of single metastases to the brain. *N Engl J Med* **322**: 494–500.
2. Hall WA, Djalilian HR, Nussbaum ES, Cho KH (2000) Long-term survival with metastatic cancer to the brain. *Med Oncol* **17**: 279–86.
3. Kalkanis SN, Kondziolka D, Gaspar LE, Burri SH, Asher AL, Cobbs CS, Ammirati M, Robinson PD, Andrews DW, Loeffler JS, McDermott M, Mehta MP, Mikkelsen T, Olson JJ, Paleologos NA, Patchell RA, Ryken TC, Linskey ME (2010) The role of surgical resection in the management of newly diagnosed brain metastases: a systematic review and evidence-based clinical practice guideline. *J Neurooncol* **96**: 33–43.
4. Kondziolka D, Parry P V., Lunsford LD, Kano H, Flickinger JC, Rakfal S, Arai Y, Loeffler JS, Rush S, Knisely JPS, Sheehan J, Friedman W, Tarhini AA, Francis L, Lieberman F, Ahluwalia MS, Linskey ME, McDermott M, Sperduto P, Stupp R (2013) The accuracy of predicting survival in individual patients with cancer. *J Neurosurg* **120**: 24–30.
5. Panciani P, Buffoni L, Ronchetti G, Spena G, Tartara F, Buglione M, Pagano M, Ducati A, Fontanella M, Garbossa D, Agnoletti A, Mencarani C (2014) Surgery in cerebral metastases: are numbers so important? *J Cancer Res Ther* **10**: 79.
6. Paek SH, Audu PB, Sperling MR, Cho J, Andrews DW (2005) Reevaluation of surgery for the treatment of brain metastases: review of 208 patients with single or multiple brain metastases treated at one institution with modern neurosurgical techniques. *Neurosurgery* **56**: 1021–33.
7. Baker CM, Glenn CA, Briggs RG, Burks JD, Smitherman AD, Conner AK, Williams AE, Malik MU, Algan O, Sughrue ME (2017) Simultaneous resection of multiple metastatic brain tumors with multiple keyhole craniotomies. *World Neurosurg* **106**: 359–67.
8. Hassaneen W, Levine NB, Suki D, Salaskar AL, de Moura Lima A, McCutcheon IE, Prabhu SS, Lang FF, DeMonte F, Rao G, Weinberg JS, Wildrick DM, Aldape KD, Sawaya R (2010) Multiple craniotomies in the management of multifocal and multicentric glioblastoma. *J Neurosurg* **114**: 576–84.
9. Hong N, Yoo H, Gwak HS, Shin SH, Lee SH (2014) Outcome of surgical resection of symptomatic cerebral lesions in non-small cell lung cancer patients with multiple brain metastases. *Brain Tumor Res Treat* **1**: 64.
10. Teo C, Sughrue ME (2015) *Principles and Practice of Keyhole Brain Surgery*. Georg Thieme Verlag, Stuttgart.
11. Gazzeri R, Nalavenkata S, Teo C (2014) Minimally invasive key-hole approach for the surgical treatment of single and multiple brain metastases. *Clin Neurol Neurosurg* **123**: 117–26.
12. Auslands K, Apškalne D, Bicāns K, Ozols R, Ozoliņš H (2012) Postoperative survival in patients with multiple brain metastases. *Medicina* **48**: 281–5.
13. Bindal RK, Sawaya R, Leavens ME, Lee JJ (2009) Surgical treatment of multiple brain metastases. *J Neurosurg* **79**: 210–16.
14. Stark AM, Tscheslog H, Buhl R, Held-Feindt J, Mehdorn HM (2005) Surgical treatment for brain metastases: prognostic factors and survival in 177 patients. *Neurosurg Rev* **28**: 115–19.
15. Pollock BE, Brown PD, Foote RL, Stafford SL, Schomberg PJ (2003) Properly selected patients with multiple brain metastases may benefit from aggressive treatment of their intracranial disease. *J Neurooncol* **61**: 73–80.
16. Agboola O, Benoit B, Cross P, Da Silva V, Esche B, Lesiuk H, Gonsalves C (1998) Prognostic factors derived from recursive partition analysis (RPA) of Radiation Therapy Oncology Group (RTOG) brain metastases trials applied to surgically resected and irradiated brain metastatic cases. *Int J Radiat Oncol Biol Phys* **42**: 155–9.
17. Lacroix M, AbiSaid D, Fourney DR, Gokaslan ZL, Shi W, DeMonte F, et al. (2001) A multivariate analysis of 416 patients with glioblastoma multiforme: prognosis, extent of resection, and survival. *J Neurosurg* **95**: 190–8.

18. Buckner JC (2003) Factors influencing survival in high-grade gliomas. *Semin Oncol* **30** (6 Suppl 19): 10–14.

19. Laws ER, Parney IF, Huang W, Anderson F, Morris AM, Asher A, et al. (2003) Survival following surgery and prognostic factors for recently diagnosed malignant glioma: data from the Glioma Outcomes Project. *J Neurosurg* **99**: 467–73.

20. Bonney PA, Conner AK, Boettcher LB, Cheema AA, Glenn CA, Smitherman AD, Pittman NA, Sughrue ME (2017) A simplified method of accurate postprocessing of diffusion tensor imaging for use in brain tumor resection. *Oper Neurosurg* **13**: 47–58.

21. Burks JD, Conner AK, Bonney PA, Glenn CA, Smitherman AD, Ghafil CA, Briggs RG, Baker CM, Kirch NI, Sughrue ME (2018) Frontal keyhole craniotomy for resection of low- and high-grade gliomas. *Clin Neurosurg* **82**: 388–96.

22. McGirt MJ, Chaichana KL, Gathinji M, Attenello FJ, Than K, Olivi A, et al (2009) Independent association of extent of resection with survival in patients with malignant brain astrocytoma. *J Neurosurg* **110**: 156–62.

23. Walker MD, Green SB, Byar DP, Alexander E Jr, Batzdorf U, Brooks WH, et al. (1980) Randomized comparisons of radiotherapy and nitrosoureas for the treatment of malignant glioma after surgery. *N Engl J Med* **303**: 1323–9.

24. Laperriere N, Zuraw L (2002) Cairncross G: radiotherapy for newly diagnosed malignant glioma in adults: a systematic review. *Radiother Oncol* **64**: 259–73.

25. Arvold ND, Lee EQ, Mehta MP, Margolin K, Alexander BM, Lin NU, Anders CK, Soffietti R, Camidge DR, Vogelbaum MA, Dunn IF, Wen PY (2016) Updates in the management of brain metastases. *Neuro Oncol* **18**: 1043–65.

26. Tsao MN, Lloyd NS, Wong RK, Rakovitch E, Chow E, Laperriere N (2005) Supportive Care Guidelines Group of Cancer Care Ontario's program in evidence-based care. Radiotherapeutic management of brain metastases: a systematic review and meta-analysis. *Cancer Treat Rev* **31**: 256–73.

27. Salvati M, Oppido PA, Artizzu S, Fiorenza F, Puzzilli F (1991) Orlando ER: Multicentric gliomas. Report of seven cases. *Tumori* **77**: 518–22.

28. Synowitz M, von Eckardstein K, Brauer C, Hoch HH, Kiwit JC (2002) Case history: multicentric glioma with involvement of the optic chiasm. *Clin Neurol Neurosurg* **105**: 66–68.

29. Chadduck WM, Roycroft D, Brown MW (1983) Multicentric glioma as a cause of multiple cerebral lesions. *Neurosurgery* **13**: 170–5.

30. Ampil F, Burton GV, Gonzalez Toledo E, Nanda A (2007) Do we need whole-brain irradiation in multifocal or multicentric high-grade cerebral gliomas? Review of cases and the literature. *J Neurooncol* **85**: 353–5.

31. Showalter TN, Andrel J, Andrews DW, Curran WJ Jr, Daskalakis C, Werner Wasik M (2007) Multifocal glioblastoma multiforme: prognostic factors and patterns of progression. *Int J Radiat Oncol Biol Phys* **69**: 820–4.

32. Patchell RA (1991) Brain metastases. *Neurol Clin* **9**: 817–24.

33. Galicich JH, Arbit E (1990) Metastatic brain tumors, in Youmans JR, ed., *Neurological Surgery*, 3rd ed. Philadelphia, WB Saunders, pp. 3204–22.

Chapter 20

Combined Microsurgical and Endovascular Treatment of Cerebrovascular and Skull Base Pathology

Brian M. Howard, Jonathan A. Grossberg, Daniel L. Barrow, and C. Michael Cawley

Introduction

While the history of cerebrovascular and skull base microsurgery is relatively short, advances since the inception of the field have been dramatic and have expanded the spectrum of pathologies that cranial base surgeons treat. Innovations include skull base approaches, dissection techniques, and positioning, but the single most important innovation to stoke the progress of skull base microsurgery is the advent of the operating microscope. The microscope provides illumination and magnification to allow visualization of regions of the cranial vault that are otherwise unable to be seen in sufficient detail to operate safely. Dr. Theodore Kurze first used the operating microscope in the neurosurgical theatre in the late 1950s, but it was not until Dr. M. Gazi Yasargil developed counterbalancing, joint braking, and the mouth switch that the full potential of intraoperative microscopy was realized (1).

Since the inception of the operating microscope, the field of skull base surgery has continued to heavily rely on technology and innovation by virtue of the tools and skills required to perform such cases effectively. The early part of the twenty-first century has ushered in a new era of technologically dependent, less-invasive skull base procedures and techniques that have increased efficacy while mitigating risk. For example, indications for endoscopic skull base surgery – which began primarily with transsphenoidal approaches to the anterior and central skull base – have grown tremendously, and techniques continue to be honed. Similarly, as endoscopic techniques have transformed skull base tumor surgery, endovascular treatment of cerebrovascular pathology has been the largest paradigm-disrupter for cerebrovascular skull base surgery.

Endovascular therapy, though once viewed with skepticism by skull base surgeons as a less invasive but potentially less effective alternative to surgery, has recently been embraced as an adjunct to cranial base surgery and, in many ways, can improve surgical outcomes while reducing operative risk (2). As much as skull base surgery has benefitted from multidisciplinary contribution and collaboration among neurosurgeons, head and neck surgeons, otologists, and maxillofacial surgeons; together, interventional neuroradiologists, interventional neurologists, and vascular neurosurgeons, along with a host of allied subspecialists in related fields now work to deliver effective, cutting edge care to patients with cerebro- and spino-vascular disease as well as vascular, traumatic and oncologic disorders of the head and neck (3). As such, comprehensive cerebrovascular and skull base teams now consist of combinations of providers from interventional neuroradiologists and neurologists to dually trained neurosurgeons, traditionally and endoscopically trained neurooncological surgeons, and specialized head and neck surgeons.

The reach of the neurointerventional surgeon has never been greater. Flow diverters have revolutionized the treatment of intracranial aneurysms (IAs). Liquid embolic agents have made the treatment of dural arteriovenous fistulas (dAVFs) safer and less invasive. Preoperative embolization of intracranial arteriovenous malformations (AVMs) and certain intracranial and head and neck tumors has decreased surgical morbidity. Although in some cases endovascular therapy has supplanted traditional open skull base approaches to cerebrovascular pathology, many pathologies require synergistic, multidisciplinary management that combines endovascular techniques and skull base surgery. The focus of this chapter is to describe the indications for, and technical nuances of, combined microsurgical and endovascular treatment of cerebrovascular and skull base disease. In particular, three major disease states will be parsed: intracranial aneurysms, arteriovenous malformations of the brain and dura, and skull base tumors.

Indications and Technique

Intracranial Aneurysms

Microsurgical management of IAs can be challenging. The skills required to successfully perform aneurysm surgery are exacting, and clip-ligation of IAs is associated with risks, due to the proximity of such lesions to surrounding neurovascular structures. Many IAs are more safely approached using skull base surgical techniques to improve exposure and minimize or eliminate the need for brain retraction. Such aneurysms include internal carotid artery (ICA) aneurysms at the ophthalmic, superior hypophyseal, or posterior communicating artery origins and vertebral artery (VA) aneurysms at the posterior inferior cerebellar artery origin. Gaining sufficient exposure to clip such aneurysms and obtaining proximal control often requires skull base techniques such as anterior clinoidectomy or far lateral/transcondylar exposure, which are associated with added technical difficulty, associated risk, and increased morbidity. The introduction of endovascular treatment of IAs has made a large proportion of these complicated aneurysms more easily and safely treatable. However, not all IAs are amenable to endovascular intervention, and those remaining aneurysms often challenge the skills of the microsurgeon.

Broadly speaking, the field of endovascular management of IAs can be divided into two epochs: the pre- and post-flow diverter eras. Although the indication for flow diversion in the United States is limited to the treatment of unruptured aneurysms of the ICA between the petrous and supraclinoid segments, numerous series detailing the advantages and risks of off-label use of flow diverters have been published (4,5). Before the introduction of flow diversion, the primary indication for combined open skull base and endovascular treatment of skull base IAs was the inability to safely treat using either method alone. This combined approach typically involved one of several strategic approaches, such as

- surgical aneurysm exploration followed by endovascular coiling (particularly in the era prior to stent-assisted coiling, wherein partial aneurysm clipping was used to make wide-neck IAs more favorable for subsequent endovascular coiling);
- extracranial-to-intracranial (EC-IC) bypass followed by endovascular parent vessel or aneurysm occlusion;
- partial coiling to protect the dome of a ruptured aneurysm followed by delayed clipping;
- temporary parent artery occlusion by endovascular balloon during clipping; and
- permanent vessel occlusion with subsequent surgical aneurysm deflation to reduce the mass effect on surrounding skull base structures, particularly cranial nerves (2,6–9).

A number of these techniques have been obviated by flow diversion in many circumstances. Most clinoidal and proximal supraclinoid ICA aneurysms are now amenable to elective treatment with flow diverters, as are many vertebral artery aneurysms (5,10,11). More importantly, many of the extremely wide-neck or fusiform aneurysms that previously required complex combined approaches are now effectively managed with flow diversion (12,13). Even ruptured IAs can be managed by flow diversion despite the need for dual antiplatelet therapy (DAPT) and when the surgical risk is extremely high, as in the case of ruptured blister aneurysms of the dorsal proximal ICA. Although surgical strategies are time-honored and durable, these cases carry risk, and flow diversion may be preferable in select cases (14).

Although rare, the indication for combined microsurgical and endovascular management of IAs has not changed in the modern endovascular era, as such combined approaches are saved for complex aneurysms with no safe or complete surgical or interventional solution. A combined treatment strategy is typically considered for patients with large or giant saccular IAs that have a wide neck or branch vessels that originate from either the aneurysm neck or fundus. For similar reasons, fusiform IAs may require staged open and endovascular surgery.

Presurgical screening and work-up should always be conducted by a multidisciplinary team with experience in managing challenging intracranial vascular pathology. Before a treatment paradigm can be established and executed, it is of the utmost importance to perform a diagnostic cerebral angiogram with computer-assisted three-dimensional reconstruction. Depending on the particular circumstance, adjunctive axial imaging such as computed tomography (CT) or magnetic resonance imaging (MRI) is often required to gauge the relationship of the aneurysm to surrounding neurovascular and skull base structures. Balloon test occlusion (BTO) with both clinical testing and radionucleotide uptake imaging are typically recommended to assess circulation and the potential need for bypass, in case surgical or endovascular sacrifice of the ICA or vertebral artery is required as a bailout strategy.

Combined microsurgical and endovascular management of IAs usually incorporates a deconstructive and reconstructive component. Whether surgery is performed before endovascular treatment or vice versa is dependent on the goals of the specific operation as determined by the patient's anatomy (15). Combined approaches to IAs in the post-flow diversion era fall into three broad categories:

1. Giant saccular aneurysms, the neck of which incorporates a relatively long segment and/or large circumference of the parent vessel, in patients where flow diversion or simple vessel sacrifice are not feasible due to anatomy, contraindication to DAPT, or failed BTO. These patients require parent vessel and aneurysm sacrifice with bypass distal to the aneurysm to supply sufficient downstream revascularization.
2. Aneurysms with a large branch vessel originating from either the neck or fundus of a saccular aneurysm or the affected segment of a fusiform or dissecting pseudoaneurysm, in which case bypass to the affected branch vessel is required prior to myriad combinations of endovascular treatment strategies. Endovascular management of such aneurysms may include standard coiling, stent-assisted coiling (including coiling in combination with flow diversion), or parent vessel sacrifice (Figure 20.1, Video 20.1).
3. Aneurysms for which open microsurgical clip ligation is incomplete and adjunctive endovascular treatment is required to completely obliterate the aneurysm (Figure 20.2).

The combined microsurgical and endovascular approach has the same technical nuances and intraoperative considerations as microsurgery and endovascular treatment of IAs individually. Those details are described elsewhere; however, combined surgical approaches to IAs frequently include a bypass for revascularization followed by a deconstructive component, and it is imperative to ensure that the bypass is patent at the time of surgery. This can be achieved with indocyanine green video angiography, conventional digital subtraction angiography (DSA), or both. If a purely deconstructive approach is taken endovascularly and the intraoperative angiogram (IOA) reveals that the goals for revascularization have been achieved, long-term imaging follow-up is typically unnecessary. In cases where the endovascular portion requires flow diversion, coiling, or stent-/balloon-assisted coiling, the prescribed follow-up imaging regimen most often parallels that for endovascularly treated aneurysms. This may include both short- and long-term imaging using both CT and MR angiography or DSA, given the well-established increased rate of recurrence of endovascularly treated IAs relative to those that are microsurgically clip ligated.

Video 20.1 Bypass technique for the case described in Figure 20.1. 00:00–00:37; the Sylvian fissure is split and the MCA aneurysm is explored. The branch originating from the fundus is identified and a temporary aneurysm clip is applied to that branch. 00:38–01:08; An indocyanine green video angiogram is completed and after the surface arteries opacify, the temporary aneurysm clip is removed to identify the cortical branch that opacifies in a delayed fashion to reveal that branch that requires bypassing prior to occlusion at the aneurysm fundus. 01:09–02:42; STA to MCA bypass. 02:43–02:56; A temporary clip is reapplied to the treated branch at the aneurysm fundus to occlude antegrade flow from the M1. A repeat indocyanine green video angiogram confirms patency of the bypass. 02:57–03:16; permanent clipping of the bypassed M2 branch.

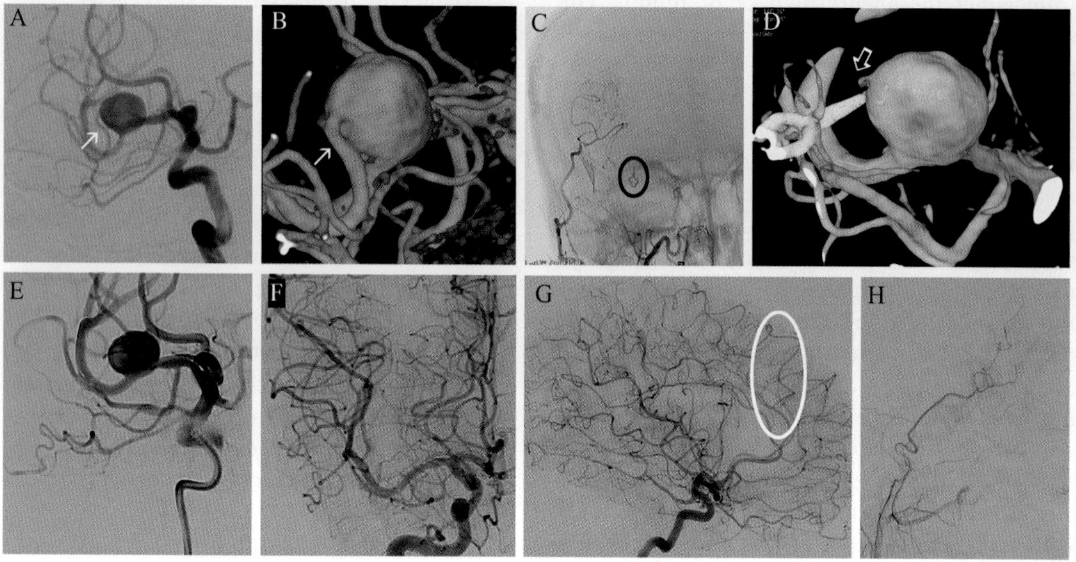

Figure 20.1 A 17-year-old man with a right MCA bifurcation aneurysm, from which a large superior division M2 branch originates from the aneurysm fundus (A and B, white arrows). The patient was brought to the operating room for a superficial temporal artery to middle cerebral artery bypass to the branch that originates from the aneurysm (Video 20.1). Postoperative angiography reveals a patent bypass (C) and aneurysm clip on the bypassed vessel at the aneurysm fundus (C black circle and D open white arrow). (E) A Pipeline embolization device was later placed across the aneurysm neck. (F and G) Follow-up right ICA angiography reveals complete occlusion of the aneurysm, but an anterior MCA distribution filling defect in the late arterial into capillary phase (white circle). (H) Selective right ECA angiography reveals a patent bypass and capillary blush in the region not opacified on the ICA injection.

Arteriovenous Malformations

Combined endovascular and microsurgical treatment of arteriovenous malformations is common in neurosurgical practice and is best accomplished by a multidisciplinary treatment team. Considerations regarding whether to preoperatively embolize an intracranial AVM are the same whether the AVM is in the middle of the right frontal lobe or involves the inferolateral margin of the cerebellum, necessitating a skull base approach. The first consideration is whether the AVM can be embolized with a risk profile that is sufficiently low to achieve commensurate risk-reduction for microsurgical extirpation of the lesion. Before the advent of ethylene vinyl alcohol (EVOH) copolymer liquid embolic agents, such as Onyx or Squid, N-butyl-2-cyanoacrylate (NBCA) glue was the mainstay of embolic treatment of AVMs. Studies have demonstrated that, in appropriately selected cases, intracranial AVMs can be safely embolized with Onyx with a corresponding reduction in blood loss and reduced operative time for surgical removal (16,17).

The sine qua non for safe preoperative endovascular embolization of intracranial AVMs is having an appropriate route of access to the AVM that is free of branches that supply blood to the normal brain. Arterial feeders with proximal branches that run en-passage to the normal brain are typically not safe to embolize, as reflux around the delivery catheter may cause embolization of embolic material into normal brain vessels, resulting in infarction. For particularly eloquent areas with little tolerance for reflux, provocative testing with intraarterial lidocaine or Amytal is often recommended. Several newer technological advances, such as detachable tip microcatheters and dual-lumen balloon microcatheters, have mitigated this consideration to some extent by allowing the interventionist more leeway in driving the embolic material forward toward the AVM while limiting reflux on the delivery catheter. Not only do such catheters aid in safer embolization, but they also limit the risk of "gluing the catheter in." Ultimately, meticulous endovascular technique is required to limit the risk of AVM embolization, and perinidal microcatheter position and slow, controlled delivery of the embolisate are of utmost importance. While transvenous embolization of intracranial AVMs is increasingly described in literature, this technique is most

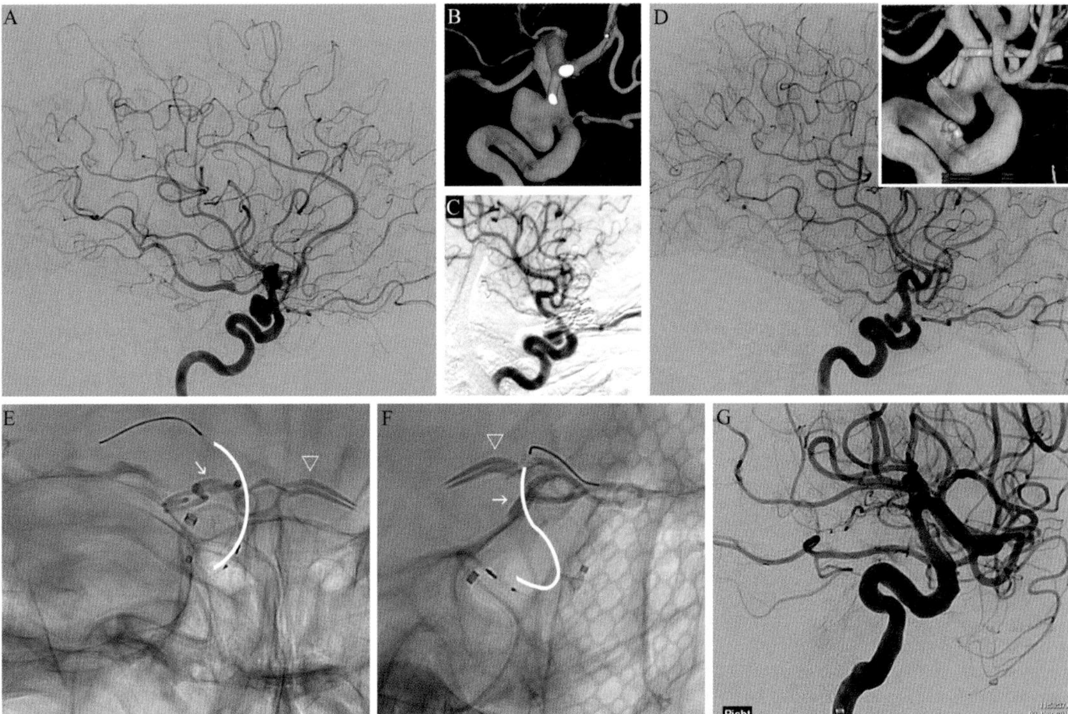

Figure 20.2 A 54-year-old man with bilateral superior hypophyseal artery (SHA) origin ICA aneurysms. A right craniotomy was completed and both aneurysms were clipped. The left SHA aneurysm was completely occluded on intraoperative angiography (IOA, not shown). The right SHA aneurysm could not be entirely clipped, despite removal of the anterior clinoid, opening of the falciform ligament and distal dural ring. (A) Lateral preoperative 2-D angiogram showing the SHA origin ICA aneurysm. (B) 3D right ICA reconstruction. (C) Right ICA IOA revealing partial clipping of the aneurysm, but residual filling via the portion of the neck within the cavernous sinus. (D) Postoperative 2D and 3D (inset) right ICA angiograms confirming residual filling of the aneurysm. (E and F) AP and lateral skull X-rays showing the two 45-degree angled aneurysms clips, one on the left SHA aneurysm (open arrow) and the other on the right SHA aneurysm (white arrow). The residual aneurysm was treated with a Pipeline embolization device as outlined in white. (G) Post-Pipeline angiography reveals occlusion of the right SHA aneurysm.

commonly used in the setting of attempted endovascular cure of the AVM rather than as a surgical adjunct (18).

Many factors are of importance when considering multimodal treatment of intracranial AVMs. The major goals of limiting blood loss, defining the nidus, and increasing the safety of the surgical resection should remain at the forefront of the interventionist's mind when performing a preoperative embolization. Embolization is most helpful if the deepest feeders and the nidus at the furthest point from the surgical approach can be safely embolized. More often than not, if a safe transarterial route to the AVM is identified, such embolization can be achieved in a single session. However, particularly in the setting of large AVMs, multiple sessions spaced over a few days or weeks can be scheduled to most safely achieve the goals of the preoperative embolization (16,17,19,20). In general, larger and higher-grade AVMs are the best candidates for a multimodal approach, as are AVMs where the predominant feeding vessels will not be controlled by the surgeon until late in the operation after significant dissection of the AVM nidus. Smaller AVMs and those with predominant feeding arteries near the surface of the surgical approach are often treated easily with surgery alone, and the added risk of endovascular embolization is not justified. Lastly, great care must be taken not to push embolic material into the predominant draining vein(s), as shutting down the venous outflow of the AVM without complete cure may pressurize the malformation and lead to hemorrhage before the electively planned surgical portion of the case can be completed. To this end, it is prudent to schedule embolization on the day of, or a day or two before, surgical resection to limit the time that the AVM

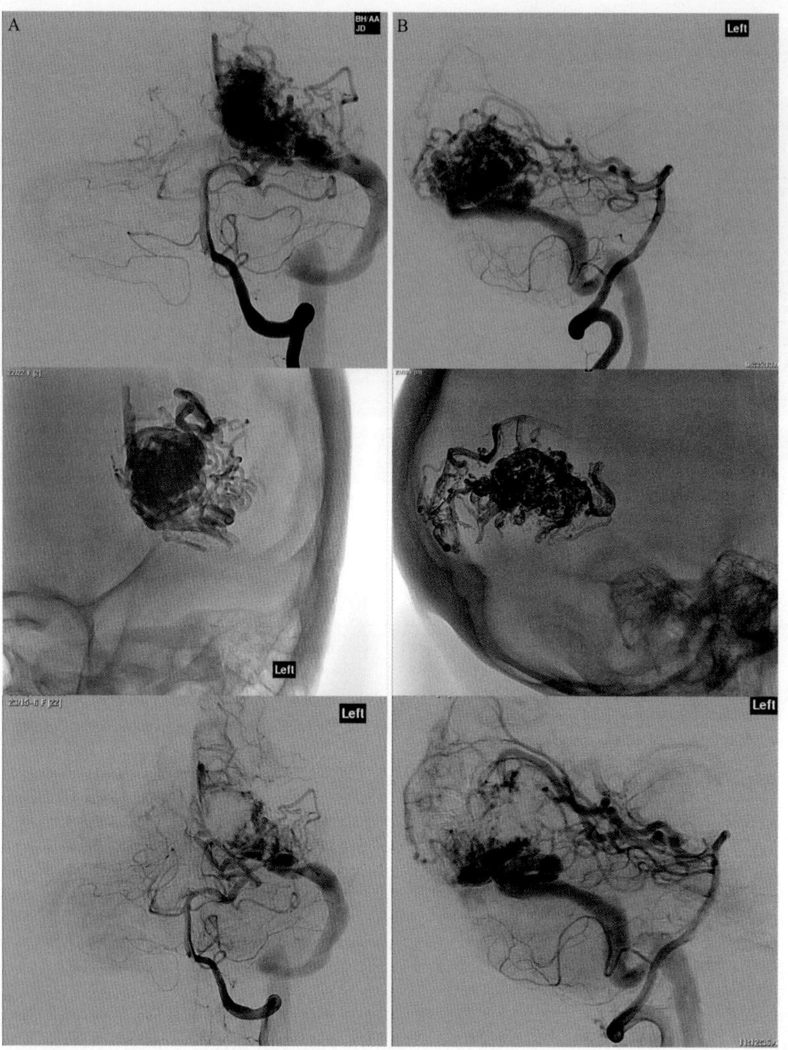

Figure 20.3 A 25-year-old female presented for elective resection of a left mesial occipital AVM centered immediately above the tentorium. She initially came to attention due to subarachnoid hemorrhage from a ruptured basilar artery apex flow-related aneurysm from which she completely recovered. A and B, top panels show AP and lateral angiograms that reveal the AVM. Of note, a single draining vein originated from the antero-infero-lateral aspect of the malformation. A and B, middle panels show the onyx case which demonstrates several of the principles of intracranial vascular malformation embolization discussed above. The PCA pedicle at the anterior-most aspect of the lesion was embolized, as was the pedicle coming over the top of the lesion. In so doing, the depth of the AVM nidus was fully embolized to assist the surgeon at the time of resection. A and B, bottom panels) Near-complete embolization of the nidus is shown; however, the antero-infero-lateral aspect of the AVM was left untreated as this would have risked embolization into the solitary draining vein. In addition, this region was somewhat less critical to embolize in terms of limiting surgical blood loss as the undersurface of the lesion was accessible from a supratentorial corridor, which avoided dissection of normal brain and from the lateral aspect of the embolized nidus more posteriorly which helped to define the surgical plane.

is left with altered hemodynamics prior to removal. The principles described herein are illustrated in Figure 20.3.

Dural Arteriovenous Fistula

dAVFs are arteriovenous malformations, the nidus of which is located within the leaflets of the pachymeninges, with arterial supply primarily from dural branches of the external carotid artery (ECA), the VA, or the ICA, and drainage into a dural venous sinus, leptomeningeal veins, or both (21–23). Additionally, dAVFs can acquire or parasitize pial arterial supply. The underlying cause of these acquired lesions remains unclear. Two main classification systems (Cognard et al. (22) and Borden et al. (21)) are widely used to describe dAVFs and predict their risk of aggressive behavior. While the Cognard system is more versatile in its descriptive power in that it contains many subcategories of fistulae, it is also more complicated. The Borden system is simpler and, in many ways, captures the most clinically important aspect of dAVFs more succinctly. The Borden scale is broken into three main subtypes based on venous drainage: type 1, wherein the venous drainage is entirely antegrade into a dural venous sinus; type 2, involving both antegrade dural venous sinus outflow and retrograde leptomeningeal venous drainage; and type 3, where the venous drainage is either entirely retrograde via leptomeningeal veins or into a trapped, defunctionalized dural venous sinus with reflux into leptomeningeal veins. The latter two types are of most concern, as leptomeningeal venous drainage, sometimes referred to as cortical venous reflux (CVR), is predictive of an aggressive natural history, including progressive neurological deficits and intracranial hemorrhage. dAVFs with CVR confer upwards of 10% mortality and a 15% overall neurological event rate per annum (24). Consequently, any patient who presents with CVR warrants relatively urgent treatment of the dAVF barring extenuating considerations. Since Borden type 1 dAVFs present no risk of intracranial hemorrhage, treatment is controversial and typically reserved only for cases of extreme intolerance to symptoms (pulsatile tinnitus in particular) that has not been addressed by all conservative measures and that is adversely affecting the patient's daily life.

Currently, the majority of dAVFs are treated endovascularly with EVOH via a transarterial route (23,25). Whether an endovascular, surgical, or combined approach is taken, the goal of treatment is the same: to disconnect the recipient vein(s) from the arterial supply. Regarding the safety of the use of liquid embolic agents, the principles outlined previously with intracranial AVMs also apply to the treatment of dAVFs. Transvenous embolization is usually reserved for fistulas that cannot be treated transarterially due to tortuous or complex anatomy, but is the first line of treatment for particular anatomic locations, such as the cavernous sinus.

The surgical management of dAVFs is largely applied to anterior fossa lesions with primary supply via the ethmoidal arteries due to the risk of reflux-induced blindness or stroke associated with endovascular therapy. In addition, surgery is commonly reserved for dAVFs that have failed endovascular treatment and have no additional endovascular access, or for which incomplete endovascular treatment has rendered the lesion high-risk for continued interventional treatment. Again, the surgical management of dAVFs is centered on disconnection of the arterial supply from the venous outflow and typically falls into one of three broad categories: coagulation and division of the solitary draining vein(s), skeletonizing the involved dural sinus if the sinus remains functional, or ligation or packing of a defunctionalized sinus. Alternatively, in rare cases, a combined surgical endovascular approach is chosen to surgically provide access to the recipient venous pouch for direct catheterization and transvenous embolization (Figure 20.4).

Skull Base Tumors

Embolization

Preoperative embolization of tumors is another indication for combined endovascular and microsurgical management of skull base pathology. The predominant tumor types for which preoperative embolization is recommended are meningiomas and hemangiopericytomas; however, any potentially heavily vascularized mass is a candidate for embolization. As with AVMs, the indication for preoperative embolization is to limit intraoperative blood loss and make surgery safer. The principles surrounding safe embolization of AVMs generally apply to the embolization of tumors with some minor differences. The most commonly used agents for embolization of skull base masses are polyvinyl alcohol (PVA) and absorbable gelatin powder (Gelfoam). Additionally, Gelfoam sponges can be formed into pledgets and delivered via a microcatheter to provide proximal arterial feeder occlusion. The size of the Gelfoam or PVA particles used for embolization ranges from approximately 40 to 1,000 microns. To afford the surgeon the best possible hemostasis, embolization of the tumor bulk is more useful than proximal arterial occlusion, as the tumor capsule in many cases parasitizes surrounding microvasculature. Smaller particles (<150 microns) will more deeply penetrate the tumor but will also risk embolization to the surrounding microvasculature, which may result in occlusion of the neurovasorum of the cranial nerves at the skull base or more easily traverse common ECA-to-ICA or VA anastomoses and result in inadvertent intracranial embolization and stroke. To avoid such complications, 150–250 or 250–350 micron PVA, in most cases, will provide sufficient tumor penetration but will minimize the risk of embolization to the microvasculature (Figure 20.5).

Stenting

Stenting of the ICA or VA prior to head and neck surgery for resection of skull base tumors that encase the aforementioned arteries is uncommon

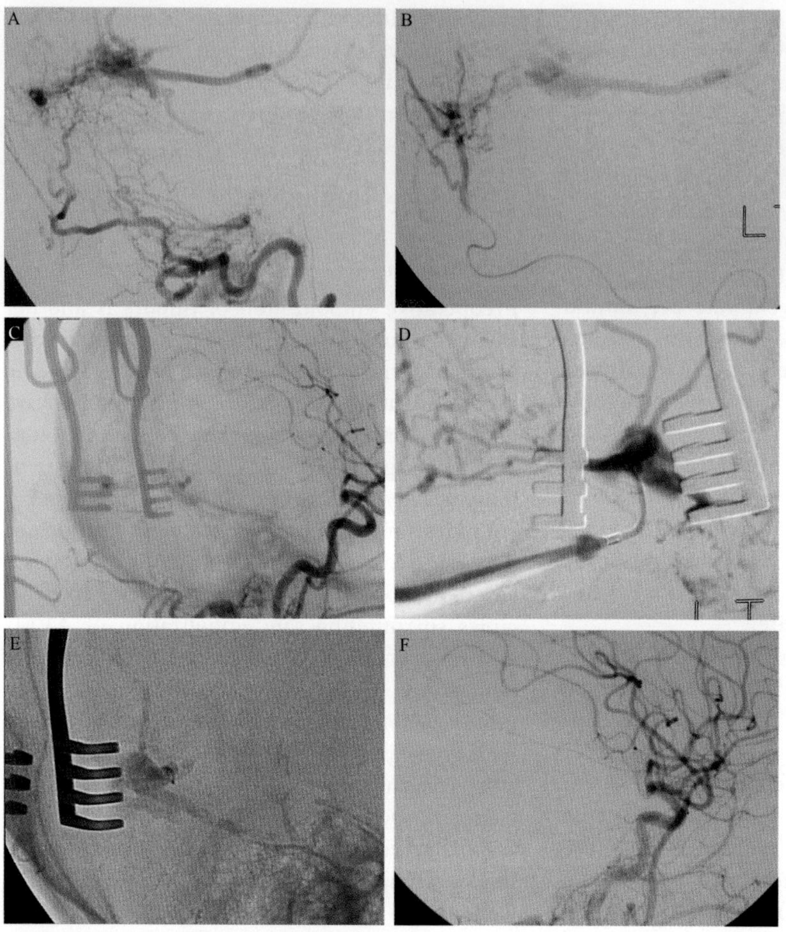

Figure 20.4 A 68-year-old woman with a Borden type 3 dural arteriovenous fistula fed by the left occipital artery. (A) Selective occipital artery injection reveals numerous small, tortuous transosseous branches that supply the fistula and trapped transverse sinus with cortical venous reflux. (B) Catheterization of multiple occipital artery pedicles (one depicted here) did not provide deep enough access to the fistulous site making transarterial embolization with either nBCA or EVOH liquid embolic challenging. Given the trapped sinus, transvenous access was rendered impossible endovascularly. The patient thus underwent surgical placement with a burr hole directly over the trapped left transverse sinus localized by angiography and fluoroscopy. (C) Intraoperative imaging reveals the fistula with a Weitlaner self-retaining retractor positioned over the left transverse sinus. (D) After a burr hole was made, the left transverse sinus was directly accessed and a dimethyl sulfoxide compatible catheter was inserted into the sinus. (E) An Onyx cast is noted within the trapped sinus and draining veins of the shunt. (F) Post embolization angiography shows that the fistula has been occluded.

but potentially beneficial in select cases. The aim in such cases is to provide added structural integrity to the ICA or VA when the tumor surrounds a large proportion of the entire circumference of the vessel. Preoperative stenting is most commonly considered for complex paragangliomas or head and neck cancers that involve the ICA (Figure 20.6; 26–28). The vertebral artery can also be stented prior to tumor resection, but circumstances that require preservation of the vertebral artery are much less common, as surgical or endovascular sacrifice of a unilateral vertebral artery is typically well tolerated, given most patients' anatomy. In addition, surgical access both proximal and distal to the involved vertebral artery is often achievable, which renders preoperative endovascular intervention unnecessary. However, in cases where access to either the proximal or distal vertebral artery is made difficult due to the tumor or patient anatomy, coil sacrifice of the involved VA is an option.

Summary

Interventional neuroradiology techniques can be applied in combination with traditional surgical skull base cerebrovascular and neurosurgical oncology procedures to provide patients with otherwise difficult or seemingly impossible-to-treat problems with potentially curative solutions. In this chapter, we reviewed the indications for and technical nuances surrounding combined interventional neuroradiological and open surgical techniques to skull base pathology.

- Combined interventional neuroradiology techniques can provide a supplement to traditional skull base approaches to improve surgical outcomes.

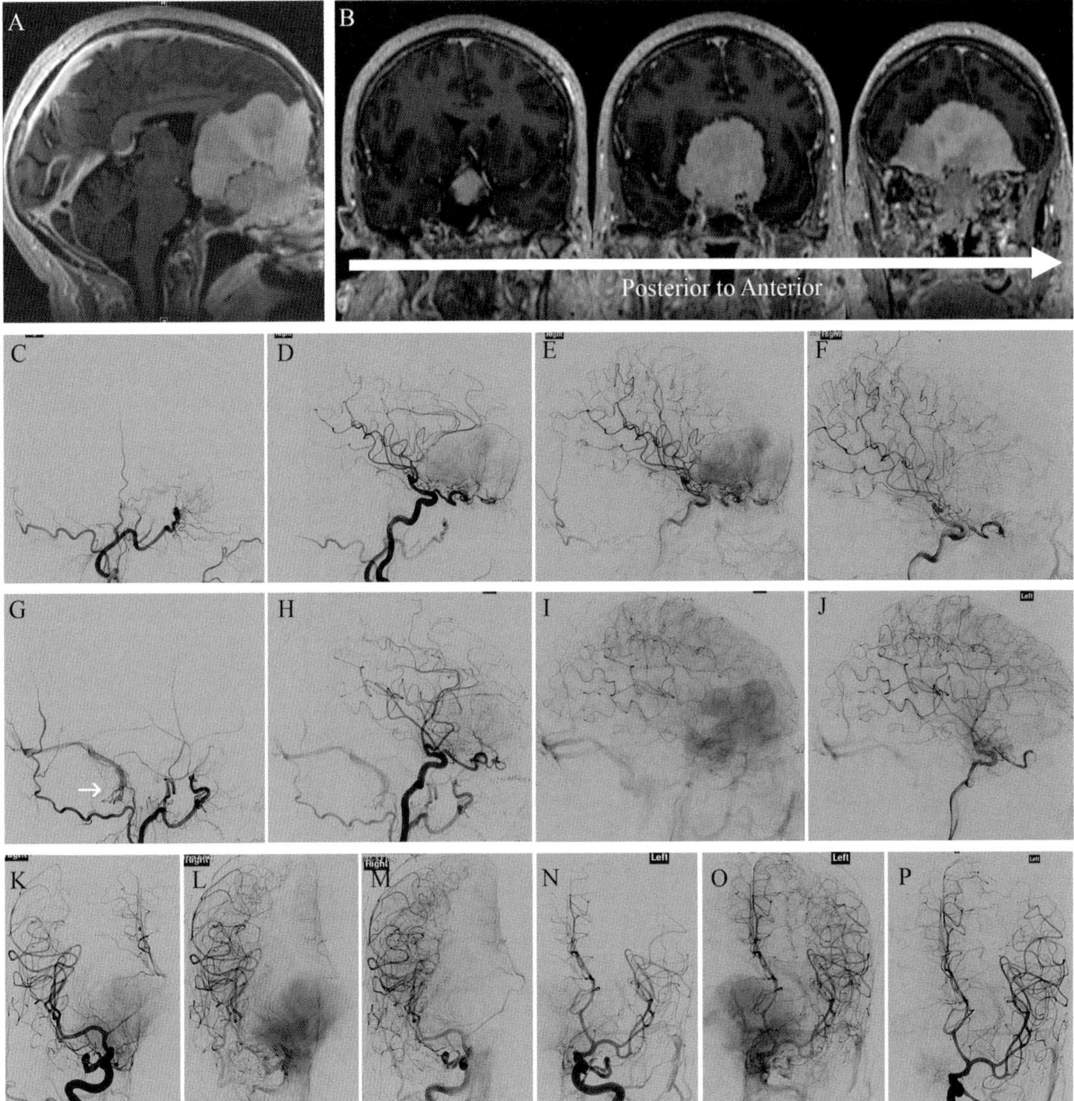

Figure 20.5 A 63-year-old female with a large anterior skull base meningioma. Sagittal (A) and coronal (B) MRI reveal a large planum sphenoidale meningioma with mass effect on the underlying frontal lobes. Diagnostic angiography showed minimal blood supply from the ECA on the right (C) with major blood supply from the anterior and posterior ethmoidal arteries on the selective ICA run (D and E). A microcatheter was advanced into the ophthalmic artery distal to the origin of the central retinal artery and 250–350 micron PVA was used to embolize the tumor with near-complete obliteration of the tumor blush. (G–J) Left ECA and ICA angiograms reveal a similar pattern. An incidental left skull base dural arteriovenous fistula supplied by the ascending pharyngeal artery was noted (white arrow). (K–P) AP angiograms of the right and left ICA before and after PVA embolization.

- Multidisciplinary teamwork and planning are critical to effectively treat these often challenging disease processes effectively.
- Combined interventional neuroradiology and skull base techniques are most often applied to intracranial aneurysms, AVMs, dAVFs, and skull base tumors.

References

1. Uluc K, Kujoth GC, Baskaya MK. Operating microscopes: past, present, and future. *Neurosurg Focus.* 2009;**27**(3):E4.

2. Lawton MT, Quinones-Hinojosa A, Sanai N, Malek JY, Dowd CF. Combined microsurgical and endovascular management of complex intracranial

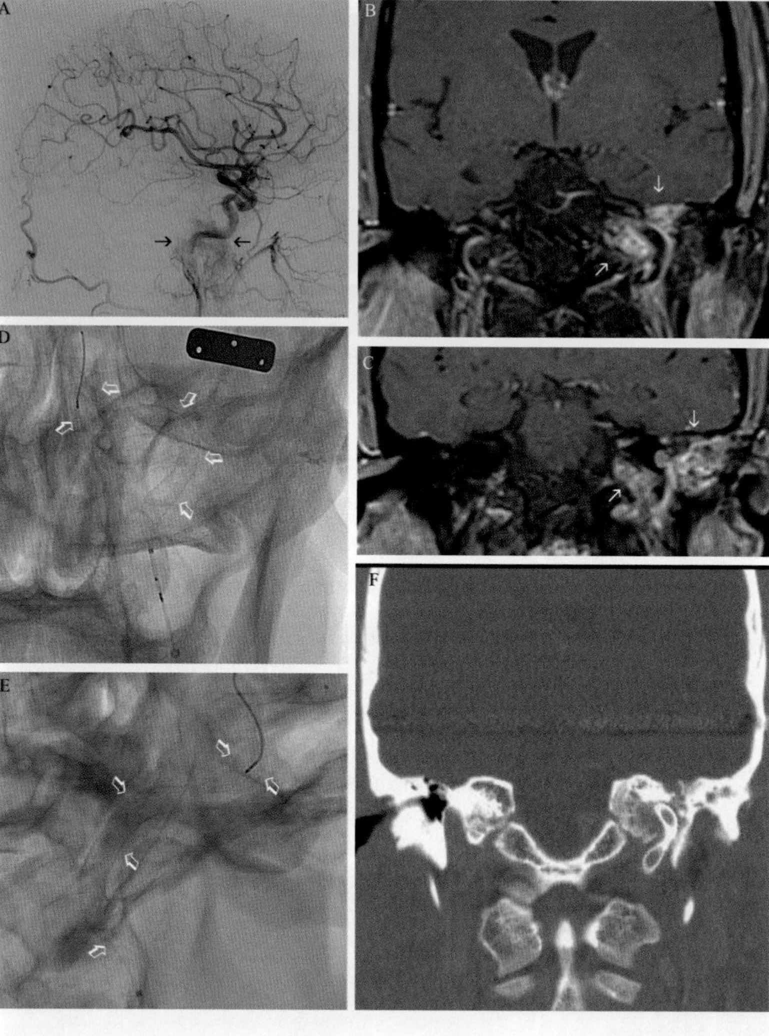

Figure 20.6 A 42-year-old male with a multiply recurrent glomus tympanicum tumor. He underwent three previous resections. He presented to the head and neck surgery clinic with a recurrent tumor in the mastoid and petrous bone, encasing the petrous ICA and invading foramen spinosum, as shown on angiography (A, black arrows) and MRI (B and C, white arrows). Telescoping Pipeline stents were placed from the vertical petrous segment through the distal cervical ICA 6 months prior to surgery to bolster the wall of the ICA prior to surgical resection of the tumor. (D and E) Angiography shows good apposition of the stents to the vessel walls (open white arrows) and delayed CT of the skull base for surgical planning shows the stent within the petrous ICA (F).

aneurysms. *Neurosurgery*. 2003;**52**(2):263–74; discussion 74–5.

3. Mack WJ. Casting a wide net: the unique diversity of neuroendovascular surgery. *J Neurointerv Surg*. 2015;7(8):549–50.
4. Patel PD, Chalouhi N, Atallah E, Tjoumakaris S, Hasan D, Zarzour H, et al. Off-label uses of the Pipeline embolization device: a review of the literature. *Neurosurg Focus*. 2017;**42**(6):E4.
5. Zammar SG, Buell TJ, Chen CJ, Crowley RW, Ding D, Griessenauer CJ, et al. Outcomes after off-label use of the pipeline embolization device for intracranial aneurysms: a multicenter cohort study. *World Neurosurg*. 2018;**115**:e200–e205.
6. Hacein-Bey L, Connolly ES Jr., Mayer SA, Young WL, Pile-Spellman J, Solomon RA. Complex intracranial aneurysms: combined operative and endovascular approaches. *Neurosurgery*. 1998;**43** (6):1304–12; discussion 12–13.
7. Barnett DW, Barrow DL, Joseph GJ. Combined extracranial-intracranial bypass and intraoperative balloon occlusion for the treatment of intracavernous and proximal carotid artery aneurysms. *Neurosurgery*. 1994;**35**(1):92–7; discussion 7–8.
8. Barakate MS, Fisher CM, Appleberg M, Farrar MA, Tse RV, Harrington TJ, et al. Combined endovascular and open surgery for four-vessel cerebrovascular occlusive disease. *J Endovasc Ther*. 2001;**8**(1):62–6.
9. Matsumoto K, Masaki H, Hirai M, Tsujino H, Hashimoto N, Mineura K. Combined surgical and intraoperative endovascular approach for a giant internal carotid artery aneurysm in the high cervical region. *Minim Invasive Neurosurg*. 2002;**45**(2):112–13.
10. Wallace AN, Kamran M, Madaelil TP, Kayan Y, Osbun JW, Roy AK, et al. Endovascular treatment of posterior inferior cerebellar artery aneurysms

with flow diversion. *World Neurosurg*. 2018;**114**: e581–e587.

11. Wallace AN, Madaelil TP, Kamran M, Miller TR, Delgado Almandoz JE, Grossberg JA, et al. Pipeline embolization of vertebrobasilar aneurysms – a multicenter case series. *World Neurosurg*. 2019;S1878-8750(18):32939-5.
12. Becske T, Kallmes DF, Saatci I, McDougall CG, Szikora I, Lanzino G, et al. Pipeline for uncoilable or failed aneurysms: results from a multicenter clinical trial. *Radiology*. 2013;**267**(3):858–68.
13. Becske T, Potts MB, Shapiro M, Kallmes DF, Brinjikji W, Saatci I, et al. Pipeline for uncoilable or failed aneurysms: 3-year follow-up results. *J Neurosurg*. 2017;**127**(1):81–8.
14. Mokin M, Chinea A, Primiani CT, Ren Z, Kan P, Srinivasan VM, et al. Treatment of blood blister aneurysms of the internal carotid artery with flow diversion. *J Neurointerv Surg*. 2018;**10**(11):1074–8.
15. Sato K, Endo H, Fujimura M, Endo T, Matsumoto Y, Shimizu H, et al. Endovascular treatments in combination with extracranial-intracranial bypass for complex intracranial aneurysms. *World Neurosurg*. 2018;**113**:e747–60.
16. Natarajan SK, Ghodke B, Britz GW, Born DE, Sekhar LN. Multimodality treatment of brain arteriovenous malformations with microsurgery after embolization with onyx: single-center experience and technical nuances. *Neurosurgery*. 2008;**62**(6):1213–25; discussion 25–6.
17. Loh Y, Duckwiler GR, Onyx Trial I. A prospective, multicenter, randomized trial of the Onyx liquid embolic system and N-butyl cyanoacrylate embolization of cerebral arteriovenous malformations. Clinical article. *J Neurosurg*. 2010;**113**(4):733–41.
18. Rangel-Castilla L, Shallwani H, Siddiqui AH. Transvenous embolization of thalamic arteriovenous malformation under transient cardiac standstill. *Neurosurg Focus*. 2019;**46**(Suppl 1):V10.
19. Del Maestro M, Luzzi S, Gallieni M, Trovarelli D, Giordano AV, Gallucci M, et al. Surgical treatment of arteriovenous malformations: role of preoperative staged embolization. *Acta Neurochir Suppl*. 2018;**129**:109–13.
20. Luzzi S, Del Maestro M, Bongetta D, Zoia C, Giordano AV, Trovarelli D, et al. Onyx embolization before the surgical treatment of grade iii spetzler-martin brain arteriovenous malformations: single-center experience and technical nuances. *World Neurosurg*. 2018;**116**: e340–e53.
21. Borden JA, Wu JK, Shucart WA. A proposed classification for spinal and cranial dural arteriovenous fistulous malformations and implications for treatment. *J Neurosurg*. 1995;**82**(2):166–79.
22. Cognard C, Gobin YP, Pierot L, Bailly AL, Houdart E, Casasco A, et al. Cerebral dural arteriovenous fistulas: clinical and angiographic correlation with a revised classification of venous drainage. *Radiology*. 1995;**194**(3):671–80.
23. Natarajan SK, Ghodke B, Kim LJ, Hallam DK, Britz GW, Sekhar LN. Multimodality treatment of intracranial dural arteriovenous fistulas in the Onyx era: a single center experience. *World Neurosurg*. 2010;**73**(4):365–79.
24. van Dijk JM, terBrugge KG, Willinsky RA, Wallace MC. Clinical course of cranial dural arteriovenous fistulas with long-term persistent cortical venous reflux. *Stroke*. 2002;**33**(5):1233–6.
25. Howard BM, Grossberg JA, Prater A, Cawley CM, Dion JE, Tong FC. Incompletely obliterated cranial arteriovenous fistulae are safely and effectively treated with adjuvant epsilon-aminocaproic acid. *J Neurointerv Surg*. 2018;**10**(7):698–703.
26. Piazza P, Di Lella F, Bacciu A, Di Trapani G, Ait Mimoune H, Sanna M. Preoperative protective stenting of the internal carotid artery in the management of complex head and neck paragangliomas: long-term results. *Audiol Neurootol*. 2013;**18**(6):345–52.
27. Markiewicz MR, Pirgousis P, Bryant C, Cunningham JC, Dagan R, Sandhu SJ, et al. Preoperative protective endovascular covered stent placement followed by surgery for management of the cervical common and internal carotid arteries with tumor encasement. *J Neurol Surg B Skull Base*. 2017;**78**(1):52–8.
28. Bacciu A, Prasad SC, Sist N, Rossi G, Piazza P, Sanna M. Management of the cervico-petrous internal carotid artery in class C tympanojugular paragangliomas. *Head Neck*. 2016;**38**(6):899–905.

Chapter 21

Combined Transsylvian-Subtemporal Approach to Anterior Circulation and Basilar Apex Aneurysms

James G. Malcolm and Daniel L. Barrow

Introduction

Over the past several decades, outcomes in the open surgical treatment of posterior circulation aneurysms have steadily improved. This progress has been largely due to the development of microsurgery and its many adjuncts, such as advances in neuroanesthesia and brain protection, temporary clips, modern permanent aneurysm clips, intraoperative imaging, bypass techniques, skull base surgery, and specialty training of individuals allowing them to concentrate on cerebrovascular disease. Posterior circulation aneurysms, including those of the basilar apex, have been among the most challenging to treat. Surgery in this area is especially treacherous due to the deep location, as well as the close proximity of perforators to the brainstem. Basilar tip aneurysms are also less frequently encountered than aneurysms of the anterior circulation, making it more difficult to master the nuances of their surgical treatment. With advances in endovascular tools and techniques, more of these aneurysms can be treated without the morbidity of an open craniotomy, which has further reduced the experience and exposure of trainees in recent decades.

The first description of a BA aneurysm dates back to 1779, when Morgagni presented a case of an aneurysm involving the basilar artery and both posterior cerebral arteries (PCAs) (1). Little progress was made concerning the identification and treatment of posterior circulation aneurysms until the mid-twentieth century. In the 1950s, the subtemporal approach was developed, and it was during this time that Charles Drake emerged as a pioneer in the surgical management of basilar tip aneurysms (2). In 1959, he presented his experience with four patients presenting with subarachnoid hemorrhage (SAH) from basilar bifurcation aneurysms (3). Although two of his patients succumbed to complications due to their initial hemorrhage, his case description laid the groundwork for standards of BA aneurysm treatment. Review of the literature over two decades prior to the publication of Drake's paper had identified 38 cases of aneurysms involving the vertebrobasilar (VB) circulation. Following Drake's publication, additional literature was published concerning the treatment and outcome of basilar aneurysms. In 1964, Jamieson reviewed his operative experience of 19 patients with VB aneurysms (4). Only four of those patients made a sufficient enough recovery to return to work. As Drake's experience with BA aneurysms grew, his results also improved in parallel.

Part of his success was attributable to advances in microinstruments and microsurgical technique, including the use of the surgical microscope. Ultimately, these factors culminated in improved surgical outcomes for Drake's patients harboring BA aneurysms. In a 1968 report, Drake described his experience after treating 17 basilar artery aneurysms with only one fatality (5). As part of his legacy, in 1996, two years prior to his death, Drake published his 25 years of experience treating 1,767 aneurysms of the VB system (6). The vast majority of these patients (72%) harbored aneurysms at the basilar bifurcation or PCAs. Drake reported excellent outcomes in 70–80% of his patients who initially presented with a good-grade SAH and those who harbored non-giant BA aneurysms. Drake's chapter continues to be the standard against which other series involving basilar artery aneurysms are judged.

The approach to posterior circulation aneurysms has been significantly impacted by endovascular techniques with the introduction of detachable coils in 1991 (7). The current era of minimally invasive procedures for the treatment of VB circulation aneurysms is uniquely different from what Drake and his colleagues experienced. This chapter focuses on those aneurysms that are not amenable to endovascular management and thus require open microsurgical treatment. This also includes patients with multiple aneurysms where one or more are not suitable for endovascular therapy but can be addressed by a single surgical procedure.

Traditionally, the two approaches used to expose the rostral BA for clipping aneurysms were the subtemporal approach introduced by Drake and the transsylvian or pterional approach popularized by Yasargil. Both of these approaches have assets and liabilities, and both have modifications to expand the field of view (Table 21.1).

For isolated basilar tip aneurysms, the relationship of the aneurysm neck to the posterior clinoid process typically dictates which of these approaches is selected. Aneurysms with a low bifurcation relative to the posterior clinoid are often best visualized through an anterior subtemporal approach, whereas those with a high bifurcation are better visualized through a transsylvian approach. With particularly high bifurcations, an orbitozygomatic extension of the transsylvian approach provides an enhanced view of the upper limits of the interpeduncular cistern (11). Also, removal of the posterior clinoid process can provide exposure of the more proximal basilar artery for temporary occlusion if necessary. Aneurysms arising at or below the middle depth of the sella are best approached via a subtemporal craniotomy, often combined with additional skull base techniques such as removal of the petrous apex (Kawase approach) (8). We have employed all of these techniques in treating BA aneurysms at our institution. For select basilar aneurysms, and particularly when patients harbor both anterior and posterior circulation aneurysms, the advantages of the pterional transsylvian craniotomy, in combination with some elements of the subtemporal craniotomy (half-and-half approach), provide optimal exposure and allow for the management of multiple aneurysms with a single microsurgical procedure.

Indications and Contraindications

The transsylvian-subtemporal (half and half) approach is designed for specific rostral BA aneurysms where the use of both transsylvian and subtemporal exposures may provide better visualization than either approach alone or, more commonly, when concurrent aneurysms of the anterior (transsylvian) and posterior (subtemporal) circulation can be treated with one procedure. Clinical decision-making must be individualized, and it is not possible to outline every indication for the decision to treat a BA aneurysm by surgical clip ligation. If a BA aneurysm is treatable by endovascular techniques, that is often the best choice for individual patients and is usually preferred. For those patients who are poor operative candidates, observation alone may be considered, or endovascular management of the ruptured aneurysm and delayed management of an unruptured aneurysm may be appropriate. For patients who are not ideal candidates for endovascular therapy, surgical clip ligation should

Table 21.1 Benefits and risks of the transsylvian and subtemporal approaches

Transsylvian		Subtemporal	
assets	**Liabilities**	**assets**	**Liabilities**
Familiarity	Low bifurcation	Proximal control	Inability to trap
Proximal control/trap	Poor perforator visualization	Improved visualization and access to perforators	Narrow operating field
Increased operating space	Not recommended for anterior/posterior projected aneurysms	Widened exposure by tentorial division	Poor visualization of the contralateral P1
Blood evacuation		Best for anterior/posterior projected aneurysms	Risk of CN III palsy
No retraction			Risk of injury to temporal lobe
Best for non-anterior or posterior projected aneurysms			Not recommended for obese patients

be considered. This includes younger patients; patients with another aneurysm that is not amenable to endovascular therapy but who are otherwise good surgical candidates for the elimination of all aneurysms with a single procedure; patients with an acute subarachnoid hemorrhage whose endovascular therapy would require the use of dual antiplatelet therapy; or patients with a large hematoma requiring surgical evacuation.

The introduction of detachable coils for the treatment of saccular aneurysms introduced a new chapter in the field of cerebrovascular surgery. No longer was it necessary to treat every aneurysm with a major craniotomy, including challenging cases in the posterior circulation. Coiling did not gain wide acceptance until the milestone publication of the International Subarachnoid Aneurysm Trial (ISAT) (9). The data from ISAT helped make the use of endovascular therapy for the treatment of saccular aneurysms mainstream. Ninety-seven percent of the patients enrolled in the ISAT trial harbored aneurysms that were in the anterior circulation, so we learned little about the outcome of posterior circulation aneurysms from that study. The International Study of Unruptured Intracranial Aneurysms in 2003 further supported endovascular therapy as a treatment modality for cerebral aneurysms (10). The investigators concluded that for any posterior circulation aneurysm 12 mm or larger, the chance of poor outcome was significantly greater in the surgical group compared with the endovascular group. Successful endovascular therapy for the treatment of BA aneurysms has been well documented in the literature, with the procedural morbidity and mortality rates ranging from 3–9% (11–13). This has made coil embolization of these aneurysms the first line of treatment at many institutions. However, with reported recurrence rates as high as 17.5%, coiling of these aneurysms may not be the definitive treatment in every instance. In addition, with recurrence rates greater than 50% for large and giant BA aneurysms, endovascular therapy is not always suitable for larger lesions.

Wide-neck aneurysms of the BA have posed another challenge for endovascular techniques. Initially, these aneurysms were difficult to embolize due to their poor dome-to-neck ratio (less than 2:1). To address some of these limitations, several new devices have been developed to stent and divert flow from the aneurysm. These devices have enabled neuro-interventionalists to treat aneurysms that were not previously amenable to coil embolization. There have been limitations to the use of these devices, however. For example, their use is limited in patients with SAHs because of the need for dual antiplatelet therapy to prevent parent vessel thrombosis (14).

Review of Relevant Anatomy

The basilar tip and PCAs are located in the confined space of the interpeduncular cistern. They are enclosed by the posterior clinoids and clivus anteriorly, mesial temporal lobes laterally, cerebral peduncles posteriorly, and mammillary bodies superiorly. The BA is approximately 15 mm posterior to the internal carotid artery (ICA) (15). The termination of the BA gives rise to bilateral PCAs. The superior cerebellar arteries (SCAs) arise immediately proximal to the basilar bifurcation. The oculomotor nerve exits between the PCAs and the SCAs and is therefore vulnerable to injury during surgery. The segment of the PCA from its origin from the BA to the ostium of the posterior communicating artery (PCOM) is referred to as the P1 segment of the PCA. The PCA distal to the PCOM is also known as the P2 segment. The P2 segment extends from the PCOM to the posterior edge of the midbrain. Flow to the PCA territory may run predominantly from the PCOM in cases of a fetal PCOM that occurs in 15–40% of the population. Anterior thalamoperforators typically arise from the PCOM. These vessels supply a portion of the cerebral peduncles, posterior thalamus, subthalamic nucleus, optic chiasm, tuber cinereum, and mammillary bodies. The posterior thalamoperforators usually arise from the BA or the proximal P1 segments. These vessels supply the thalamus, hypothalamus, posterior limb of the internal capsule, and subthalamic nucleus. There may be considerable variation in the configuration and areas supplied by the anterior and posterior thalamoperforators. Due to the extent of the vascular territories supplied by these vessels, the compromise of any of these perforators can lead to devastating results.

Surgical Technique

The half-and-half is a hybrid approach combining the advantages of both the transsylvian and subtemporal approaches. The transsylvian approach is familiar to most neurosurgeons, since it is utilized for many standard aneurysms of the anterior circulation and for tumors in the suprasellar region. Exposure of both the basilar trunk and the bilateral P1 segments is straightforward, allowing for temporary clip placement if needed for aneurysm trapping. The primary disadvantage of the transsylvian approach is that there is poor access to the posterior aspect of the interpeduncular fossa, where the thalamoperforators are located. With the subtemporal approach, the posterior perforators are more readily visualized than they are in a frontotemporal approach. A lateral trajectory facilitates visualization and dissection of posterior perforators, especially for posteriorly projecting aneurysms. Preservation of these perforators is perhaps the most crucial objective of these procedures. Proximal control is also easy to obtain with this approach. As the surgeon is working along the axis of the aneurysm neck, aneurysm clips can be placed with optimal visualization of the aneurysm neck as well as of the thalamoperforators. Lastly, division of the tentorium and even removal of the petrous apex through this approach allows for exposure of the upper third of the clivus for access to low-lying bifurcations. The subtemporal craniotomy does have some disadvantages. There is poor visualization of the contralateral P1 through the narrow corridor; cranial nerve III (CN III) is centered in the field, which often leads to postoperative oculomotor nerve palsies; and excessive retraction may lead to temporal lobe injury.

The half-and-half approach has many similarities to the standard pterional craniotomy pioneered by Yasargil (16). In addition to the pterional craniotomy, an extensive subtemporal craniectomy is performed, providing exposure of the anterior temporal tip and the floor of the middle cranial fossa. The additional bone removal allows the surgeon to mobilize the temporal lobe superiorly and laterally, providing the surgeon with a wider corridor for approaching BA aneurysms. Alternatively, this approach provides for separate transsylvian and subtemporal exposures during the same procedure for clip ligation of separate aneurysms.

Neuroanesthesia

Brain relaxation is crucial for maximum exposure of the surgical site and minimization of retraction during the operation. In addition to CSF drainage through the sequential opening of the basilar cisterns, intracranial relaxation is achieved by administration of 50–100 g of mannitol (0.5–1 g per kilogram of body weight) prior to entering the cranium. If further relaxation is necessary, furosemide (0.5–1 mg/kg) is given intravenously. If necessary, sympathetic agonists are used to maintain mean arterial pressure (MAP) within 20% of the patient's baseline pressure. Respiratory parameters are adjusted to keep the $PaCO_2$ between 32 and 44 mm Hg, with a PaO2 target greater than 100 mm Hg. Continuous assessment of fluid status is facilitated by closely monitoring hourly urine output and central venous pressure.

When temporary clip occlusion of a parent vessel is necessary, a set of standard steps is initiated prior to clip placement. The MAP is kept above 90 mm Hg to augment collateral blood flow. Burst suppression for cerebral protection is achieved by supplementing the anesthetic with intravenous pentobarbital or propofol. Permissive hypothermia is closely monitored, and the patient is cooled to maintain a body temperature of at least 32°C. Temporary vessel occlusion is limited to as short an interval as possible to prevent ischemic injury. This technique softens the aneurysm sac, facilitating clip placement at the neck. As the aneurysm sac softens, identification of perforator vessels is also achieved more easily. To lower the risk of recurrent hemorrhage prior to surgery, we routinely place our SAH patients on the lysine analog ε-aminocaproic acid (Amicar, Xanodyne Pharmaceuticals) with a 5 g intravenous bolus followed by a 1 g/hr maintenance dose. We stop this infusion following clip placement.

We do not routinely perform electroencephalography or brain stem auditory evoked potentials (BAEPs) when treating BA aneurysms. An exception is made when treating giant or complex BA aneurysms using deep hypothermic circulatory arrest. This technique is a useful adjunct in the treatment of complex intracranial aneurysms, particularly when prolonged cerebral hypoperfusion is needed (17). In these situations, we use electroencephalography, spontaneous somatosensory evoked potentials (SSEPs), and BAEPs in conjunction with deep hypothermic (18°C) circulatory arrest. The suppression of electroencephalogram activity by barbiturates is used to titrate an effective dose for cerebral protection. The SSEPs are an indicator of intact sensory pathway conduction and persist despite burst suppression.

Positioning and Scalp Incision

The outlined procedure assumes a right-sided craniotomy. Where there is flexibility in choice, a right-sided approach is used to avoid injury to the dominant temporal lobe. A left-sided approach is used when there is a preexisting left CN III palsy or right hemiparesis or if aneurysmal anatomy favors a left-sided approach. In addition, for right-handed neurosurgeons, the trajectory afforded by a right-sided approach is more familiar and intuitive.

The patient is placed supine on the operating room table with a right shoulder roll and the head placed in rigid pin fixation. We use a radiolucent headrest and adapter that allows unobstructed, zero-artifact views during intraoperative angiography. A single pin is placed over the left frontal region, and additional pins are placed in the right mastoid and occipital regions, respectively. The head is rotated approximately 30 degrees to the left with slight neck extension, placing the malar eminence at the highest point of the operating field. Although fixed retractors are rarely used for the transsylvian approach, we routinely secure the Budde Halo retraction system to the headrest in the event it is urgently needed and utilize gentle retraction for the subtemporal portion of the procedure. The microscope and surgical chair are also draped and ready for use prior to skin incision. The incision begins 1 cm anterior to the tragus at the root of the zygomatic arch. The incision curves forward gently past the midline to where the hairline intersects with the contralateral midpupillary line. The scalp flap is elevated anteriorly with blunt and sharp dissection, leaving the fascia of the temporalis muscle intact. The skin flap is retracted using fishhooks connected to a Leyla bar. The subgaleal fat pad is identified in the pterional region. The temporalis muscle and fascia are divided posterior to the fat pad and perpendicular to the zygomatic root, to avoid injury to the frontalis branch of the facial nerve. The muscle is also divided along the superior temporal line, leaving a fascial cuff to facilitate reapproximation of the muscle later in the procedure. The posterior limb of the muscle is retracted posteriorly and is secured using a 2-0 Vicryl suture. The anterior limb of the dissected muscle is retracted anteriorly with the scalp flap and secured using the fishhook-Leyla bar construct (Figure 21.1).

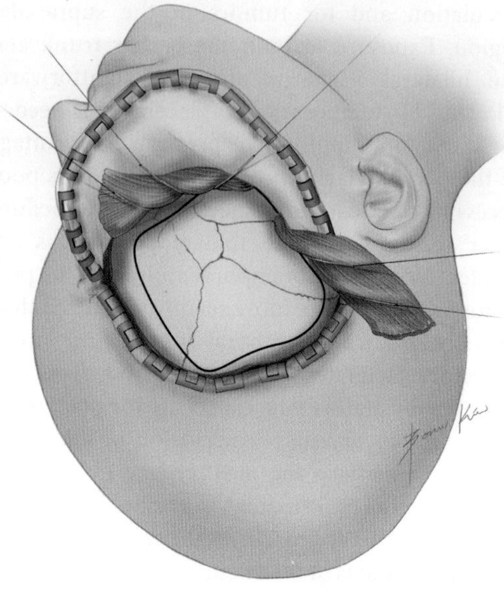

Figure 21.1 Muscular exposure for a transsylvian approach

Craniotomy

Burr holes are placed at the posterior extent of the superior temporal line, the keyhole, and the root of the zygoma. A craniotome is used to connect the burr holes, making a circular bone flap with its superior edge extending to the level of the ipsilateral midpupillary line. The posterior edge extends to the edge of the scalp flap. The inferior edge is marked by the root of the zygoma, and the anterior border is marked by the sphenoid ridge. A round cutting burr is used to drill inferiorly until flush with the floor of the middle fossa, allowing for visualization of the anterior temporal tip. The superior rim of the zygomatic arch may be drilled to achieve bone removal flush with the floor of the middle fossa. The same drill attachment is used to generously drill the lateral sphenoid wing flat to the level of the superior orbital fissure (Figure 21.2). Once the bone work is complete, hemostasis is achieved using bone wax and oxidized cellulose.

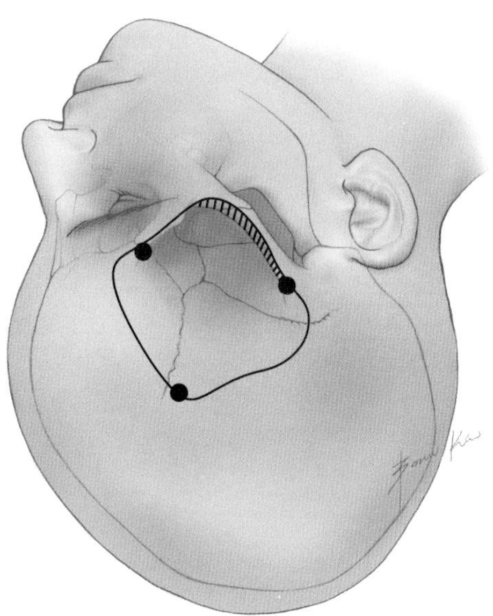

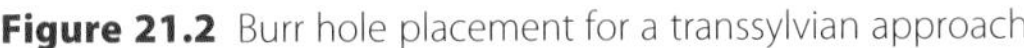

Figure 21.2 Burr hole placement for a transsylvian approach

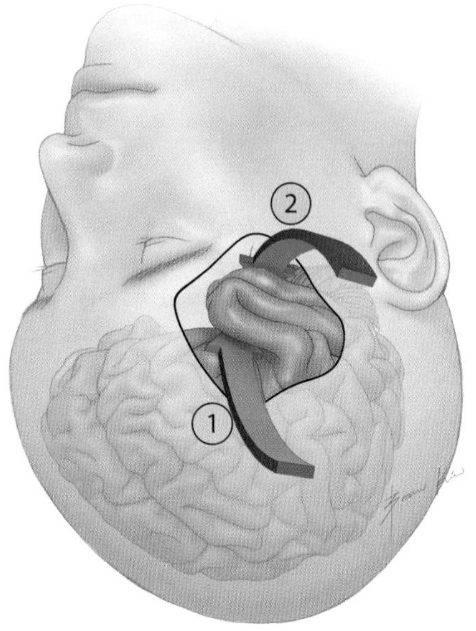

Figure 21.3 Brain exposure allowed via a right-sided transsylvian approach

Subarachnoid Dissection and Clip Application

The dura is opened in a curvilinear fashion with an anteriorly based flap and secured anteriorly using a 3–0 Vicryl suture. If further relaxation is needed and a ventriculostomy is not in place, a ventriculostomy is inserted at Paine's point, allowing CSF drainage from the lateral ventricles (18). The surgical microscope is brought into the field at this time. The use of a mouthpiece on the microscope frees the surgeon's hands and allows subtle angle and focus adjustments during the dissection that optimize visualization during clip application. The operating table is lowered, and the surgical chair is positioned for optimal comfort.

Generally, no fixed retractors are used for the transsylvian portion of the procedure; dynamic retraction with microinstruments is used to gain exposure. As the cisterns are progressively opened, brain relaxation enhances exposure. The Sylvian fissure is opened, and the middle cerebral artery is followed to the carotid bifurcation, proximal ICA, and optic nerves. The fissure is typically opened distal-to-proximal, but this can vary based on individual Sylvian fissure anatomy and the presence of anterior circulation aneurysms. This exposure and approach provide the option of exposing the rostral basilar artery through either the Sylvian fissure or an anterior subtemporal route (Figure 21.3). The opticocarotid and pre-chiasmatic cisterns are opened sharply to free the frontal lobe further. There are three anatomic triangles through which the rostral BA may be exposed: the opticocarotid, the carotid-oculomotor, and the supracarotid. The carotid-oculomotor is the most often used. Any aneurysms of the anterior circulation are addressed through the transsylvian approach, including ICA and anterior communicating or MCA aneurysms. If the BA artery aneurysm is well visualized through the Sylvian fissure approach, it can be clipped without the subtemporal exposure. If there are anterior circulation aneurysms, we attempt to clip the BA aneurysm first so that the clips on the anterior circulation aneurysm(s) do not obscure the view of the BA.

The membrane of Liliequist is opened to provide clear visualization of the interpeduncular cistern and facilitate potential clot removal. The PCOM is followed to its junction with the PCA (P1-P2 junction). The SCA is identified and followed around the curve of the cerebral peduncle

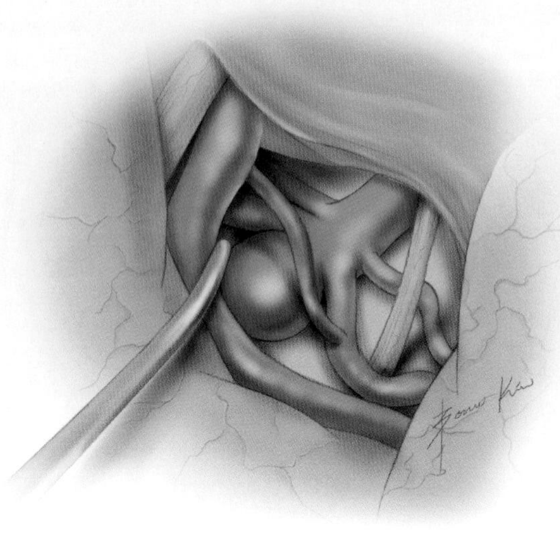

Figure 21.4 View of the vascular anatomy allowed via a transsylvian approach

to its junction with the basilar trunk. The BA is dissected free of its arachnoid adhesions in preparation for temporary clipping. The P1 segment is then identified above CN III and followed medially to the BA. Dissection of the arachnoid around the BA also brings the contralateral P1 into view (Figure 21.4). Visualization of the basilar trunk, bilateral P1 segments, and SCAs allows trapping of the aneurysm if needed. Occasionally, removal of the posterior clinoid process is required to expose the BA for proximal control and temporary clipping. In recent years, we have used an ultrasonic drill rather than a pneumatic drill for this purpose.

In the traditional half-and-half approach, the temporal lobe is retracted laterally to expand the view to include an anterior temporal approach, thus creating a more panoramic view of the rostral basilar artery. This usually requires the sacrifice of draining veins at the tip of the temporal lobe to retract the temporal lobe away from the tentorium. We have used the combined approach more often in recent times to clip anterior circulation aneurysms through the transsylvian approach and rostral basilar aneurysms through an anterior subtemporal approach. The latter typically requires gentle elevation of the temporal lobe with fixed retractors but does not require sacrificing of the anterior temporal veins.

If the BA aneurysm is better exposed through a subtemporal approach, the anterior temporal lobe is gently elevated with multiple fixed retractors to avoid the potential injury from a single retractor attempting to lift the temporal lobe from the floor of the middle fossa. Every attempt is made to preserve all veins. CN III is identified, and all efforts are made not to dissect the III nerve from its arachnoid encasement, if possible. It is helpful at this point to place a small suture into the free edge of the tentorium, anchoring it to the floor of the middle cranial fossa, avoiding the trochlear nerve running in the free edge of the tentorium. This maneuver provides 3 to 4 mm of additional exposure in the surgical field (Figure 21.5). With exposure of the BA from either the transsylvian or subtemporal approach, it is imperative that the surgeon identify both PCAs and the thalamoperforating arteries that may be adherent to the back wall of the aneurysm. Proximal control is usually more straightforward with the subtemporal exposure. If temporary occlusion is used, we typically ask our anesthesiologist to initiate burst suppression and increase blood pressure at this time. A temporary clip is placed across the basilar trunk. Gentle traction with the microsuction can be placed on the fundus of the aneurysm to displace it anteriorly. This maneuver allows better visualization of the posterior thalamoperforators that need to be dissected off of the aneurysm and

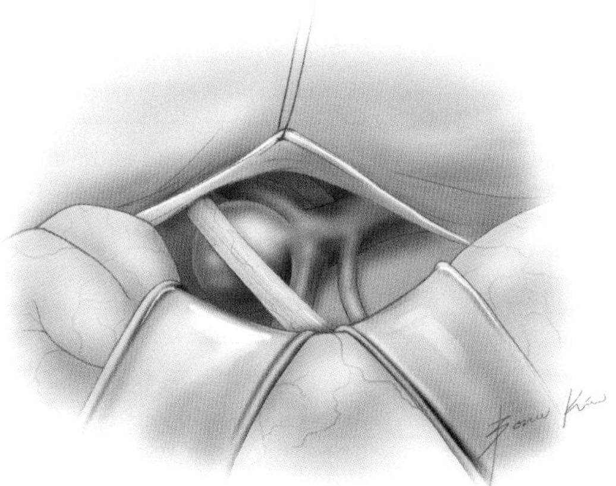

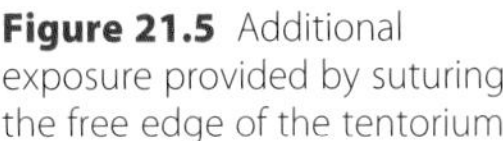
Figure 21.5 Additional exposure provided by suturing the free edge of the tentorium

displaced posteriorly, as they often adhere to the neck and dome of the aneurysm. Through the transsylvian approach, a straight clip is most often utilized for basilar apex aneurysms, but clip choice is dictated by the particular anatomy. For wide-necked aneurysms, the tandem clipping technique is often used, where a fenestrated clip is placed so the blades obliterate the distal neck and a straight clip is used to occlude that portion of the neck passing through the aperture. Through the subtemporal approach, it is often necessary to use a fenestrated clip with the fenestration encircling the ipsilateral PCA and the blades obliterating the neck. Smaller aneurysms can typically be clipped using standard straight clips placed in tandem. We typically use clips that are similar in size to the length of the aneurysm neck. The use of a longer clip may compromise perforators on the contralateral P1. Using the suction tip, the aneurysm may be retracted anteriorly to better visualize the thalamoperforating arteries. Once the initial clip is applied, it may be necessary to place a second clip above the initial one to completely secure the aneurysm. We routinely use intraoperative indocyanine green videography and intraoperative angiography following clipping to evaluate perforators, larger vessels, and any residual aneurysm.

Conclusions

The young history of basilar tip aneurysms is interesting. In the early nineteenth century, the diagnosis of a ruptured basilar tip aneurysm ultimately led to certain mortality. The pioneering work of Drake paved the way for the successful treatment of these treacherous aneurysms. With each passing decade, as microsurgical techniques and endovascular methods have improved, so have patient outcomes. The presence of a BA aneurysm no longer carries the ominous prognosis it bore just a few decades earlier.

Despite the development of endovascular methods, not all aneurysms are amenable or ideal for endovascular techniques, and so every cerebrovascular surgeon must be prepared to navigate these treacherous corridors through eloquent anatomy. This chapter provides a roadmap pointing out one such pathway and the hazards to keep in mind.

Summary

- For selected cases of BA aneurysms or simultaneous anterior and posterior circulation aneurysms not amenable to endovascular treatment, the half-and-half approach provides a viable option.

- Success depends on adequate exposure of the aneurysm, knowledge of the complex anatomy, identification and preservation of perforating arteries, and venous drainage.
- Surgical adjuncts include a coordinated neuroanesthesia team for blood pressure management and brain protection, skull base techniques to expand exposure, minimizing or eliminating fixed retraction, use of temporary clips, safe clip placement, and intraoperative angiography to confirm aneurysm obliteration and preservation of normal vasculature.

References

1. Morgagni J. *De sedibus et causis morborum per antomen indagatis libri quinque*. 1779.
2. Höök O, Norlén G, Guzmán J.Saccular aneurysms of the vertebral-basilar arterial system: a report of 28 cases. *Acta Neurol Scand.* 1963;**39**(4):271–304.
3. Drake CG. Bleeding aneurysms of the basilar artery: direct surgical management in four cases. *Can J Neurol Sci.* 1999 Nov 2;**26**(4):335–40.
4. Jamieson KG. Aneurysms of the vertebrobasilar system: surgical intervention in 19 cases. *J Neurosurg.* 1964;**21**(9):781–97.
5. Drake CG. Further experience with surgical treatment of aneurysms of the basilar artery. *J Neurosurg.* 1968;**29**(4):372–92.
6. Drake CG, Peerless SJ, Hernesniemi JA. *Surgery of Vertebrobasilar Aneurysms: London, Ontario Experience on 1767 Patients.* Vienna: Springer-Verlag; 1996.
7. Guglielmi G, Viñuela F, Dion J, Duckwiler G. Electrothrombosis of saccular aneurysms via endovascular approach. Part 2: preliminary clinical experience. *J Neurosurg.* 1991;**75**(1):8–14.
8. Kawase T, Toya S, Shiobara R, Mine T. Transpetrosal approach for aneurysms of the lower basilar artery. *J Neurosurg.* 1985;**63**(6):857–61.
9. Molyneux AJ, Kerr RSC, Yu L-M, Clarke M, Sneade M, Yarnold JA, et al. International subarachnoid aneurysm trial (ISAT) of neurosurgical clipping versus endovascular coiling in 2143 patients with ruptured intracranial aneurysms: a randomised comparison of effects on survival, dependency, seizures, rebleeding, subgroups, and aneurysm occlusion. *Lancet.* 366(9488):809–17.
10. Wiebers DO et al. Unruptured intracranial aneurysms: natural history, clinical outcome, and risks of surgical and endovascular treatment. *Lancet.* 2003;**362**(9378):103–10.
11. Klein GE, Szolar DH, Leber KA, Karaic R, Hausegger KA. Basilar tip aneurysm: endovascular treatment with Guglielmi detachable coils–midterm results. *Radiology.* 1997;**205**(1):191–6.
12. Eskridge JM, Song JK. Endovascular embolization of 150 basilar tip aneurysms with guglielmi detachable coils: results of the food and drug administration multicenter clinical trial. *J Vasc Interv Radiol.* 1999;**10**(1):112.
13. Peluso JPP, van Rooij WJ, Sluzewski M, Beute GN. Coiling of basilar tip aneurysms: results in 154 consecutive patients with emphasis on recurrent haemorrhage and re-treatment during mid-and long-term follow-up. *J Neurol Neurosurg Psychiatry.* 2008;**79**(6):706–11.
14. Tumialán LM, Zhang YJ, Cawley CM, Dion JE, Tong FC, Barrow DL. Intracranial hemorrhage associated with stent-assisted coil embolization of cerebral aneurysms: a cautionary report. *J Neurosurg.* 2008 **Jun;108**(6):1122–9.
15. Samson DS, Hodosh RM, Clark KW. Microsurgical evaluation of the pterional approach to aneurysms of the distal basilar circulation. *Neurosurgery.* 1978;**3**(2):135–41.
16. Yasargil MG. Microsurgical pterional approach to the aneurysms of the basilar bifurcation. *Surg Neurol.* 1976;**6**:83–91.
17. Spetzler RF, Hadley MN, Rigamonti D, Carter LP, Raudzens PA, Shedd SA, et al. Aneurysms of the basilar artery treated with circulatory arrest, hypothermia, and barbiturate cerebral protection. *J Neurosurg.* 1988;**68**(6):868–79.
18. Paine JT, Batjer HH, Samson D. Intraoperative ventricular puncture. *Neurosurgery.* 1988;**22**(6P1-P2):1107–9.

Index